Adult-Gerontology Acute Care Nurse Practitioner:

A Case-Based Approach

Adult-Gerontology Acute Care Nurse Practitioner:
A Case-Based Approach

Paula McCauley, DNP, ACNP-BC, CMC, CSC, FAANP
Acute Care Nurse Practitioner Cardiology/Cardiothoracic Surgery
University of Connecticut Health Center
Farmington, Connecticut
Associate Professor
University of Connecticut School of Nursing
Storrs, Connecticut

Angela Starkweather, PhD, ACNP-BC, CNRN, FAAN, FAANP
Professor and Associate Dean for Academic Affairs
University of Connecticut School of Nursing
Storrs, Connecticut
Affiliate Professor
University of Connecticut School of Medicine
Farmington, Connecticut

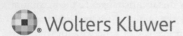. Wolters Kluwer

Philadelphia • Baltimore • New York • London
Buenos Aires • Hong Kong • Sydney • Tokyo

Not authorised for sale in United States, Canada, Australia, New Zealand, Puerto Rico, and U.S. Virgin Islands.

Vice President and Publisher: Julie K. Stegman
Acquisitions Editor: Jamie Blum
Director of Product Development: Jennifer K. Forestieri
Development Editor: Robyn Alvarez
Senior Editorial Coordinator: Lindsay Ries
Marketing Manager: Linda Wetmore
Production Project Manager: Sadie Buckallew
Design Coordinator: Stephen Druding
Manufacturing Coordinator: Kathleen Brown
Prepress Vendor: TNQ Technologies

9 8 7 6 5 4 3 2 1

Printed in China

Library of Congress Cataloging-in-Publication Data

ISBN-13: 978-1-9751-7367-8

Cataloging-in-Publication data available on request from the Publisher.

CCS1220

PM:

To my children, Erin, Jessica, and Curtis, and my grandchildren, Grant, Ada, and Ryleigh, who are the inspiration for all that I do.

AS:

To the inspiring mentors, who helped to shape my career as an ACNP, and the wonderful students both now and those to come, who will make up the next generation of AGACNPs.

Education for adult acute care nurse practitioners (ACNP) has evolved greatly since the role's inception in the early 1990s. Most recently, our competencies and education expanded to include more robust geriatric competencies as our aging population has grown, resulting in the adult-geriatric ACNP (AG-ACNP) credentialing. Initially, we were largely mentored and educated by physicians and followed the medical model. We as educators in acute care programs have designed curricula that embrace and emphasize the nursing component of our role as acute care nurse practitioners. In doing so, over the past several years, we developed specific learning materials we have used in our courses and seminars. Reflecting on the various teaching modalities we have employed in our academic careers, we have recognized that case-based learning was the most highly rated by our students for effectiveness. Our vision with this text was to bring those cases to print to offer others a foundation of experiential education focused on the acute and critically ill patient.

We have drawn upon the expertise of our contributors, both seasoned providers as well as newly prepared acute care nurse practitioners, to aid in delivering a variety of content and style that provides supplemental subject matter, valuable for individual or curricular application. The acute care population and problems are vast and ever changing, and we are not able to cover all of the topics within the limitations of these pages. We have attempted to incorporate several of the most commonly encountered topics, problems, and diagnoses, providing a breadth and depth of perspectives as well as application of the necessary competencies of the AG-ACNP. Our resources include key points, clinical pearls, and examination review questions.

Our hope is that this text is helpful to you whether you are a student, provider, preceptor, or educator.

ACKNOWLEDGMENTS

Thank you to our patients who have inspired us to develop these case studies, our contributors who provided their knowledge and expertise, and our students who have helped us refine them.

CONTRIBUTORS

Gloriann Albini, MSN, APRN, FNP
Hospitalist North East Medical Group
Bridgeport Hospital
Bridgeport, Connecticut

Cheryl Wainwright Anderson, EdD, APRN, ACNS-BC
Advanced Practice Provider
Department of Cardiology
Nuvance Health
Danbury, Connecticut

Sandra Barnosky, MSN, APRN, FNP-BC
Nurse Practitioner Orthopaedic surgery
UConn Health
Farmington, Connecticut

Michael Beach, DNP, ACNP-BC, PNP, FAAN
Associate Professor
Acute and Tertiary Care Department
University of Pittsburgh School of Nursing
Pittsburgh, Pennsylvania

Kristin A. Bott, DNP, APRN, ACNP-BC
Assistant Professor, Director AGACNP
 Program
University of Connecticut School of Nursing
Mansfield, Connecticut

Anna M. Bourgault, DNP, MSN, RN, CCRC
Assistant Professor
School of Nursing
University of Connecticut
Storrs, Connecticut

Julie D. Culmone, DNP, ANP-C, APRN, CCCN
Nurse Practitioner / Director Preoperative
 Care
Hartford Healthcare
Hartford, Connecticut

Jamie Gooch, DNP, APRN, ACNP-BC
Assistant Professor
School of Nursing
Storrs, Connecticut

Erin L. Hallinan, MSN, APRN, FNP-BC, AGACNP-BC, CCRN, PCCN
APRN Intensivist
Hartford Hospital at Saint Vincent's Medical
 Center Critical Care Department
Bridgeport, Connecticut

Payal M. Humbles, DNP, APRN, ACNP-BC
Clinical Service Manager
Department of Surgery and Digestive Diseases
Yale New Haven Health
New Haven, Connecticut

Arthur Kasimer-Colon, AGACNP-BC, RNFA
Orthopaedic Surgery
UConn Health
Farmington, Connecticut

Sarah E. Loschiavo, MSN, FNP-C, ACHPN
Program Director, Oncology Supportive Care
 & Survivorship
Carole and Ray Neag Comprehensive Cancer
 Center
UConn Health
Farmington, Connecticut

Anantha Sriharsha Madgula, MBBS
Resident
Department of Internal Medicine
University of Connecticut School of Medicine
Farmington, Connecticut

Bettina Magliato, APRN, MSN
Nurse Practitioner, Wound Care Specialist
Hartford Healthcare- Central Region
Hartford, Connecticut

Paula McCauley, DNP, APRN, ACNP-BC, CMC, CSC, FAANP
Nurse Practitioner Cardiology, CT Surgery
UConn Health
Farmington, Connecticut
Associate Professor
University of Connecticut School of Nursing
Mansfield, Connecticut

Cedric McKoy, ACNP-BC, MSN, RN
Neurocritical Care Nurse Practitioner
Department of Neurology
University of Chicago
Chicago, Illinois

Laura Mulka, MSN, APCNP-BC, AOCN, ACHPN, ACGN
Nurse Practitioner
Starling Physicians
Wethersfield, Connecticut

Karen Marie Petrok, MS, APRN , ACNP-BC
Nurse Practitioner
Department of Medicine, Hospitalist
NEMG, Bridgeport Hospital
Bridgeport, Connecticut

Heather L. Spear, RN, MSN, APRN-BC
Private Practice
Connecticut Anxiety and Depression Treatment Center
Farmington, Connecticut

Megan E. Speich, DNP, APRN, ACNP-BC, ACNPC-AG
Nurse Practitioner
Department of Nephrology
University of Connecticut Health Center
Farmington, Connecticut

Angela Starkweather, PhD, ACNP-BC, CNRN, FAAN, FAANP
Professor and Associate Dean for Academic Affairs
University of Connecticut School of Nursing
Storrs, Connecticut
Affiliate Professor
University of Connecticut School of Medicine
Farmington, Connecticut

Brenda C. White, DNP, APRN, ACNP-BC
Nurse Practitioner
Department of Surgery
Hartford Healthcare
Hartford, Connecticut

Heather Wilson, APRN, ACNP-BC
Advanced Practitioner Clinical Lead
Critical Care
Midstate Medical Center
Meriden, Connecticut

CONTENTS

PART 1

History and Professional Issues

1

Brief History of the Acute Care Nurse Practitioner Role, Competencies, and Impact on Health Outcomes

Paula McCauley • Angela Starkweather

INTRODUCTION

A growing need for advance practitioners in acute care occurred in the country in the mid-1900s. Throughout the early 1900s, public health nurses and nurses working in rural locations took on expanding roles in order to provide adequate care for underserved populations. During World War II, medics were trained to accompany surgeons in the field to extend physician capacity in providing basic medical care, administer medications, and assist with surgery. This role was replicated in the civilian realm through the advent of the first physician assistant program at Duke University in 1965, the same year that Loretta Ford and Henry K. Silver, MD, opened the first pediatric nurse practitioner program at the University of Colorado. Also in 1965, Medicare and Medicaid were established by the U.S. Congress to expand basic medical care services. The latter 1960s saw the emergence of the family medicine specialty with an emphasis on refocusing medical education on primary care. This, along with a decrease in residency hours in the late 1990s, resulted in a wide gap in coverage in acute care settings. This gap was initially addressed with primary care nurse practitioners (NPs). It quickly became apparent that their education lacked the knowledge and skills necessary for the acute care role, requiring additional on-the-job training and prolonged onboarding. This training led to the development of the acute care nurse practitioner (ACNP) role, education, certification, and licensure. Initially, a task force was organized to develop a consensus statement with standards and guidelines for graduate education programs. The American Nurse Credentialing Center (ANCC) and the American Association of Critical-Care Nurses (AACN) at that time also developed criteria for certification of the ACNP. The role was developed to have an immediate goal of stabilizing acutely ill patients and a long-term goal of restoring the patient to wellness or their maximum health potential. The role, along with its scope and standards, has evolved greatly over the past 2 decades.

Case Study

You are a registered nurse (RN) with 3 years' experience at the bedside in critical care and are interested in pursuing your graduate degree. You have explored programs but are not sure which track to choose. You see yourself working in acute care in the near future but do not want to limit your practice. You think you may want to work in an office setting in the future. You query advanced practice registered nurses (APRNs) you have met in the hospital and also through list serves and on social media sites. You have received quite a bit of feedback from a variety of people, including physicians, who recommend that you pursue the family nurse practitioner (FNP) certification and license because it makes you the most marketable and prepares you to work across the lifespan. However, there are other possibilities. Like an FNP, the scope of practice (SOP) of the adult gerontology primary care nurse practitioner (AGPCNP) is adult primary care. Both of these roles allow the NP to provide preventative care and manage chronic stable conditions in an office, community-based, or home setting. If you pursue a primary care program, you may have more flexibility regarding where you work and your work schedule. Those with whom you have discussed the options seem to echo the same. However, you really enjoy the fast pace, teamwork, and problem-solving required in acute care, and the past 3 years of working in the intensive care unit (ICU) has allowed you to improve your assessment and technical skills for delivering high-acuity care. So, should you apply to the FNP program?

ROLE DELINEATION, LICENSURE, ACCREDITATION, CERTIFICATION, AND EDUCATION

The Consensus Model for APRN Regulation, published in 2008, identified four regulatory elements (abbreviated as LACE): **licensure** to practice in a given state; **accreditation** of the APRN program by a national organization; **certification** by a national body that confirms the applicant's knowledge, skills, and experience; and **education** at the graduate or post-graduate certificate level (National Council of State Boards of Nursing, 2008). The APRN Consensus Model proposes that the requirements for APRNs should be framed in a way that ensures the safety of patients while expanding access to APRN care and promotes a consistent (SOP). (Kleinpell & Hudspeth).

Licensure

APRNs are licensed independent practitioners expected to practice within standards established and recognized by a licensing body (Hartigan, 2011). Licensure of APRNs is currently state regulated and includes the state's SOP. APRN education is based on a population focus, which is validated by the certification examination for that population. Potential examinations for NPs include adult gerontology acute care nurse practitioner (AGACNP), AGPCNP, FNP, pediatric (primary or acute), neonatal nurse practitioner, women's health nurse practitioner, and psychiatric-mental health nurse practitioner (across the lifespan). Traditionally, these certifications are at the master's level, but there is a national movement to require a Doctor of Nursing Practice (DNP) as entry level for all APRNs. The master's level prepares the provider for care of the individual and requires a minimum of 500 hours of clinical practice. The DNP widens the scope and education to include system-level education, incorporating a broader level of quality, outcomes, evidence-based practice, and leadership. The AACN *Essentials* documents delineate the expected outcomes for all master's level and DNP graduates.

Accreditation

All APRN education programs require accreditation through recognized national regulatory bodies, which currently are provided by the American Nurses Association through the Commission on Collegiate Nursing Education or the National League for Nursing through the Commission for Nursing Education Accreditation. Successful accreditation is achieved by meeting the standards expected of a graduate program.

Certification

Certification is offered by various organizations. The first acute care certification examination, the ACNP, was developed jointly in 1995 by ANCC and AACN. In the past several years, development of the Consensus Model has led to the recognition of the need for additional geriatric competencies of adult nurse practitioners. The national competencies, education, and certification were expanded to include a foundation that includes geriatric competence, and the examination was updated to the current AGACNP examination. All acute care programs in the country have updated the curricula to provide the AGACNP education. The ACNP examination was retired in 2014. Many ACNPs retained the title, as this was the education and certification required for practice prior to 2014 and they are able to practice with their current board certification as long as they maintain their certification status. It is no longer possible to sit for the ACNP examination. The AGACNP options for certification are through ANCC or AACN. The American Association of Nurse Practitioners does not offer acute care certification.

Education

The Consensus Model proposed that APRN education be based on one of four roles (certified registered nurse anesthetist; certified nurse midwife; clinical nurse specialist; certified nurse practitioner [CNP]) and one of six population foci (for example, the AGACNP population focus is young adult to frail elderly in acute care) be provided at a graduate level, and meet content, competencies, and clinical experience for that population. The population foci delineated in the Consensus Model include lifespan/family, adult gerontology, pediatrics, neonatal, women's health/gender-related, and psych/mental health. There must be a match with the title of the education program, the degree awarded, and the certification examination. All APRN programs must provide specific education in the three Ps (advanced pharmacology, physical assessment, and physiology/pathophysiology) as well as gerontology content. In addition, all programs must prepare graduates to assume responsibility for health promotion and maintenance as well as assessment, diagnosis, and management of common problems.

Case Study

Are you still confused about acute vs. primary care? Can you be prepared to work as an NP in acute care with a primary care education and certification?

Your role as a nurse will change as you continue your education and practice to include advanced practice. Your nursing experience is a necessary foundation, but as an RN, your SOP is limited when compared with the role you could fulfill as an APRN. On-the-job training does not replace formal education requirements. If you choose to be educated, certified, and credentialed as a primary care nurse practitioner, but accept a position in the ICU, how will you be able to justify your SOP? If any legal issues should arise, are you making yourself vulnerable to litigation?

SCOPE OF PRACTICE

Key Points

SOP of the primary care or acute care CNP is not setting specific (i.e., hospital, urgent care clinic, outpatient clinic, home) but is based on a population and patient care needs. This means that AGACNPs may be employed across different settings where their SOP is on managing adult patients with unstable, chronic, complex acute, and critical conditions; health conditions in which the patient is vulnerable to decompensation; or patients who are already dependent on healthcare interventions for survival.

The Pew Health Professions Commission (Finocchio et al., 1995) defines SOP as the "definition of the rules, the regulations, the boundaries within which a fully qualified practitioner with substantial and appropriate training, knowledge, and experience may practice" (p.1). The scope of a job is the range of operation. The American Nurses Association describes SOP as the "who, what, where, when, why, and how" of nursing practice.

The SOP for APRNs is based on state statutes. There is no consistency across all states. About 22 states and the District of Columbia give APRNs full practice authority and allow them to practice autonomously, 16 states require a collaborative agreement with a physician, and 12 states require physician supervision (American Association of Nurse Practitioners, 2019). Each state statute then controls the boundaries within which the APRN may practice.

Within each state there has begun to be closer scrutiny of providers' credentialing and restrictions based on SOP. The American Academy of Nurse Practitioners (2010), the National Panel for Acute Care Nurse Practitioner Competencies, and the AACN (2012), specifically address SOP for AGACNP practice.

FNPs have been educated to provide primary care, and AGACNPs have been educated to provide acute care for their patients. This educational difference is what defines each of the NP roles. The ACNP provides care for patients with unstable, chronic, complex acute, and critical conditions. Initially, the work of ACNPs was focused on critically ill patients, but it has expanded to include the breadth of all critical and acute care services such as care of patients in cardiothoracic surgery, cardiology, medical, neurosurgical, and surgical ICUs (Kleinpell & Hudspeth, 2013). Other areas of practice for ACNPs include working on a hospitalist service, in the emergency department or urgent care clinic, and in specialties such as hematology/oncology, or transplant services on an inpatient or outpatient basis, across the continuum of care. However, it is important to note that the role of the primary care and the acute care provider will sometimes overlap. For example, if a patient shows up at a clinic in a hypertensive crisis, the FNP has a legal duty to provide stabilization measures for the patient and then arrange immediate transport to a hospital where an AGACNP (or other acute care provider) would then treat the patient until discharge.

In 2012, the National Organization of Nurse Practitioner Faculties (NONPF) and the AACN collaborated on a document that outlines acute care adult and gerontology competencies (NONPF, 2012), and in 2013, NONPF published a document delineating the population-focused nurse practitioner competencies. Currently, the publication of these national guidelines and supportive terminology for population-focused nurse practitioners distinguishes and validates the role of AGACNPs as those who are recognized as trained and educated to care for acutely, chronically, and critically ill patients, typically but not limited to the inpatient hospital setting (NONPF, 2013).

Before the advent of acute care educational programs and currently in states where ACNP programs or graduates are lacking, primary care–prepared providers were hired to work within hospital settings, often on the basis of the patient population and acuity. However, there is a growing recognition of the various APRN roles and delineation in SOP. As a consequence, there has been an increase in the number of malpractice claims related to providers practicing outside their SOP (Nurses Service Organization, 2017).

It is important for the provider to appreciate and respect their SOP in order to provide the best available and appropriate health care. To practice across the lifespan in any setting would require, *at minimum*, education and certification in both primary and acute care. This does not include the pediatric acute care or neonatal populations. Informing prospective students about the implications of SOP for their career goals is paramount for educational programs and must include understanding of the components of the Consensus Model and the SOP of the state(s) where their student wishes to practice (Standards for educational programs: preparing students as ACNPs, from the Preparing Nurses for Advanced Practice in Acute Care Consensus Conference, 1993). Lack of understanding of the NP SOP can lead to malpractice against the hiring agency or facility for credentialing an NP inappropriately. The NP may be disciplined by the State Board of Nursing and potentially lose certification or licensure as an RN.

Case Study

You are favoring the AGACNP role over the FNP but would like more information about the AGACNP role and responsibilities, population, and outcomes. Let us explore this and help define what you can do as an AGACNP.

ROLES AND RESPONSIBILITIES

AGACNPs focus on care of patients across the acute care continuum. Initially the majority of ACNPs practiced in critical care and supplemented the medical residency work hour gaps. Their value was quickly recognized and expanded to include both inpatient and outpatient settings. Haut and Madden (2015) provide specific job description components. Specific job description components are listed in Box 1.1.

BOX 1.1 The AGACNP Job Description

- Independently elicits, selects, and integrates information concerning patients with acute, critical, and/or complex chronic illnesses. Assesses the complex, acute, critical, and chronically ill patient for urgent and emergent conditions (Haut & Madden, 2015; Kleinpell & Hudspeth, 2013)
- Conducts pharmacological assessment to include pharmacogenetic risks, complex therapies, drug interactions between prescribed and over-the-counter (OTC) medications, and other adverse events (Haut & Madden, 2015)
- Analyzes and synthesizes assessment data to determine differential diagnoses for adult patients with acute, critical, and/or complex chronic illness (Kleinpell & Hudspeth, 2013)
- Determines plan of care that incorporates rapidly changing pathophysiology in acute and critical illness, responds to urgent and life-threatening events, and develops and implements outcome-based management plan and prescribes evidence-based interventions (Haut & Madden, 2015; Kleinpell & Hudspeth, 2013)
- Functions in a leadership role to identify individualized goals and outcomes for patients with acute, critical, and/or complex chronic illnesses (Kleinpell & Hudspeth, 2013)
- Collaborates with individuals, their families, and caregivers to address educational needs, evaluate care, and support evidence-based interventions (Haut & Madden, 2015)

Magdic and Rosenzweig (1997) describe integration of the ACNP into various practice settings such as cardiology and transplant with primary responsibilities as frontline providers. The role encompasses management of the patient from admission to discharge, including diagnostic workup, admission history and physicals, diagnostic and therapeutic procedures, management, and coordination of discharge planning with social services as well as patient and family teaching.

Outcomes

Several documents are now available that emphasize the value of AGACNPs in various settings. Holliday et al. (2017) describe how AGACNPs have become an integral part of providing acute care trauma services. Utilization of AGACNPs has consistently been shown to improve quality of care and length of stay (LOS), transitions of care, and cost of care (American Association of Nurse Practitioners, 2015). Coordination of care, patient and family counseling, and education are important aspects of care provided by AGACNPs and improve patient and family satisfaction as well as team coordination and efficiency (Sidani & Doran, 2010). We will explore outcomes of AGACNP practice in another section of this book.

Case Study

As part of your preparation and decision-making process, additional recommendations would include further exploration of the Consensus Model and other available references. Explore your state nurse practice act, various job descriptions, SOP, and practice bylaws (Kleinpell & Hravnak, 2005). As an AGACNP, you may practice under the medical staff bylaws within the system or facility of employment. A recent article by Miller (2019) reflects the current state of our profession and offers guidance in your decisions.

REVIEW QUESTIONS

1. Licensure for nurse practitioners is obtained at which level?
    a. Employer
    b. State
    c. National
    d. Federal

2. SOP for nurse practitioners is determined by which of the following?
    a. federal regulations
    b. national competencies
    c. state statutes
    d. professional organizations

3. The Consensus Model for APRN Regulation published in 2008 identified four regulatory elements, which include the following:
    a. population foci, certification, licensure, SOP
    b. education, national certification, SOP, state regulations
    c. setting, population care needs, certification, licensure
    d. licensure, accreditation, certification, education

Answers: 1, b; 2, c; 3, d

REFERENCES

American Academy of Nurse Practitioners. (2010). *Scope of practice for nurse practitioners, 2010.* American Academy of Nurse Practitioners.

American Association of Critical-Care Nurses. (2012). *Scope and standards of practice for the acute care nurse practitioner.* American Association of Critical-Care Nurses.

American Association of Nurse Practitioners. (2015). *Quality of nurse practitioner practice.* American Association of Nurse Practitioners.

American Association of Nurse Practitioners. (2019). *State practice environment.* American Association of Nurse Practitioners.

Finocchio, L. J., Dower, C. M., McMahon, T., Gragnola, C. M. and Task Force on health Care Workforce Regulation. 1995. *Reforming Health Care Workforce Regulation: Policy Considerations for the 21st Century.* San Francisco, CA: Pew Health Professions Commission.

Hartigan, C. (2011). APRN regulation: The licensure-certification interface. *AACN Advanced Critical Care*, 22(1), 50-65.

Haut, C., & Madden, M. (2015). Hiring appropriate providers for different populations: Acute care nurse practitioners. *Critical Care Nurse*, 35(3), e1–e8.

Holliday, A., Samanta, D., Budinger, J., Hardway, J., & Bethea, A. (2017). An outcome analysis of nurse practitioner in acute care trauma services. *Journal of Trauma Nursing*, 24(6), 365–370.

Kleinpell, R. M., & Hravnak, M. M. (2005). Strategies for success in the acute care nurse practitioner role. *Critical Care Nursing Clinics of North America*, 17(2), 177–181.

Kleinpell, R. M., & Hudspeth, R. S. (2013). Advanced practice nursing scope of practice for hospitals, acute care/critical care, and ambulatory care settings: A primer for clinicians, executives, and preceptors. *AACN Advanced Critical Care*, 24(1), 23–29.

Magdic, K., & Rosenzweig, M. Q. (1997). Advanced practice nursing. Integrating the acute care nurse practitioner into clinical practice: Strategies for success. *Dimensions of Critical Care Nursing*, 16(4), 208–214.

Miller, K. (2019). Setting or patient care needs: Which defines advanced practice registered nurse scope of practice. *Journal for Nurse Practitioners*, 15, 494–495.

National Council of State Boards of Nursing. (2008). *Consensus model for APRN regulation: Licensure, accreditation, certification and education.* National Council of State Boards of Nursing.

National Organization of Nurse Practitioner Faculties. (2012). *Statement on acute care and primary care certified nurse practitioner practice 2012.* National Organization of Nurse Practitioner Faculties.

National Organization of Nurse Practitioner Faculties. (2013). *Primary care and acute care certified nurse practitioners.* National Organization of Nurse Practitioner Faculties.

Nurses Service Organization. (2017). *Nurse practitioner claim report: 4th edition—a guide to identifying and addressing professional liability exposures*. Nurses Service Organization.

Sidani, S., & Doran, D. (2010). Relationships between processes and outcomes of nurse practitioners in acute care: An exploration. *Journal of Nursing Care Quality*, 25(1), 31-38.

Standards for educational programs: Preparing students as acute care nurse practitioners, from the preparing nurses for advanced practice in acute care consensus conference. (1993). *AACN Clinical Issues in Critical Care Nursing*, 4(4), 593–598.

2

Acute Care Nurse Practitioner Role as Leader, Innovator, and Systems-Level Change Agent

Paula McCauley • Kristin A. Bott

INTRODUCTION

When practicing to the full extent of their license, ACNPs bring a valuable resource to healthcare. The impact of the use of ACNPs on quality and outcomes has expanded significantly over the past 2 decades. With the rapid growth of the AGACNP role comes data to support that NPs provide a cost-effective quality resource that impacts LOS, consistent evidence-based standards of care, and high-quality clinical care, as well as providing leadership, teaching, and coaching.

Case Study

You are nearing the end of your AGACNP education and considering potential employment once you finish. You are currently employed as an RN in your hospital's intermediate unit and have recognized what you perceive as a need for an AGACNP on the cardiology service. You have noted gaps in care within the system, protocols that need revisions, breakdown in the transitions of care from admission to discharge, and limited referrals for cardiac rehabilitation in your patients with acute coronary syndrome (ACS). You foresee how an AGACNP would be a valuable asset to the service and how this could potentially be your dream job. You approach your administrator and the medical director of cardiology about the possibility of creating such a role. They are both intrigued by the idea but need to justify the value and cost of the position to the healthcare system. They ask you to write a proposal along with a job description for further consideration. You do not know where to begin. With your newfound competencies from your graduate education, you decide to do a literature review to research the role of the AGACNP as a leader, innovator, and systems-level change agent. To help guide your research, you ask yourself several questions:

- How would my new role and competence impact care, including clinical and fiscal outcomes?
- What preparation and competence do I bring that will impact quality of care?
- As an AGACNP, what is my role in policy and process?
- How do I facilitate transitions in care?

AGACNP COMPETENCIES

ACNP professional practice domains include education, research, management, leadership, and consultancy. Educational preparation includes promotion of health, treatment of disease, teaching, coaching, and management and negotiation of healthcare delivery systems and quality care (AACN, 2006). The AGACNP focuses on restorative care that is characterized by rapidly changing clinical conditions as well as providing care for unstable chronic conditions, complex acute illnesses, and critical illnesses. The Standards of Professional Performance of the AGACNP describe a competent level of behavior in the professional role, including activities related to professional practice, education, collaboration, ethics, systems thinking, resource utilization, leadership, collegiality, quality, and clinical inquiry (AACN, 2017).

Your formal educational preparation qualifies you as an ACNP to independently

- perform comprehensive health assessments,
- order and interpret the full spectrum of diagnostic tests and procedures,
- formulate a differential diagnosis to reach a diagnosis, and
- order, provide, and evaluate the outcomes of interventions.

(National Organization of Nurse Practitioner Faculty, 2014).

OUTCOMES

Key Points
The ACNP can affect clinical, psychosocial, functional, and fiscal outcomes and satisfaction.

Several studies have evaluated the AGACNP's impact on outcomes. Ruth Kleinpell is among the most widely recognized scholars who have conducted surveys of AGACNP practice. She has written several articles and books dedicated to advance practice outcomes. In the fourth edition of *Outcome Assessment in Advanced Practice Nursing* (2017), she provides a comprehensive compilation of examples of outcomes in multiple areas, such as *effectiveness research*, which encompasses cost, access to care, and patient satisfaction; *care-related outcomes* including LOS, readmission, and procedure complication rates; and *performance-related outcomes* such as clinical competence, procedure complication rates, and adherence to best practice guidelines. Let us review some specific ways in which AGACNPs have demonstrated impact on these outcomes.

David et al. (2015) evaluated a cardiology service in which an AGACNP was incorporated into a multidisciplinary team and affected several outcomes, including clinical, fiscal, and patient satisfaction. The NP provided a strong relationship with the other caregivers and established a consistent point of contact and a stable presence on the team with a deep understanding of the barriers to improving patient outcomes. The NP developed several effective solutions to these barriers and documented improvements in patient care.

Bissonnette (2011) evaluated outcomes of transplant patients with kidney disease managed by NPs. They had a positive impact on fiscal and clinical outcomes including reduction in hospital admissions and ED visits by successfully implementing guideline-based treatments. Kilpatrick et al. (2013) developed a program that used NPs in their cardiology service, including a tool to evaluate effectiveness. They found that involving NPs decreased hospital LOS, and NPs implemented measures to improve clinical and functional outcomes through patient education and adherence to discharge medications. Sung et al. (2011) impacted clinical and process outcomes and improved time to CT scan, time to initial neurologic evaluation, and initiation of thrombolytic therapy. Sole et al. (2001) used NPs in the trauma service to improve functional outcomes of rehabilitation and discharge planning as well as nutrition-based orders.

Many studies illustrate a direct fiscal impact and have shown that the use of AGACNPs can help decrease costs and improve revenue for the hospital. Kapu and Jones (2012) evaluated the addition of AGACNPs to hospitalist and ICU teams and after only 3 months reported savings of $4,656 per case through a reduction in LOS. Another study by Meyer and Miers (2005) found that the addition of ACNPs to surgical teams for a cardiac surgery program had a statistically significant (p = .039) lower mean LOS compared with a group of surgeons working alone. After accounting for the salaries of the four AGACNPs, the estimated savings to the healthcare system was $3,388,015.20 per year. Vanhook (2000) incorporated NPs in an acute stroke team and improved fiscal outcomes of mortality rate, LOS, hospital charges, and improved process time. Gracias et al. (2003 to 2008) evaluated how NPs positively influenced compliance with practice guidelines for venous thromboembolism (VTE), stress ulcer, and anemia. These studies illustrate how the ACNP is well positioned to decrease costs and improve revenue for the hospital as well as benefit the patient.

Case Study

Your thoughts for a proposal are coming together. You envision how the role will incorporate your presence into daily rounds with the cardiology service, where you will review the daily roster with the attending and fellow. You will identify the patients who will be discharged and assist with their transition to home. Your literature review is expanded to investigate further how NPs have impacted quality in acute care and you discover multiple examples, such as reducing rates of urinary tract infections (UTIs) and skin breakdown (Albers-Heitner et al., 2012) and ventilator weaning (Burns et al., 2003). You are most interested in the impact within cardiology service settings and discover outcome assessments in reduction of cardiac risk factors such as hypertension (HTN) and lipid control, readmission rates, and symptom management with heart failure (HF) populations, and functional status of patients who have undergone coronary interventions and bypass surgery (Kilpatrick, 2011; Kleinpell, 2017; Lowery et al., 2012).

You find this information supportive of your proposed role but now would like to expand it to incorporate innovative ways to support the cardiology population and improve the system. As noted before, you have identified gaps in care that your newfound competence can address. You appreciate that administration will identify most with those that will impact fiscal outcomes, so you need to identify innovative ways that this newly developed role will do so. You compile a significant number of articles that used AGACNPs in efforts to standardize evidence-based care and guideline-based treatments and strengthen interprofessional teams. Areas you have identified with data to support are transitions of care, especially with the discharge, and follow-up processes for patients with HF and ACS.

SYSTEMS-LEVEL CHANGE PROVIDED BY AGACNPS

Sidani and Doran (2010) evaluated coordination of patient care and provision of counseling and education, as provided by AGACNPs, were associated with improvement in functioning and satisfaction with care. Overall, the study findings supported the relationships between selected processes and outcomes of care provided by AGACNPs.

David, Britting and Dalton (2015) conducted a study on the effectiveness of cardiology AGANCPs in a retrospective comparison of a cardiology service with two teams, one with and one without a cardiology AGACNP. Patient selection included those with a primary diagnosis of ST- or non–ST-segment elevation myocardial infarction (72.4%) or heart failure (27.6%). The addition of an AGACNP to a multidisciplinary inpatient medical team caring for myocardial infarction and heart failure patients was associated with lower 30-day emergency department readmission and 30-day hospital readmission rates. The cardiology AGACNP added a stable presence to a team that included fellows and attending physicians, rotating on and off the service. This provided continuity for patients, nursing staff, case managers, and other staff. The AGACNP provided staff with a consistent point of contact that allowed for strong relationships to develop and enhanced communication. The AGACNP developed expertise for a specific group of patients and can become an expert in the day-to-day care of these patients and develop a deep understanding of barriers and solutions to patient care problems such as the intricacies of insurance coverage, prescription reimbursement, and specialized services that were available.

Case Study

Using the information you have discovered, you develop a specific proposal that will include HF and ACS patients. Your plan will include establishing guideline-based care goals at the time of discharge for the HF patients. You will develop and provide a specific program of education incorporating diet, daily weights, and diuretics that will be addressed prior to discharge with each patient. Along with this, they will have a scheduled visit with you within a week of discharge to examine, weigh, and discuss progress once home. You also have identified a gap with advanced HF patients who need inotropic support for palliative care at home and have a proposal for follow-up with them as outpatients through telehealth. You propose a detailed process for acute myocardial infarction (AMI) teaching, medication review, and review of their medication coverage so that dual antiplatelet therapy (DAPT) is instituted and continued with the best available coverage. This will include education of the cardiology team and nursing staff on the unit.

Of course, implementing a new role and process will require evaluation, and along with your proposed job description and implementation of the role, you would evaluate the impact. Your hypothesis is that the addition of a cardiac ACNP to medical teams caring for myocardial infarction and heart failure patients will have a positive impact on reducing 30-day emergency department return and hospital readmission rates. You will use the programs and evaluation methods already developed as your blueprint (David et al., 2015; Kilpatrick et al., 2012).

Your evaluation will include two groups, one where patients received care from a medical team that included a cardiac AGACNP vs. those who received care from a medical team alone. You will collect 6 months of data including patient history, cardiac assessment, medical interventions, discharge disposition, discharge time, and three outcomes (LOS, 30-day readmission, and time of discharge). You will compare the two treatment groups using logistic regression to identify predictors of 30-day readmission. Based on data, you will determine if the outcomes for your patients are different from the control group.

Decreasing hospital admission can be a significant cost savings for the institution making this a valuable role for your unit. The only other aspect you need to explore is reimbursement and how this will impact the service and institution as well as your own professional advancement. You go back to your literature review and various organizations to explore this.

REIMBURSEMENT

The ACNP must have an understanding of billing mechanisms and policy-related restrictions and guidelines that dictate billing practices. The institution where the nurse practitioner is employed will often offer billing services assistance that can be helpful in understanding the arduous and complex process of billing.

> ### Key Points
>
> Whether an NP can bill for services delivered in the hospital inpatient setting depends on how the salary is listed on the hospital's Medicare cost report. This is an important question for the employer as to whether the NP is considered a provider, as the answer directly impacts whether the NP may bill.

The ACNP can bill for services rendered as long as they fall within the nurse practitioner's SOP (Hoffman & Guttendorf, 2017). The individual Medicare/Medicaid number for the NP can be used to bill both inpatient and outpatient services. Medicare refers to NPs and physician's assistants as nonphysician providers (NPPs).

Specific information related to billing and coding is readily available. A claims processing manual is available through the Centers for Medicare & Medicaid Services (CMS) with Chapter 12 specifically addressing NPPs. *Coding for Chest Medicine* (Chest, 2016) and *Coding and Billing for Critical Care—A Practice Tool* (Dorman et al., 2014) are helpful references for detailed information on this topic. The Current Procedural Terminology (CPT) provides codes for inpatient and adult critical care services.

Inpatient NPs may bill in one of two ways: direct or shared. When billing direct, services are billed under the NP's own National Provider Identifier (NPI) number regardless of setting. Shared billing occurs in the inpatient hospital setting and may either be done under the NP's or physician's NPI number but not both. There needs to be documentation from both to support shared billing, often where the NP sees the patient and the collaborating physician may link their documentation to the NP's note and include one or more elements of the history, physical examination, and decision-making (Magic, 2103).

Critical care services are time-based codes, and the initial critical care time (CPT code 99291) must be met by a single physician or qualified NPP. Additional critical care time (CPT code 99292) in the same calendar day can be billed by another provider in the same practice following the guidelines outlined by the CMS. Separate progress notes are required to support claims made on the two calendar dates, and the critical care time documented must match what was submitted on each claim (Dorman et al., 2014; Munro, 2013).

Prolonged services may occur when the patient has just been informed of a serious diagnosis that requires considerable discussion related to complex treatment options. Use of prolonged service codes can be used to capture the extended face-to-face time spent with the patient in the inpatient hospital (99356, 99357) setting. Prolonged service codes are considered companion codes to the usual Evaluation and Management (E&M) codes. For inpatient hospital settings, code 99356 is used when there is a medically necessary, direct, face-to-face patient encounter that requires 1 hr beyond the usual service threshold time. This code may only be used once in a calendar day, and the time does not have to be continuous but must be performed by the same provider. Code 99357 is used to report each additional 30 min beyond the first hour of prolonged services. In addition to the required documentation for the primary or daily visit, the medical record must also include documentation of time spent face-to-face with the patient and the content of the medically necessary prolonged service (Magdic, 2013).

Institutional regulations may dictate how the billing process occurs, but the ACNP should recognize the benefits of billing under their own provider number. As a profession, we need to provide evidence of our value and worth to the healthcare system.

Key Points

By billing under our own provider numbers, we are able to quantify the financial contribution of our work to the system.

Billing with the ACNP's provider number allows for an aggregate collection of data to create a profile of the financial contribution and patient outcomes produced by the ACNP. Without utilizing our provider number, these data are unable to be obtained. Through evaluation of services billed by ACNPs at the national level, an aggregate profile of ACNP practice with respect to billable direct patient care activities can be developed (Magdic, 2006). This information can be used to advance policy in relation to ACNP practice and help guide future policy.

Case Study

You present your job description, program goals, and research proposal to your administrative team along with recommendations for billing and coding based upon the information you have discovered through your research of the hospital bylaws as well as interviews with the other neonatal nurse practitioners (NNPs) and your medical record coding experts. Your administrators are impressed by your work and potential value you will bring to the service. An Full time equivalent (FTE) is created, and you are hired upon completion of your program, certification, and licensure. Your credentialing process and orientation include workshops for billing and coding. You request additional time with your program director of quality to review current indicators collected as well as options to expand for a more comprehensive program that will incorporate specific cardiology metrics. Congratulations, you have demonstrated your competence as a leader, innovator, and system s-level change agent. Good luck in your new position!

REVIEW QUESTIONS

1. Studies have documented the AGACNP impact on various outcomes, including
   a. clinical outcomes such as symptom relief.
   b. fiscal outcomes such as reduction in length of stay and readmissions.
   c. patient satisfaction.
   d. all of the above.

2. AGACNP billing is directly impacted by
   a. Centers for Medicare and Medicaid Services.
   b. the salary listing on the institution's roster and cost report.
   c. individual insurance organizations.
   d. the state of licensure.

3. The AGACNP may bill
   a. for services that fall within the NP's scope of practice.
   b. only under the physician's NPI number.
   c. without using their provider number.
   d. for undocumented services, such as counseling.

   Answers: 1, d; 2, b; 3, a

REFERENCES

Albers-Heitner, C. P., Joore, M. A., Winkens, R. A., Lagro-Janssen, A. L. M., Severens, J. L., & Berghmans, L. C. M. (2012). Cost-effectiveness of involving nurse specialist for adult patients with urinary incontinence in primary care compared to care-as-usual: An economic evaluation alongside a pragmatic randomized controlled trial. *Neurology Urodynamics*, 31(4), 526–534.

American Association of Colleges of Nursing. (2006). *The essentials of doctoral education for advanced nursing practice*. American Association of Colleges of Nursing.

American Association of Critical-Care Nurses. (2017). *Scope and standards of practice for the acute care nurse practitioner*. American Association of Critical-Care Nurses.

Bissonnette, J. (2011). *Evaluation of an advanced practice nurse led interprofessional collaborative chronic care approach for kidney transplant patients: The TARGET study* (doctoral dissertation). University of Ottowa.

Burns, S. M., Earven, S., Fischer, C., Lewis, R., Merrell, P., Schubart, J. R., Truwit, J. D., Bleck, T. P., & FCCM University of Virginia Long Term Mechanical Ventilation Team. (2003). Implementation of an institutional program to improve clinical and financial outcomes of mechanically ventilated patients; One-year outcomes and lessons learned. *Critical Care Medicine*, 31(12), 2752–2763.

Centers for Medicare & Medicaid Services (CMS). (2019). *Physicians/nonphysician providers*. In *Medicare claims processing manual*. Chap. 12, Sec. 30.6. Accessed January 4, 2020. https://www.cms.gov/Regulations-and-Guidance/Guidance/Manuals/Internet-Only-Manuals-IOMs-Items/CMS018912

CHEST. (2016). *Coding for chest medicine 2016: A coding and billing update*. Accessed January 4, 2020. https://www.chestnet.org/Publications/Other-Publications/Coding-for-Chest-Medicine

David, D., Britting, L., & Dalton, J. (2015). Cardiac acute care nurse practitioner and 30-day readmission. *Journal of Cardiovasc Nursing*, 30(3), 248–255.

Dorman, T., Britton, F. M., Brown, D. R., & Munro, N. (2014). *Coding and billing for critical care—a practice tool* (6th ed.). Society of Critical Care Medicine.

Gracias, V. H., Sicoutris, C. P., Stawicki, S. P., Meredith, D. M., Horan, A. D., Gupta, R., Haut, E. R., Auerbach, S., Sonnad, S., Hanson, C. W. III, & Schwab, C. W. (2008). Critical care nurse practitioners improve compliance with clinical practice guidelines in "semiclosed" surgical intensive care unit. *Journal of Nursing Care Quality*, 23(4), 338–344. https://doi.org/10.1097/01.NCQ.0000323286.56397.8c

Hoffman, L., Guttendorf, J. (2017). Preparation and evolving role of the acute care nurse practitioner. *Chest*, 152(6), 1339–1345.

Kapu, A, & Jones, P. (2012). Financial impact of adding acute care nurse practitioners (ACNPs) to inpatient models of care. *Critical Care Medicine*, 40(12), 1–328.

Kilpatrick, K. (2011). Development and validation of a time and motion tool to measure cardiology acute care nurse practitioner activities. *Canadian Journal of Cardiovascular Nursing*, 21(4), 18–26.

Kilpatrick, K., Lavoie-Tremblay, M., Ritchie, J. A., Lamothe, L., Doran, D., & Rochefort, C. (2012). How are acute care nurse practitioners enacting their roles in healthcare teams? A descriptive multiple-case study. *International Journal of Nursing Studies*, 49(7), 850–862.

Kilpatrick, K, Lavoie, TM, Lamothe, L, Ritchie, J. A., & Doran, D. (2013). Conceptual framework of acute care nurse practitioner role enactment, boundary work, and perceptions of team effectiveness. *Journal of Advanced Nursing*, 69(1), 205–217.

Kleinpell, R. M. (2017). *Outcome assessment in advanced practice nursing* (4th ed.). Springer.

Lowery, J., Hopp, F., Subramanian, U., Wiitala, W., Welsh, D. E., Larkin, A., Stemmer, K., Zak, C., & Vaitkevicius, P. (2012). Evaluation of a nurse practitioner disease management model for chronic heart failure: A multi-site implementation study. *Congestive Heart Failure*, 18(1), 64–71.

Magdic, K. (2006). Acute care billing: Shared visits. *Nurse Practitioner*, 31, 9–10.

Magdic, K. S. (2013). Billing for NPs in acute care: Do you know the rules? *The Nurse Practitioner*, 38(3), 10–14. Accessed June 7, 2020. https://doi.org/10.1097/01.NPR.0000425833.20930

Meyer, S. C., & Miers, L. J. (2005). Cardiovascular surgeon and acute care nurse practitioner: Collaboration on postoperative outcomes. *AACN Clinical Issues*, 16(2), 149–158.

Munro, N. (2013). What acute care nurse practitioners should understand about reimbursement: Critical care issues. *AACN Advanced Critical Care*, 24(3), 241–244.

National Organization of Nurse Practitioner Faculties. (2014). *Nurse practitioner core competencies content*. National Organization of Nurse Practitioner Faculties.

Sidani, S., & Doran, D. (2010). Relationships between processes and outcomes of nurse practitioners in acute care: An exploration. *Journal of Nursing Care Quality*, 25(1), 31–38.

Sole, M. L., Hunkar-Huie, A. M., Schiller, J. S., & Cheatham, M. L. (2001). Comprehensive trauma patient care by non-physician providers. *AACN Clinical Issues*, 12(3), 438–446.

Sung, S. F., Huang, Y. C., Ong, C. T., & Chen, Y. W. (2011). A parallel thrombolysis protocol with nurse practitioners as coordinators minimized door-to-needle time for acute ischemic stroke. *Stroke Research and Treatment*, 2011, 198518.

Vanhook, P. (2000). *Presence of nurse practitioner on stroke team reduced morbidity, mortality. American heart association 25th international stroke conference report.* Reuters Medical News.

PART 2

Foundational Skills

3 Patient- and Family-Centered Care in the Process of Diagnosis and Selection of Treatment Options

Brenda C. White   •   Payal M. Humbles

INTRODUCTION

Many patients and families unexpectedly are placed in situations where they are unable to understand the diagnosis or conditions encountered during their acute illness. There have been myths and misconceptions generated throughout the years by the healthcare delivery team secondary to fear of consequences and failure to understand the importance of families (Table 3.1). Family is defined as a group of individuals with a continuing legal, genetic, and/or emotional relationship. The patient defines who his family is and to what extent he wants them to be involved. Family presence at the bedside is seen as a privilege, not as a necessary component of the patient's care. One of the biggest predictors of family dissatisfaction occurs due to communication that is commonly inconsistent, inadequate, and of poor quality (Fox, 2014).

As the foundation of healthcare delivery moves toward a patient- and family-centered care (PFCC) paradigm (Society for Critical Care Medicine, n.d.), it has become crucial to maintain therapeutic relationships based on communication and trust. This allows for shared decision-making and timely decisions regarding their loved one. According to the

TABLE 3.1 MYTHS AND FACTS REGARDING FAMILY INVOLVEMENT IN CARE

MYTH	FACT
Family presence spreads infection.	The predominant risk of infection is the transfer of nosocomial infections from patient to patient by caregivers (Burchardi, 2002).
Family presence is a burden to families.	Actively involving families increases feelings of security and satisfaction and decreases anxiety and confusion (Davidson et al., 2017).
Family presence interferes with care delivery.	Family members have a positive influence on the patient's care and recovery from their acute illness (Adams et al., 2017). Actively involving families decreases patient falls, anxiety, confusion, agitation, CV complications, and ICU length of stay (Davidson et al., 2017).
Family presence exhausts the patient.	Family members may help the patient to endure the difficult period of their acute illness (Burchardi, 2002).

CV, cardiovascular; ICU, intensive care unit.

American Association of Retired Persons (AARP), family members give over $450 billion worth of care and they should be considered a crucial member of the team surrounding the patient (AARP, 2020).

PFCC is defined as an approach to health care that is respectful of and responsive to individual families' needs and values (Davidson et al., 2017). It involves patients and their families in planning, delivery, and evaluation of healthcare services (Bamm & Rosenbaum, 2008).

Case Study

You are an advanced provider (AP) working in the ED of a teaching hospital. Mrs. S is an obese female, who speaks mostly Spanish and appears to be in her 40s. She is presenting with 3 days of abdominal pain, nausea and bloating after eating, and lack of appetite, which has worsened over the past few hours and is most significant for sharp pain in the right upper quadrant. Through the use of fragmented English with the resident and the AP, she tells him that "husband work, scared."

Her history and physical reveal the following:

- **Allergies:** no known drug allergies
- **Past medical history:** hypothyroidism, hypertension (HTN), hyperlipidemia
- **Past surgical history:** none
- **Home meds:** Levothyroxine 125 µg daily, Toprol 25 mg daily, Crestor 40 mg daily
- **Family Hx:** unaware of all family history, but aware her father had HTN and died of colon cancer, and unknown reason why mother died. No siblings.
- **Social Hx:** married with two children, does not smoke, drinks socially
- Review of systems (**ROS**): She denies chills, night sweats, and weight loss. She endorses fatigue, fever, abdominal distention, abdominal pain, nausea, and right upper quadrant pain. She denies palpitations, orthopnea, or urinary symptoms.
- **Physical examination:** heart rate (HR), 102; blood pressure (BP), 128/72; respiratory rate (RR), 14; oxygen saturation (SpO_2), 98%; temp, 100.6 °F. The patient appears mildly uncomfortable and is constantly changing positions. She is alert and oriented to person, place, and time. Her lungs are clear and her cardiac examination is consistent with a regular rhythm. There is moderate epigastric tenderness and guarding throughout the abdomen, with no peritoneal signs noted. She has a positive Murphy sign. No other acute or abnormal findings are noted on physical examination.
- **Labs/diagnostic/consults:** Emergency general surgery (EGS) consult, basic metabolic panel (BMP), complete blood count (CBC) with diff, lactate, and right upper quadrant ultrasound secondary to concerns for acute cholecystitis.

Key Points

Key characteristics of PFCC include keeping patients and families:

1. **Informed** by early effective communication.
2. **Involved** by providing informed and shared decision-making.

3. **Engaged** by encouraging family presence.
4. **Supported** via physical comfort/emotional support to patient and family.
5. **Feeling respected with sensitivity** toward cultural differences and view belief on illness.

EARLY EFFECTIVE COMMUNICATION

Meeting the needs of families is the primary responsibility of healthcare providers, which allows for perception of high-quality care (Auerbach, 2005). Families are the main social and personal support for a patient and a key link to the healthcare team. The most significant, documented need of the patient's family is access to clear, understandable, and honest communication on information about the patient's medical condition (Fox, 2014). Communication can be defined as the exchange of information and dialogue between the two parties, but within the healthcare system, it can also be viewed as an ensemble of relationships that allows for autonomy and the ability to make better decisions. Many times, because of lack of time, personal attributes (e.g., lack of cultural sensitivity, personal biases), and patient overload, accurate communication is not timely, leading to decreased satisfaction (Auerbach, 2005). Evidence through literature has supported good and effective communication, shared decision-making, and the patient's wishes as predictors of satisfaction and the ability to make good decisions. The Society of Critical Care Medicine (SCCM) and Association of Critical Care Nurses (AACN) have dedicated resources toward development of effective communication via guidelines and important interventions regarding effective communication (Davidson et al., 2017). When Hinkle and Fitzpatrick (2011) used the Critical Care Family Needs Inventory (CCFNI) survey, the three major needs that were addressed through communication were responses to their questions, reassurance that their loved one was getting the best care, and feeling that the healthcare team actually cared about the patient and family (Hinkle & Fitzpatrick, 2011). In addition, the delivery of information and development of trusting relationships were found to be crucial factors in helping families adjust to traumatic events. When communication is effective, it helps patients and families accept prognosis and illness realities, make better decisions, and improve their quality of life. Box 3.1 describes how to effectively communicate with patients and families.

BOX 3.1 How to Effectively Communicate

- Start the conversation regarding goals of care and advance directives early in the hospitalization (Bernacki & Block, 2014).
- Standardize the timing and conduct of early communication techniques that are unit specific (ICU vs. medical/surgical stepdown vs. medical/surgical floor).
- Obtain communication training in interactive case-based sessions.
- Develop unit-based criteria that may trigger an earlier conversation.
- Start conversations with an understanding of the patient's and family's knowledge of the illness. This can be done with an open-ended question, such as "What is your understanding of the current status of your loved one?"
- Provide open, honest, clear, and noncontradicting information.
- Sit down in a conference-like setting at eye level to assure no authority and to level the playing field for an open discussion.

(continued)

> ### BOX 3.1   How to Effectively Communicate (*continued*)
>
> - Make the language understandable, avoid technical language, and explain on a level appropriate to the relatives' understanding.
> - Check understanding at various points throughout the discussion to ensure full transparency and understanding of information being delivered (Gauntlett & Laws, 2008).
> - Providers should learn their own feelings toward the situation being discussed and learn to be self-aware (Gauntlett & Laws, 2008).

Fundamental Models of Communication

There are four fundamental models that have been researched through communication literature that can be applied during the dialogue with the family (Institute for Healthcare Improvement, 2019):

- Ask-tell-ask
- Tell me more
- Reflections rather than questions
- Responding to emotion

Ask-Tell-Ask

First, *ask* the family/patient to describe their understanding of the current issues (Lilly et al., 2000). This allows providers to gain knowledge about how much information still needs to be relayed and if any misperceptions need to be addressed during the conversation. Prior to the discussion with the family and the patient, identify concerns, needs, and the most important issue from the family's point of view. This develops trust and rapport and allows for open communication. Next, *tell* the family, in simple, straightforward language, what needs to be communicated about the current illness, prognosis, current treatment options, and recommendations. Develop two or three take-home statements and messages rather than overwhelming them with too much information. Finally, *ask* families if they understood and have any further questions, knowing that families are experiencing some element of stress and anxiety. Clarify misperceptions and answer questions not yet answered. Confirm that the family has a source to contact for follow-up questions.

Tell Me More

Sometimes in conversations, it is easy to get sidetracked (Institute for Healthcare Improvement, 2019). Redirection may be required and can be done by asking the family to explain their current understanding. This also allows an understanding of current emotional status, aiding in navigating the conversation.

Reflections Rather Than Questions

Reflections are restatements to paraphrase what the family is trying to express. Restatements should be clear and accurately portray what a family is experiencing. The downfall is that a provider may get the interpretation wrong, although this may allow the family to reflect on what they are saying or feeling. Reflecting provides empathy and empowerment, and families feel they are being heard through this discussion.

> **BOX 3.2** Responding to Emotion Using the NURSE Mnemonic
>
> **N**aming the emotion: suggestive not declarative
> **U**nderstanding: sensitive appreciation for families' emotions
> **R**especting: nonverbal gestures, making their emotions important
> **S**upporting: expressing concern and developing partnership
> **E**xploring: allowing families to talk through the emotions, exploring the background
> and story of the family member

Responding to Emotion

While the loved one is in an acute care setting, most patients and families experience emotions related to loss of physical function, social function, and/or quality of life. Many families have strong emotions of anger, frustration, sadness, and hopelessness. Provider acknowledgment of these emotional reactions allows the family to be receptive to information discussed during the meeting. A common mnemonic used in this model is *NURSE* (Back et al., 2005). Refer to Box 3.2.

Ultimately, facilitating early effective communication skills will give providers, RNs, and ancillary services the ability to successfully help families and their patients to make better decisions via the use of informed shared decision-making.

Case Study

The most crucial aspect of healthcare delivery is building a trusting relationship with good communication. Having someone who speaks the patient's and family's language will facilitate open dialogue and can ultimately make communication easier. Although the patient spoke some fragmented English, using an interpreter will help make conversation regarding her health more effective. You also want to talk to her husband in order to help build the relationship. You ask her via the interpreter if she wants to wait for her husband to go over everything, or if it would be okay to have a discussion with her regarding the situation and update her husband once he arrives. Ideally, you want to start the conversation early; the ED is the perfect place to start the effective open communication.

You want to use the principle of responding to emotions to help improve your communication. You address her fears of being "scared" to help her to feel more at ease and make better decisions. You ask her what is making her scared. The fear of a terminal diagnosis due to her father dying from colon cancer, finding someone to watch her kids, and dealing with the financial implications of hospitalization are all reasons for her fear.

Next, you apply NURSE to Mrs. S's case.

Naming the fact she stated she was scared in a suggestive tone
Understanding what she means by feeling scared
Respecting her nonverbal gestures, and her wailing as a sign of how she
expresses emotions

Supporting her through her fears and providing a feeling of rapport and partnership

Exploring through the emotion and helping to navigate through potential barriers

Mrs. S's laboratory and diagnostic workup revealed the following pertinent positives: white blood cell (WBC) count, 17.5/µL; lactate, 4.2 mg/dL; bicarb, 18 mEq/L. Her imaging was consistent with acute cholecystitis.

SHARED DECISION-MAKING

More recently, studies have shown that clinicians ask for patient and family preferences in medical decisions only about 50% of the time. In a study of 1,057 patient encounters with over 3,000 decisions, only 9% defined it as informed shared decision-making (Elwyn et al., 2012). Shared decision-making is defined as "an approach where clinicians and patients share the best available evidence when faced with the task of making decisions, and where patients are supported to consider options, to achieve informed preferences" (Elwyn et al., 2012). The current reimbursement system does not incentivize clinicians to engage in informed shared decision-making except during procedures and surgeries. Effective communication is highly valuable as the concepts of shared and informed decision-making take place within the acute care setting. Shared decision-making ties in the importance of communication and information sharing in order to facilitate appropriate decisions to be made between the family and healthcare team for the patient. The challenges that the healthcare team experience are the ability to minimize patient's misunderstanding, misinterpretation of risks and benefits of treatment options, and avoiding imposing personal biases and preferences onto families and patients.

Along with effective communication is the ability to maintain autonomy for patients and their families. Autonomy conceptually protects patients and families and is emphasized on overcoming problems that arise from paternalistic decision-making. When maintaining autonomy, patients and families can exercise the right of self-determination and accept the outcome of decision-making. To perform informed decision-making, clinicians should present evidence and summarize the problems and make an effort to explain risk and benefits of each treatment option, thus allowing for active decision-making and patient and family satisfaction, and ultimately improving compliance. Lastly, decision-making should be family and patient centered, although this could be difficult if clinicians do not examine individuals' decision-making capabilities and coping styles (Bae, 2017).

Assess the Other Person's Decision-Making and Coping Style

Although some family members are involved in depth, others are less involved. Many families, given different experiences and cultural backgrounds, view family involvement differently and thus have multiple ways to make decisions and cope. Research shows that there are two types of major coping styles: monitors and blunters (Luce, 2010). Monitors seek information, plan ahead, and are problem focused. Helping them move toward acknowledging their emotions is fundamental in helping them cope and make better decisions. Blunters are emotionally focused and cope by avoiding information and practical planning. For this type of family member, moving toward a concrete planning stage is essential. This can be achieved by applying the ask-tell-ask model. Family members can also be a mix of both styles and can change over the course of the illness.

Key Points

Avoid common pitfalls during family meetings and shared decision-making with families. Do not give a pathophysiology lesson; maintain the big picture and keep the information simple. Make sure to stay on topic during shared information delivery. Not being informed regarding a family's needs and coping styles can result in losing control of the situation. Do not rush a family to make decisions that ultimately have an implication on their overall emotional state and quality of life post illness.

BOX 3.3   Examples of Questions for Shared Decision-Making

- If your loved one was unable to participate and could hear what we are saying, what would he/she say? (What would be the patient's wishes?)
- What did your loved one enjoy doing? Would he/she be okay never doing that again?
- What would be most important to your loved one right now given the current situation?
- Have you ever discussed what your loved would have wanted?
- How are you doing? What can we help you with during this time?
- Can you tell me what you are feeling right now?

Box 3.3 lists some examples of questions that can be asked during shared decision-making.

The questions listed in Box 3.3 and others used in patient communication can be grouped into the mnemonic VALUE in order to improve clinical-family communication (Box 3.4). This mnemonic was studied in 126 patients in 22 intensive care units (ICUs). When practitioners applied the mnemonic to their communication with patients, the patients showed higher satisfaction of communication at end of life vs. the group using traditional methods of communication (95% vs. 75%, respectively) (Luce, 2010).

Shared decision-making increases family satisfaction and benefits the patient. It all comes down to treating others as you would want to be treated. Take the time for families and patients to understand and value their emotional and practical thought processes through these difficult times.

BOX 3.4   VALUE

Value and appreciate what the family says
Acknowledge their emotions
Listen effectively
Understand the patient as a person
Elicit and ask questions of the family to keep the family involved

> **Key Points**
>
> There are several goals to strive for in implementing family-centered care, including the following:
>
> - Shared planning/decision-making
> - Doing things with patients' families, not for or to them
> - Partnership = patient + family + ICU team
> - Full disclosure of patient's status
> - Regular meetings within 24–48 hours during acute care management
> - Staff training in these areas:
>   - Good communication skills for facilitation of family-centered care
>   - Conflict management skills

Case Study

Mr. S has arrived and is at the bedside anxiously waiting to hear the results.

You, the EGS team, and a Spanish interpreter inform Mrs. and Mr. S that she has acute cholecystitis and needs an operation to remove her gallbladder. She starts crying and showing strong emotions over this. You identify her as someone who is a blunter when it comes to coping styles. This makes the treatment team focus on concrete planning while allowing for emotions and shared decision-making to be used. Using the interpreter, the team explains in a manner that the patient and family would understand what acute cholecystitis is, what the surgery will entail, the risks and benefits of her treatment options, and what her postoperative course will look like. At this time, she will be admitted into the general surgical floor unless the surgical team has concerns for complications intraoperatively.

Allowing Mrs. and Mr. S time to ask questions and make an informed decision is imperative, especially at a time that may be very scary for individuals. It is essential to address the concerns for anesthesia as well as any further fears, which will ultimately help them have shared decision-making in an informed manner. Mrs. S signs the informed consent and is taken to surgery 1 hour later.

FAMILY ENGAGEMENT

PFCC focuses on keeping patients and families engaged by encouraging family presence during the patient's acute illness. Davidson et al. (2017) recommends family to be offered (1) open or flexible family presence at the bedside, (2) the option of participating in interdisciplinary team rounds to improve satisfaction and communication and increase family engagement, and (3) the option of being present during resuscitation efforts with a staff member assigned to support the family.

Family presence is necessary for family engagement at the bedside. Because family members want to be near their loved ones during any hospitalization, open family visitation can increase family presence and participation in care. Open visiting with flexibility accounting for the need of the patient and family increases patient, family, and nurse satisfaction, as the policy allows the family to give emotional support to the patient, decreases patient boredom, and provides more valuable information to the family regarding their loved one and about the patient to the healthcare team (Ciufo et al., 2011).

Encouraging family members' participation in interdisciplinary team rounds can enhance family presence. According to Davidson et al. (2017), family members who participate in family-centered rounds report improvement in understanding and involvement in decision-making and satisfaction with provider communication than those who do not. Another way to increase family presence is the option of being present during resuscitation efforts with a staff member assigned to support the family. According to the AACN practice alert, there has been no adverse psychological effect among family members who witnessed resuscitation, no patient disruption, and no negative outcome (AACN, 2016). Similarly, a multicenter randomized trial by Jabre et al. (2013) revealed that family members who were invited by emergency medical services personnel to witness resuscitation efforts had lower rates of posttraumatic stress disorder (PTSD)–related symptoms and did not interfere with medical efforts, increase stress in the healthcare team, or result in medicolegal conflict. Family presence during this crucial time should only be allowed when the family members are escorted by a designated person who has the knowledge to explain to the family what is happening, as it is essential for families to have support while witnessing the resuscitation. Additional ways to engage family members in the care of the patient are listed in Box 3.5

BOX 3.5   Strategies to Promote Family Engagement

- Provide education and role modeling
- Provide brochures that give information regarding the specific setting to reduce family members' anxiety and stress (Davidson et al., 2017)
- Suggest ways that family members can help the patient
- Speak softly to patients and use simple words
- Reorient the patient (who, what, when, where, why, and how [5 Ws + 1H]).
- Talk about family and friends
- Bring patient's sensory aids (eyeglasses, hearing aids)
- Decorate the room with reminders of home
- Allow family to participate in mobilizing the patient
- Provide an open or flexible visitation policy
- Encourage participation in interdisciplinary team rounds
- Encourage family presence during resuscitation efforts
- Document the patient's stay in a diary. Diaries are effective in aiding psychological recovery and reducing the incidence of new PTSD (Jones et al., 2010)

Key Points

Allowing family presence at the bedside is the most important way to enhance family engagement.

Case Study

Given intraoperative findings, the surgical team wants to admit the patient to the ICU for postoperative monitoring. With ongoing use of early effective communication and shared decision-making with Mr. and Mrs. S regarding her acute cholecystitis, you will now focus on orienting the patient and family to the surgical ICU. You provide a brochure regarding the logistics of the unit; information includes a description of the unit, visitation hours, and times of multidisciplinary rounds. You provide postoperative teaching to both and encourage Mr. S to participate in care by repositioning and ambulating with the patient. Mr. S has expressed that he would be unable to miss work. Given that information, flexible visitation hours should be considered to meet family needs and encourage family presence.

PHYSICAL COMFORT/EMOTIONAL SUPPORT

Families need ongoing support from the healthcare team; without this, it can lead to poor adaptability, diversion toward unhealthy behaviors, and an inability to make decisions for themselves and their loved ones. Dissatisfaction in turn comes with uncertainty, which leads to a lack of confidence in decision-making and feeling unsupported (Majesko et al., 2012). Families also experience psychological disorders related to their loved one's hospitalization, including anxiety, PTSD, and depression. Meeting the needs of families has been shown to relieve such symptoms and improve satisfaction (Gay, 2009). A multidisciplinary approach by early consultation of social workers, case coordinators, pastoral services, and palliative care services is key in providing physical and emotional support.

Inpatient palliative care services are intended to meet many of these needs. The goals of these services are to improve pain and symptom management; discuss the patient's illness, prognosis, and treatment options; and develop goals of care. Palliative care can also include provision of spiritual support from a spiritual advisor or chaplain. Family members report discussion with the inpatient palliative care team results in improved communication and knowledge, which contributes to decision-making ability (Enguidanos et al., 2014). Early involvement of social workers for counseling, support, and case management can be helpful along with care coordinators to help families navigate the healthcare system and assess their options. An ethics consultation should be considered if there is a value-related conflict between clinicians and the patient and/or family members.

Key Points

Emotional support for families improves decision-making ability.

Case Study

As the AP, you are providing physical comfort and emotional support from the time the patient and family arrive. You recognize that Mr. and Mrs. S are working parents and missing work has created anxiety that can preclude them from currently focusing on the acute problem. In an attempt to alleviate anxiety, you consult a social worker and case coordinator for counseling and to help them navigate the system. You ask Mr. S what the best way is to communicate on daily goals, as he is unable to attend rounds. You agree to call him at a set time each morning to update him on her status and daily goals. Additionally, you encourage Mr. S to bring familiar items from home that can provide a sense of comfort to Mrs. S.

CULTURAL SENSITIVITY AND BELIEFS SURROUNDING ILLNESS

In the United States, ethnic minorities of different cultures and backgrounds make up at least one-third of the population (Searight & Gaffort, 2005). Society and the medical community have placed emphasis on legal requirements, informed consent, and shared decision-making. This means the value of having a community and being culturally sensitive have taken a back seat. Many different ethnic groups have cultural factors that influence reactions, decisions, and involvement in their care, especially during end-of-life discussions. Healthcare clinicians can seek to incorporate cultural values by providing an opportunity for the patient and family to voice their preferences and make modifications in the plan of care based on the values they hold. This may entail asking the patient if there are any cultural practices that the healthcare team should be aware of so that the clinicians can provide respectful and dignified care.

The challenge of providing health care to different ethnicities in the United States requires being culturally sensitive and learning the differences that exist regarding healing and suffering (Searight & Gaffort, 2005). The American Academy of Family Physicians (AAFP) has published guidelines to assist with cultural sensitivity, although few resources are available to apply these principles. The fundamental goal is to be sensitive toward different cultures without stereotyping. The NP can begin by asking the patient who should be involved in receiving information about her status and decision-making and who she would prefer to make decisions for her in the case of her care (patient, loved one, or head of household). In other situations, there may be cultural differences in how communication of terminal diagnosis or poor prognosis is carried out or attitudes toward advance directives and end-of-life care that providers need to be aware of prior to discussing with the patient (Bae, 2017). Initial discussion about the potential sensitivity of certain topics and the desire for the patient's care to be performed with respect and dignity can go a long way in building trust between the patient and family, and the healthcare team. It is important that no assumptions are made and that the NP enters into conversation with the patient and/or family in a nonjudgmental tone. Asking the patient and family whether there are any cultural beliefs or practices that are important to them and ways that they want to include these practices in their care would be one strategy to open the conversation.

Provider practices need to encompass the general paradigm of allowing different ethnic groups to practice with autonomy, beneficence, nonmaleficence, and justice (Searight & Gafford, 2005). In the United States, autonomy typically takes precedence over beneficence, whereas other cultures prioritize beneficence over autonomy. Some cultures view autonomy as "isolating rather than empowering" (Searight & Gaffort, 2005) and believe solely in a community rather than individuals alone. Many Asian cultures believe it is the

TABLE 3.2 HOW CAN WE AS CLINICIANS BE MORE SENSITIVE?	
ISSUES	SOLUTIONS
Decisions should be made by the appointed responsible party deemed by patient.	Clinicians should ask patients who will be making decisions and how treatment decisions should be made.
Do patients or the family want the information about potential terminal disease?	Ask directly to patients if they want the results or if it should be given to the family.
What language do they prefer for primary communication?	Have accessible, reliable, and trained interpreters.
What are patients' thoughts on goals of care, advance directives, and resuscitation efforts?	Clinicians should provide education and accessibility to fill these forms out and discuss them openly.
Clinicians treat patients from many different ethnic backgrounds.	Become knowledgeable about cultural norms in patients with ethnic backgrounds commonly treated in your area.
Nonverbal cues can be interpreted differently among different cultures.	Educate yourself on nonverbal cues seen in ethnic backgrounds commonly treated in your area.

BOX 3.6 Key Recommendations Toward Cultural Sensitivity

- Emphasis on individualism vs. community
- What individuals define as family (extended, nuclear, and so forth)
- Views of different relationships that exist
- Communication patterns (direct vs. indirect, eye contact vs. no eye contact, and meaning of nonverbal gestures)
- Views of suffering and afterlife along with common religious and belief systems
- Views of the value of providers

provider's responsibility and obligation to make decisions on the welfare of the patient. Being sensitive to different cultures and values (Table 3.2; Box 3.6) improves quality of care delivery and acceptance. This hopefully in turn allows family discussions to be effective and well received. Overall, being sensitive to different cultures and values will improve the quality of care delivery and acceptance. This, in turn, hopefully will allow end-of-life discussions to be effective and well received.

Case Study

Through discussion with the family, you must apply cultural sensitivity. As the AP, you realize that the patient and family originate from Puerto Rico and consider themselves to be Hispanic. Using a Spanish interpreter was the first step in being culturally sensitive. You have learned that many Hispanics feel like they are having an anxiety attack when given news that something is wrong with them; they call it *ataque de nervios* (Juckett, 2008). It is usually an intense but brief explosion of emotions as Mrs. S experienced once she was told she had acute cholecystitis in the ED. Additionally, Hispanics traditionally value the concept of support via family. Mrs. S. wanted to wait for her husband to arrive before discussing what was going on. Collectively with family, including extended family, making decisions collaboratively although paternalistic behaviors is prominent in the Hispanic culture. Furthermore, Hispanics believe in "hot" and "cold" illnesses, and this would be considered "hot" given the need for surgery. Because of this association, certain foods and behaviors are avoided.

However, as a provider, you know that some of those old ways of thinking may differ and you try not to stereotype all Hispanic individuals into the same category. Generally speaking, keeping informed on cultural differences that may change communication patterns and health decisions is important for the beneficence of patients and families. When asking Mrs. S whether there is anything she needs, she points to a bracelet made of red and black stone beads that was removed from her wrist prior to surgery. With the interpreter, she explains that the bracelet is an amulet to protect her from the *mal de ojo*, or evil eye, and that she would like to wear it as she recovers in the hospital. With this information, the NP can inform the nursing staff of the patient's preference to keep the bracelet on as it does not interfere with care. Acceptance of the patient and family's cultural beliefs and allowing the patient to carry out her cultural practices build trust and a therapeutic environment where they can feel that their care is respectful and responsive to their needs.

Mrs. S has an uncomplicated recovery, she is fully ambulating, and her pain is under control. While preparing her for discharge home, the NP once again asks Mrs. S if there are any healing practices that she would like to include in her plan of care. Mrs. S regularly uses a homemade ointment on her skin to prevent dryness; however, she is unsure if she should also apply it to the wound. The NP explains to Mrs. S the need to keep the surgical wound clean and dry until the staples are removed and reviews signs and symptoms of infection and who and when to call for immediate concerns. Mrs. S states that she is comfortable with the information and does not have any further questions. She is discharged home with her husband to continue her recovery and provided with a follow-up appointment in 2 weeks.

CONCLUSION

The primary goals of patient- and family-centered care are to keep patients and families informed by early effective communication, involved through the use of informed and shared decision-making, and engaged by encouraging family presence; to provide support via physical and emotional comfort; and to provide culturally sensitive care. It is essential for the healthcare team to be respectful and supportive of all patient and family decisions. This entails realizing that the patient's and family's knowledge, values, cultural backgrounds, and beliefs influence their decision capacities.

CLINICAL PEARLS

- The most significant, documented need of patient's family is access to clear, understandable, and honest communication on information about the patient's medical condition (Fox, 2014).
- Use the four methods to help communicate with your families and patients: ask-tell-ask, tell me more, reflections rather than questions, and responding to emotions.
- Shared decision-making ties in the importance of communication and information sharing in hopes to facilitate appropriate decisions to be made between the family and healthcare team for the patient.
- To perform informed decision-making, clinicians should present evidence and summarize the problems and make an effort to explain risk and benefits of each treatment option.
- Two coping styles that affect decision-making are monitors, who seek information, plan ahead, and are problem focused, and blunters, who are emotionally focused and cope by avoiding information and practical planning.
- Keep families engaged via participation in multidisciplinary team rounds, being present during resuscitation efforts, and an open visitation policy.
- Provide emotional support via the use of ancillary services (social work, case coordinator, pastoral care, and palliative care).
- Be culturally competent toward others and sensitive to individual's needs.

REVIEW QUESTIONS

1. The most fundamental need identified by the Family Needs Inventory is:
   a. To have culturally competent care
   b. Effective early communication
   c. Open visitation policy

2. Mr. P is a 34-year-old male admitted to the intensive care unit after a motorcycle crash. He is expressing his concerns on his inability to work, going to church, and ongoing pain needs. What ancillary services should be consulted (select all that apply)?
   a. Ethics committee
   b. Social work
   c. Pastoral care
   d. Palliative care
   e. Pain consult

3. A 24-year-old female who speaks only Chinese presents with acute appendicitis and needs an appendectomy. Select all that apply for this patient.
   a. Use an interpreter for communication
   b. Ensure parents are notified to help with decision-making
   c. Inform patient and family of treatment option along with risk and benefits
   d. Tell family because she is of age, they cannot help her with the decisions
   e. Skip the details of the operation because it does not matter in the decision-making
   f. Engage social work given their need for social interconnection

Answers: 1, b; 2, b, c, and e; 3, a, c, and f

REFERENCES

Adams, A., Mannix, T., & Harrington, A. (2017). Nurses' communication with families in the intensive care unit, a literature review. *Nursing in Critical Care*, 22(2), 70–80.

American Association of Critical-Care Nurses. (2016). *AACN practice alert: Family presence during resuscitation and invasive procedures*. www.aacn.org/wd/practice/docs/practicealerts/fam-pres-resusc-pa-feb2016ccn-pages.pdf

American Association of Retired Persons (AARP). (2020). *About AARP*. https://www.aarp.org/about-aarp/

Auerbach, S. (2005). Optimism, satisfaction with needs met, interpersonal perceptions of the healthcare team, and emotional distress in patients' family members during critical care hospitalization. *American Journal of Critical Care*, 14, 202–210.

Back, A., Arnold, R., Baile, W., Tulsky, J., & Fryer-Edwards, K. (2005). Approaching difficult communication in oncology. *Cancer Journal for Clinicians*, 55(3), 164–177.

Bae, J. (2017). Shared decision making: Relevant concepts and facilitating strategies. *Epidemiology and Health*, 39, e2017048.

Bamm, E. L., & Rosenbaum, P. (2008). Family-centered theory: Origins, development, barriers, and supports to implementation in rehabilitation medicine. *Archives of Physical Medicine and Rehabilitation*, 89(8), 1618–1624.

Bernacki, R., & Block, S. (2014). Communication about serious illness care goals: A review and synthesis of best practices. *JAMA Internal Medicine*, 174(12), 1994–2003.

Burchardi, H. (2002). Let's open the door! *Intensive Care Medicine*, 28(10), 1371–1372.

Ciufo, D., Hader, R., & Holly, C. (2011). A comprehensive systematic review of visitation models in adult critical care units within the context of patient- and family-centered care. *International Journal of Evidence-Based Healthcare*, 9(4), 362–387.

Davidson, J. E., Aslakson, R. A., Long, A. C., Puntillo, K. A., Kross, E. K., Hart, J., Cox, C. E., Wunsch, H., Wickline, M. A., Nunnally, M. E., Netzer, G., Kentish-Barnes, N., Sprung, C. L., Hartog, C. S., Coombs, M., Gerritsen, R. T., Hopkins, R. O., Franck, L. S., Skrobik, Y., … Curtis, J. (2017). Guidelines for family-centered care in the neonatal, pediatric, and adult ICU. *Critical Care Medicine*, 45(1), 103–128.

Elwyn, G., Frosch, D., Thomson, R., Joseph-Williams, N., Lloyd, A., Kinnersley, P., Cording, E., Tomson, D., Dodd, C., Rollnick, S., Edwards, A., & Barry, M. (2012). Shared decision making: A model for clinical practice. *Journal of General Internal Medicine*, 27(10), 1361–1367.

Enguidanos, S., Housen, P., Penido, M., Mejia, B., & Miller, J. (2014). Family members' perceptions of inpatient palliative care consult services: A qualitative study. *Palliative Medicine*, 28(1), 42–48.

Fox, M. Y. (2014). Improving communication with patients and families in the intensive care unit: palliative care strategies for the intensive care unit nurse. *Journal of Hospice & Palliative Nursing*, 16(2), 93–98.

Hinkle, J., & Fitzpatrick, E. (2011). Needs of American relatives of intensive care patients: Perceptions of relatives, physicians and nurses. *Intensive & Critical Care Nursing*, 27(4), 218–225.

Gauntlett, R., & Laws, D. (2008). Communication skills in critical care. *Continuing Education in Anaesthesia, Critical Care & Pain*, 8(4), 121–124.

Gay, E. (2009). The intensive care unit family meeting: Making it happen. *Journal of Critical Care*, 24(4), 629.e1–629.e12.

Institute for Healthcare Improvement. (2019). *What is "ask, tell, ask"?* Ihi.org. http://www.ihi.org/education/IHIOpenSchool/resources/Pages/AudioandVideo/ConnieDavis-WhatIsAskTellAsk.aspx

Jabre, P., Belpomme, V., Azoulay, E., Jacob, L., Bertrand, L., Lapostolle, F., Tazarourte, K., Bouilleau, G., Pinaud, V., Broche, C., Normand, D., Baubet, T., Ricard-Hibon, A., Istria, J., Beltramini, A., Alheritiere, A., Assez, N., Nace, L., Vivien, B., … Adnet, F. (2013). Family presence during cardiopulmonary resuscitation. *The New England Journal of Medicine*, 368(11), 1008–1018.

Jones, C., Bäckman, C., Capuzzo, M., Egerod, I., Flaatten, H., Granja, C., Rylander, C., & Griffiths, R. (2010). Intensive care diaries reduce new onset post traumatic stress disorder following critical illness: A randomized, controlled trial. *Critical Care*, 14(5), R168.

Juckett, G. (2008). Caring for Latino patients. *American Family Physician*, 87(1), 45–54.

Lilly, C., De Meo, D., Sonna, L., Haley, K., Massaro, A., Wallace, R., & Cody, S. (2000). An intensive communication intervention for the critically ill. *The American Journal of Medicine*, 109(6), 469–475.

Luce, J. (2010). End-of-life decision making in the intensive care unit. *American Journal of Respiratory and Critical Care Medicine*, 182(1), 6–11.

Majesko, A. Y., Hong, S. B., Weissfeld, L., & White, D. (2012). Identifying family members who may struggle in the role of surrogate decision maker. *Critical Care Medicine*, 40(8), 2281–2286.

Searight, H., & Gafford, J. (2005). Cultural diversity at the end of life: Issues and guidelines for family physicians. *American Family Physician*, 71(3), 515–522.

Society of Critical Care Medicine. (n.d.). Family engagement and empowerment. https://www.sccm.org/ICULiberation/ABCDEF-Bundles/Family-Engagement

Selection and Interpretation of Diagnostic Tests

Paula McCauley

Case Study

You are the APRN working in urgent care. Mr. H is a healthy-appearing 65-year-old man who presents to you with a 1-week history of dyspnea, cough, and anterior midsternal chest pain that has become increasingly more severe this afternoon and is most significant under his right rib cage. He has had low-grade fevers of 99 °F–100 °F.

His past medical history includes HTN and coronary artery disease (CAD). His surgical history includes an appendectomy at age 12 and three-vessel coronary artery bypass and aortic valve repair last March.

His current medications include Toprol 50 mg daily and aspirin 81 mg daily.

He has no known drug allergies.

His review of systems: He denies chills, night sweats, and weight loss. He endorses fatigue, dyspnea on exertion (DOE) with difficulty climbing one flight of stairs; he has to stop to rest along the way. He denies palpitations, orthopnea, or nocturnal dyspnea. He has noted swelling to his lower extremities over the past few weeks; it appears worse at the end of the day. His cough is nonproductive. He denies abdominal pain, discomfort, or distention. He has normal bowel movements and no urinary symptoms.

His physical examination is as follows: temperature, 99.3 °F; pulse, 96 bpm; respiratory rate, 20 per min; blood pressure, 136/86 mm Hg. His lung sounds are diminished to both lower fields, and there are fine crackles to the right base with dullness on percussion to the right lower field. Cardiovascular examination reveals a regular rate and rhythm, normal S1 and S2, and no murmur, rub, or gallop. His abdomen is soft, flat, and nontender, with normal bowel sounds and no hepatosplenomegaly. His lower extremities have 1+ edema bilaterally, normal capillary refill, and no cyanosis or clubbing. His midsternal scar is well healed with no erythema, instability, or drainage. What are your next steps?

DIAGNOSTIC PROCESS AND TESTING

To diagnose is to establish an accurate and timely explanation of a patient's health problem that is communicated to the patient (National Academies of Sciences, Engineering, and Medicine, 2015). The diagnostic process is the iterative, careful critical study of a health condition to determine its nature (Carpenito-Moyet, 2007). The diagnostic process begins with the history and pertinent physical examination and incorporates information collection from the patient and family, a response to the patient's emotional state, and education of the patient. Diagnostic reasoning also includes asking "why?" within a systematic framework. You must identify a differential diagnosis or hypothesis based on signs and symptoms. Your suspected differential will guide in selection of necessary tests and additional data. Development of a differential diagnosis includes prioritizing the differential and then testing your hypothesis. This may require that you review and reprioritize your initial differential diagnosis and retest.

Key Points

Development of a complete framed differential diagnosis can be done in a variety of ways and may include an anatomic framework, an organ/system framework, a pathophysiologic framework, or combined frameworks. There are several mnemonics that can be used during this process. There are also approaches like the four Ps, which help you to prioritize your differential and include a Possibilistic approach, Probabilistic approach, Prognostic approach, or Pragmatic approach (Stern et al., 2014).

Case Study

Based on the given information, must-not-miss concerns for Mr. H are ACS, aortic dissection, and pulmonary embolus. Other top differentials might include community-acquired pneumonia (CAP), heart failure with pulmonary edema, pericarditis/effusion, and pleural effusion. Some basic questions to guide your diagnostic process for every patient include the following: Based on your patient's history and physical findings, what diagnostics will you use to test your diagnostic hypothesis? Is your review of systems comprehensive or are there additional questions you need to ask? Can you use a specific diagnostic framework? What diagnostic tests would you like to choose and why?

Diagnostic tests cover a variety of options, from diagnosis to evaluating treatment of disease. In order to test your hypothesis, you need to consider a variety of aspects, including pretest probability, potential harm of diagnostics, and test characteristics, and you need to have a basic understanding of the principles and characteristics of various tests. Principles of diagnostic tests are included in Box 4.1. Categories of tests are included in Box 4.2.

Based on the patient's characteristics, such as age and sex, and disease risk factors, such as their past medical history and family history, as well as presenting symptoms, the nurse practitioner should first examine the most likely cause. This is done by evaluating the

---

BOX 4.1 **Principles of Diagnostic Test Selection**

- Disease incidence: the rate of new cases of a disease reported as the number of new cases within a defined period of time.
- Disease prevalence: the number of cases of a disease in a specific population at a particular time.
- Potential risk factor: a variable associated with an increased risk of disease.
- Relative risk: a comparison of the risk of disease in people exposed to a potential risk factor with people who were not exposed to the risk factor.
- Cost-benefit ratio: the cost and/or health risk of performing a given diagnostic test compared with the benefit of identifying a diagnosis that will inform treatment.

---

suspected incidence, or new cases of disease in a given timeframe, and prevalence, or the number of disease cases in a given population. For instance, in this scenario of a 65-year-old male presenting with anterior midsternal pain, there is a high possibility of this being ACS or myocardial infarction because cardiovascular disease is one of the most common conditions in the United States (American Heart Association, 2020). In addition, his past medical history of HTN and CAD and a past surgical history of coronary artery bypass both increase the risk of a cardiac event. This information along with the cost-benefit ratio will help the nurse practitioner narrow in on the types of diagnostic testing to perform. For instance, in evaluating whether the etiology of his symptoms could be of cardiac origin, a blood test is less costly and with less risk compared with a coronary angiogram. However, the nurse practitioner also needs to consider other etiologies in light of his physical examination findings. Reflecting on the characteristics of the diagnostic test (Box 4.3), each diagnostic test will have a different level of accuracy to discriminate between the presence and absence of disease.

Test Characteristics

Test characteristics are listed in Box 4.3.

Understanding the sensitivity and specificity of a given diagnostic test can also help the nurse practitioner to determine which one will be most useful. For instance, a diagnostic test with sensitivity of 97.4% and a low specificity of 21.9% would provide in conclusive data of a given diagnosis, whereas a positive test with a high likelihood ratio (LR) raises the probability of disease (Box 4.4) (Stern et al., 2014). The test characteristics must be evaluated along with the clinical presentation of the patients and identification of any interfering factors that may lead to misinterpretation of the findings.

BOX 4.2 **Categories of Diagnostic Tests**

- Screening
- Evaluation of severity of the disease
- Estimation of prognosis
- Monitoring the course of the disease
- Detection of recurrence
- Selection of drugs and adjustment of therapy

BOX 4.3 Test Characteristics

- Accuracy: ability of a test to discriminate between the presence of a disease or not.
- Precision: indication of how closely a test result is reproduced.
- Reference range: the minimum and maximum threshold or limits of a laboratory test based on a group of otherwise healthy people.
- Interfering factors: variables that can cause inaccurate measurement that can lead to misinterpretation of test results.
- Sensitivity, or true-positive rate, is the likelihood of a positive test in a diseased patient. Highly sensitive tests have a low percentage of false-negative results and are useful to exclude a diagnosis.
- Specificity, or true-negative rate, is the likelihood of a positive result in a patient without disease. Tests with high specificity have a low percentage of false-positive results and are used to confirm a diagnosis.
- LR reflects how likely the test result would occur in a patient with the disease compared with a patient without the disease (Box 4.4).

Pretest Probability

The pretest probability is the evaluation of the likelihood of the presence or absence of disease before a test is performed and can help to determine the utility of the test for decision-making on the course of action or treatment. When the pretest probability is low, and the nurse practitioner is quite certain that the patient does not have the disease, a positive test has a considerable effect, whereas a negative test has little effect. In contrast, when the pretest probability is high, a positive test has little effect while a negative test has a large effect. Pretest probability will depend on the sensitivity and specificity of the test characteristics you order and the LR of the test. Using data about the patient's characteristics, risk factors, and comorbidities, along with the pretest probability, the nurse practitioner can further narrow in on the diagnostic testing that will provide the most useful information to inform the treatment plan.

Valid Clinical Decision Rules

There are several ways to determine the pretest probability of your leading hypothesis and active alternatives. Validated clinical decision rules (CDRs) use prevalence data regarding the causes or etiologies of a symptom. Examples of CDRs you may use in this case include HEART (history, electrocardiogram [ECG], age, risk factors, and troponin) score for ACS, Wells or PERC (Pulmonary Embolism Rule-out Criteria) score for pulmonary embolism (PE), and CURB65 or the pulmonary severity score for patients with CAP. These are tools to guide your diagnosis and disposition but your differential must also include your overall clinical impression. No test is perfect and rarely are there tests that will exclusively rule in or rule out a diagnosis. Knowing the gold standards for various diagnoses will assist in your choice of diagnostic tests. For ACS,

BOX 4.4 Likelihood Ratios

LR+ compares a true positive and a false positive; positive LRs are above 1.
LR− compares a false negative and a true negative; negative LRs are less than 1.
  Based on Stern et al. (2014)

the definitive diagnosis will come from a coronary angiogram. For PE, a computed tomography pulmonary angiography (CTPA) is considered the gold standard. These diagnostic tools are not without risk and the benefit needs to be considered. Are there other options that are less invasive but provide adequate data to treat? Let us explore specific examples or additional diagnostics and threshold to treat.

In patients with evidence of pulmonary edema on examination and chest x-ray (CXR), your differential would include heart failure from cardiogenic causes and other etiology that may be noncardiogenic, such as interstitial pulmonary fibrosis or adult respiratory distress syndrome (ARDS).

Cardiogenic diagnostics might include a workup for ischemia, including B-type natriuretic peptide (BNP), cardiac enzymes, and an echocardiogram. The echocardiogram will provide information regarding the left ventricular function and ejection fraction as well as wall motion abnormalities but will not give you specific information about obstructive CAD. Here, the left heart catheterization would be necessary for more definitive information for the ACS. Because it is not without risk, consider whether there are enough data to support this as your initial examination. Would a stress test provide adequate data to support or rule out your diagnosis?

Patients with noncardiogenic pulmonary edema may present with hypoxia and similar findings on radiography, so here, the etiology is often a diagnosis of exclusion. Your differential will be supported by potential precipitating causes, such as ARDS from sepsis, or history of exposure to agents that could cause inflammatory or interstitial fibrosis. If there is a mixed picture, a definitive diagnosis could be made by documenting the pulmonary capillary wedge pressure with a right heart catheterization, which would be normal or not be elevated if there is a noncardiogenic cause.

If your differential includes PE, using the PERC or Wells score will help guide additional diagnostics. Use of a highly sensitive/quantitative D-dimer in a patient with low risk for PE (after applying a Wells or PERC score) can rule out PE. If the patient is at low risk and has a d-dimer of <500, no further testing is needed because this would rule PE out. Conversely, a d-dimer is not indicated in a high-risk patient because the LR will be high, based on the data from examination and diagnostics (Stern et al., 2014). An ECG may show sinus tachycardia, an S1Q3T3 pattern, right ventricular strain, and a new incomplete right bundle branch block, but these findings only occur in 10% of PEs. An echocardiogram may provide findings that support PE, such as right heart strain, but also is not sensitive. A CT pulmonary angiogram is the gold standard and is highly sensitive. For a patient with suspected PE in whom contrast is contraindicated, a lower extremity Doppler that is positive for deep vein thrombosis (DVT) provides adequate data to treat.

Case Study

Your differentials include the must-not-miss diagnoses of ACS and PE, but the patient appears stable to you and you do not have the capability of doing a CTPA in your urgent care center. You do have laboratory and plain film capability. You decide to order a CBC with differential, basic metabolic panel, BNP, procalcitonin, d-dimer, troponin-I, ECG, and CXR. While waiting for his other diagnostics to be completed, you receive his CXR (Figure 4.1). The radiologists are not on site, so your film will be read by a remote service. You need to do a basic interpretation of the film. Where do you start?

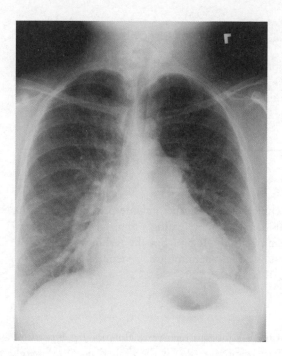

Figure 4.1 Mr. H's chest x-ray.

FUNDAMENTALS OF RADIOLOGY

The chest radiograph is one of the most frequently used radiographic studies and should be ordered as your first evaluation when there is concern for pathology in the thorax. Basic radiology interpretation is a fundamental requirement of all APRNs. All APRNs need to be comfortable doing a basic systematic interpretation of the film and be proficient in identifying normal and common pathologic findings seen on plain films. As is common with many diagnostics, use of an evidence-based process will aid in interpretation (Chen et al., 2011). There are many common systematic approaches, such as outside-in, ABC, or the five Ps. The process selected will be user-dependent, but whichever you choose, stick with it and practice, practice, practice. Use and validation of your findings with a mentor will lead to competency (Pezzotti, 2014). In acute and critical care, you will also use the plain film for appropriate placement of tubes and lines, and as the provider, you need to be comfortable with landmarks and evaluation of various devices and therapeutic lines.

Key Points

Radiology is colorful! Keep in mind that it is black and white with many shades of gray. The basic CXR also incorporates multiple body systems and can be worthwhile in diagnosing many abnormalities (Mettler, 2005).

Structures that are covered or considered in a CXR are listed in Box 4.5.

CLINICAL PEARLS

- Establishing a process for evaluation of films is important.
- Decide on a process and STICK TO IT.
- Interpretation of plain films includes technical as well as structural interpretation.
- Describe what you see.
- Compare to old films if available.

Technical Aspects

Interpretation of plain films includes technical as well as structural interpretation. The technical aspects must be reviewed and considered when evaluating a film. Digital technology has provided us with the ability to manipulate the image, but the technical quality will impact interpretation. Technical aspects include magnification, penetration, inspiration, rotation, and angulation (Chen et al., 2011; Mettler, 2005).

Magnification

Magnification refers to the position of the x-ray beam relative to the cassette. Structures closest to the cassette are magnified. Posteroanterior (PA) is the desired position, as the cassette is placed in front of the patient with the rays coming from the back. The PA film is usually done with a lateral CXR. This gives another dimension to the examination and helps determine the location of pathology or disease not evident on the frontal image, including the retrosternal space, hilar region, fissures, thoracic spine, diaphragm, and posterior costophrenic sulci (Chen et al., 2011; Mettler, 2005).

Portable films are anteroposterior (AP) films. They offer only one view and will magnify the heart; since the heart is in the forefront of the rays, it may appear or be interpreted as enlarged. Quality is usually inferior to a PA film and may also be affected by the limited inspiratory effort of the patient as well as the power of the portable machine (Chen et al., 2011).

Penetration

Penetration applies to evaluation of a properly exposed film. Consider the following questions: How well can you see the opaque parts of the film? Is the film adequate, underpenetrated, or overpenetrated? Can you visualize the outline of the vertebral bodies behind the mediastinum? With an adequately penetrated film you should be able to see the thoracic spine through the heart, but it then becomes hazy as you follow it down into the abdomen. If you cannot distinguish the vertebral bodies, then your film is underpenetrated,

BOX 4.5   Contents Viewed on a Chest Radiograph

Bony structures: ribs, clavicles, scapula, vertebra, humeral head
Heart and great vessels
Hila and lungs
Diaphragm
Soft tissue

underexposed, or white. This will create prominence of the small vessels and lung parenchyma with overinterpretation or misdiagnosis of infiltrates or pulmonary vascular congestion. An overpenetrated or overexposed film will appear dark, preventing evaluation of smaller structures such as alveolus small nodules (Chen et al., 2011; Mettler, 2005).

Inspiration

The ultimate view is done at end inspiration, providing adequate expansion of the lungs. Underexpansion can create compression or restriction of structures and cloud interpretation. Nine posterior ribs should be visible above the hemidiaphragm on the patient's right side. A PA film is preferred, as the patient will be standing and instructed to inspire, providing greater inspiratory effort. A portable or AP projection is usually done with the patient in bed, thus impacting inspiratory effort. If more than nine ribs can be seen on the CXR, it suggests hyperaeration, which will prompt you to consider whether the patient has emphysema or is hyperinflated due to mechanical ventilation. If fewer than nine ribs are seen (hyperaeration), there are several possible factors: poor inspiratory effort, a lordotic view, compromised lung health, or the diaphragm has been pushed higher than normal (Chen et al., 2011; Mettler, 2005).

Rotation

It is important to recognize existence of rotation because rotation in either direction will impact or distort normal findings. Look at the spatial relationship between the anterior ends of the clavicles. The spinous processes should fall equidistant between the medial ends of the clavicles (Chen et al., 2011; Mettler, 2005).

Angulation

A film shot at an angle will alter the appearance of the contents of the chest. In a normal or nonangulated film, the clavicle normally has an S shape and superimposes on the third or fourth rib (Chen et al., 2011; Mettler, 2005).

Process

There are several processes commonly used for interpretation (Chen et al., 2011; Pezzotti, 2014):

- The five Ps: Position, Penetration, Pleura, Parenchyma, and Plastics
- ABCs: Air, Bone, Circulation
- Outside-in: Soft tissue > bones > pleura > parenchyma > mediastinum

Key Points

Describe what you see. Do not diagnose from a CXR alone. It is part of your diagnostic process but not specific enough on its own. You may correlate the findings that are "consistent with" a differential diagnosis (Connolly, 2001). An example being in an upright film with loss of the costophrenic angle and a meniscus sign: you may say that the film is consistent with a pleural effusion. Increased interstitial edema is consistent with pulmonary edema or pulmonary fibrosis. And remember to compare with old films if available.

Case Study

Figure 4.1 shows Mr. H's CXR. Using your newfound competence and the five Ps, here is what you see.

Position: This is a portable film, so it must be an AP film. It is upright. Position is slightly rotated to the left, correlating the distance of the clavicular heads with the spinous processes. The right clavicle is closer to the spine and thus is rotated forward.

Penetration: This film is a bit underpenetrated. You cannot see his vertebrae behind his heart. You should lose this clarity when you get below the diaphragm. There is good inspiratory effort; you can count 8-9 rib spaces.

Pleura: He has symmetry to his bones/ribs/rib spaces. There is no evidence of fracture. There are lung markings out to the periphery, so there is no evidence of pneumothorax. As you travel down to the costophrenic angles, they become hazy or opacified bilaterally. The cardiac silhouette is obscured at the right base.

Parenchyma: The heart appears generous and there may be cardiomegaly but if an AP film you realize the heart is magnified. There is good aeration to the upper fields, there are interstitial changes, most evident to the right base. The cardiac silhouette is obscured on the right border. There is evidence of bilateral perihilar fullness with vascular engorgement most evident on the right and increased pulmonary vascular markings with mild cephalization. There is evidence of an air bronchogram on the left. There may be atelectasis vs consolidation at the lower right field. A gastric bubble is event under the diaphragm.

Plastics: There are no plastics or hardware evident.

Common Pathologic Conditions

Pathologic considerations exposed on CXR are listed in Box 4.6 and discussed here.

Air space disease is diffuse, lobar, interstitial, and/or unilateral and encompasses many processes, including pneumonia, pulmonary hemorrhage, contusion, or pulmonary edema (which can be blood, water, or pus). Essentially what has occurred is that the alveoli that are normally filled with air are now flooded or consolidated with fluid or pus. Linear consolidation is referred to as a reticular pattern, which may include thin to dense lines that

---

BOX 4.6 Common Pathologic Processes Seen on Chest X-ray

- Air space disease
- Atelectasis/loss of volume
- Pneumothorax
- Hemothorax
- Pleural fluid accumulation
- Pulmonary vascular changes
- Masses
- Interstitial changes
- Emphysema

may be linear or overlap, creating the appearance of a net. This is common in pathology that leads to interstitial changes, such as pulmonary edema or fibrosis (Chen et al., 2011; Mettler, 2005).

Atelectasis is often referred to as loss of volume or airlessness in the lungs (Figure 4.2). It can be a linear finding or full collapse. Collapse is often used to refer to complete atelectasis of a segment of a lobe. It can develop due to obstruction from a mass, aspiration of an object, or secretions, secondary to space-occupying processes such as pneumothorax, pleural effusion, or loss of surface tension in situations such as respiratory distress syndrome in infants (Chen et al., 2011; Mettler, 2005).

Pneumothorax is the result of a communication between the pleural linings. It will appear as an increased radiolucency of the air space within the pleural space and include the presence of air and absence of pulmonary vessels or parenchymal markings (Figure 4.3). The lung will begin to collapse away from the chest wall and may produce deviation of the mediastinum away from the affected side. In a hemothorax, as in a pneumothorax, there is communication between the two pleural linings, except the space is filled with fluid instead of air. The pleural space will become opacified (Chen et al., 2011; Mettler, 2005).

Pleural fluid accumulation can be secondary to various alterations in pressure or volume overload, as seen with cardiac or renal failure and flow related to alterations in permeability with inflammatory or infectious processes. They can be free or loculated and are categorized as transudative or exudative. Common findings include a fluid level or meniscus sign or loss of the costophrenic angle (Chen et al., 2011; Mettler, 2005).

Pulmonary vascular changes are associated with cardiogenic pulmonary edema due to the increased pulmonary capillary pressures. There is redistribution of the pulmonary blood flow from the dependent (hilar) areas of the lung, with cephalization or redistribution to the apices or periphery of the lung (Chen et al., 2011; Mettler, 2005).

Masses or nodules are often classified as single or multiple, have consistent or various sizes, may be calcified or cavitary, and may be diffuse or peripheral. They can be related to malignancy, infection, or embolic etiologies (Chen et al., 2011; Mettler, 2005).

Interstitial changes are diffuse linear lucencies or stacks of air-filled lucencies with the appearance of chicken wire or honeycombing in the lung periphery. They are consistent with pulmonary edema and fibrosis (Chen et al., 2011; Mettler, 2005).

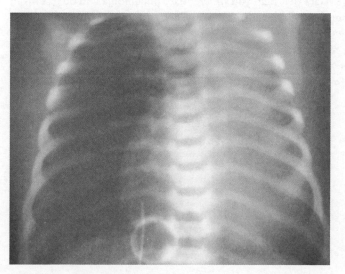

Figure 4.2 Atelectasis, loss of volume.

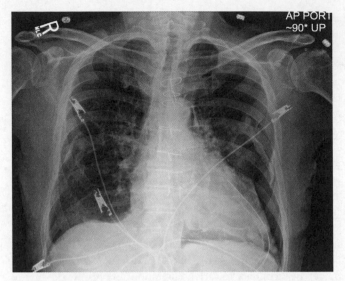

Figure 4.3 Pneumothorax.

Emphysema is seen as air-filled spaces lacking any lucency due to hyperinflation of the alveoli. The lung volumes are larger than normal and more radiolucent with flattening of the diaphragms (Chen et al., 2011; Mettler, 2005).

Technical Terms

When ordering a CXR, you will find that the radiologist interpretation will include various terms. As the provider, you need to be comfortable interpreting these findings and their association with various pathologic processes that will narrow your differential. As you began to request and interpret films, you will apply these terms. Common terms seen on CXR reports are listed in Box 4.7 (Chen et al., 2011; Mettler, 2005).

Air bronchograms result from exudative-filled alveoli surrounding air-filled bronchi. The bronchi are clearly visible. Figure 4.4 has well-defined air bronchograms.

Air bronchograms are associated with air space diseases such as pneumonia, atelectasis, or pulmonary hemorrhage. Data that help you differentiate pneumonia and atelectasis in the case of air bronchograms are included in Table 4.1 (Chen et al., 2011; Connolly, 2001; Mettler, 2005).

Batwing pattern is the appearance of wings originating from the central or hilar area extending out to the lung periphery due to consolidation of pulmonary vasculature and associated cardiogenic pulmonary edema (Mettler, 2005).

BOX 4.7   **Common Terms Used in Evaluation of Chest X-ray**

- Air bronchogram
- Batwing pattern
- Cephalization
- Honeycombing
- Kerley B lines
- Silhouette sign

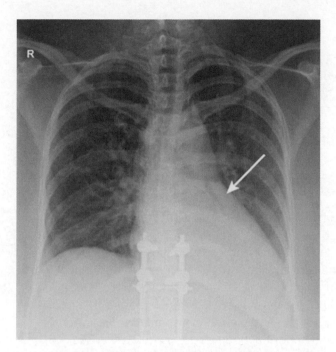

Figure 4.4 Air bronchogram.

Cephalization results when there are increased vascular markings that extend to the lung periphery. They are consistent with increased pulmonary vascular pressure associated with heart failure or pulmonary HTN (Chen et al., 2011; Mettler, 2005).

Honeycombing appears as stacked, air-filled interstitial markings and is consistent with fibrosis or pulmonary edema (Mettler, 2005).

Kerley A and B lines appear as septal thickening that results in linear opacities in the lung periphery. It is consistent with interstitial pulmonary edema (Chen et al., 2011).

Reticular pattern is a collection of linear opacities that create a netlike appearance.

Reticulonodular pattern is a collection of linear and nodular opacities together that create the appearance of a net with superimposed nodules.

Silhouette sign is the loss of a normal boarder due to an abnormality adjacent to the structure. An example is the cardiac silhouette: If the right heart border is indistinct, it would indicate a contiguous infiltrate or mass in the right middle lobe (Chen et al., 2011; Mettler, 2005).

TABLE 4.1 FACTORS DIFFERENTIATING ATELECTASIS FROM PNEUMONIA	
ATELECTASIS	**PNEUMONIA**
Volume loss	Normal or increased volume
Associated ipsilateral shift	No shift or contralateral shift
Linear, wedge-shaped	Consolidation, air space process
Air bronchograms	Air bronchograms

Key Points

You cannot diagnose from the patient's CXR alone. It will provide you with an image that will yield assistance with your differential diagnoses. Describe what you see and correlate it to your patient's history and physical and clinical findings.

Case Study

In Mr. H's film, you identified hazy costophrenic angles bilaterally. The cardiac silhouette is obscured at the bases. There is bilateral haziness to both mid- and lower lung fields, with interstitial changes and consolidation or opacification most evident to rich base. The cardiac silhouette is obscured on right and there is evidence of increased pulmonary vascular markings with cephalization. Based on the pathologic findings we have discussed thus far, our differential now includes CAP, pulmonary edema, and pleural effusion. Your laboratory test results have come back and abnormal findings are as follows: WBCs, 16.2, with elevated neutrophils on differential; H/H, platelet counts are within normal limits (WNL). His d-dimer is 125, BNP is 650, procalcitonin is 0.45, and troponin I < 0.01. ECG is normal sinus rhythm with no ST or T wave changes.

Differential Diagnosis

Correlate each with your clinical findings and defend or remove each from your differential diagnosis. His d-dimer is insignificant; he has no other findings that lead you to believe PE is the primary diagnosis. His troponin is negative and his ECG has no acute findings. Non–ST elevation myocardial infarction (STEMI) may stay on your differential and would require trending of troponins, but it is no longer on the top of your list, as he denies other symptoms consistent with an acute ischemic event. That leaves us with CAP, pleural effusion, and pulmonary edema.

Pneumonia

Mr. H has dyspnea, cough, and anterior midsternal chest pain that has become increasingly more severe and is most significant under his right rib cage, which could be pleural in nature due to inflammatory processes. He has had low-grade fevers of 99 °F–100 °F. His lung sounds are diminished to both lower fields and there are fine crackles to the right base, which could be related to consolidation. He has leukocytosis on his CBC and an elevated procalcitonin.

Radiograph findings consistent with pulmonary "infiltrates" and the differential for pneumonia include the diffuse bilateral opacification and loss of cardiac silhouette. He has no loss of volume or air bronchograms.

Pleural Effusion

Mr. H has a past medical history that includes HTN and CAD and endorses symptoms of heart failure, which could lead to a transudative pleural effusion. His chest pain has become increasingly more severe and is most significant under his right rib cage, which indicates that it could be pleural in nature. This could be an empyema if he does in fact have pneumonia. He also recently had CABG which involves entrance into the pleural space in many cases, and he may have a residual effusion post procedure. His CXR findings are consistent with or suggestive of a pleural effusion: Costophrenic angles are hazy or opacified bilaterally, and there is evidence of fluid or a meniscus sign on the right side.

Pulmonary Edema

Here again, Mr. H has a past medical history that includes HTN and CAD. He has chest pain and endorses symptoms of heart failure with his DOE and lower extremity edema, and he has fine crackles on his lung examination. His CXR findings are consistent with pulmonary edema with evidence of increased pulmonary vascular markings with cephalization, and you appreciate the vessels out toward the periphery. He has a calcified aortic arch. His troponin is not elevated and his ECG does not indicate an acute STEMI. He denies orthopnea, paroxysmal nocturnal dyspnea (PND), edema, and he does endorse DOE.

Case Study

You have successfully completed your initial evaluation of Mr. H. You have enough information at present to exclude PE and ACS but data to support CAP or pulmonary edema, and there is evidence of pleural effusion on his CXR. Have you reached a threshold to treat, or do you need more information to rule these in or out? At this point you have data to support CAP with added concern for an empyema due to his symptoms and CXR. You consider further examinations such as (but not limited to) chest ultrasound or CT scan and a diagnostic/therapeutic thoracentesis especially if you are concerned for exudative pleural effusion. Do you need to send him to the ED for admission or can you send him home after initiating antibiotic therapy? You use the CURB65 CDR to help you determine his disposition. Pulmonary edema due to heart failure is high on your differential, but his initial enzymes are negative and BNP not elevated. The changes on CXR may be secondary to infectious/inflammatory mediators. Due to his history of CAD, you decide to initiate diuresis and will pursue additional ischemic workup for his chest pain if treatment of CAP is not effective. An echocardiogram and stress test are considerations for further investigation before a cardiac catheterization.

Plastics

There are many plastics, such as lines and tubes, you may encounter in acute care. You will be evaluating films for placement of endotracheal tubes (ETTs), central line and pulmonary artery catheters, gastrostomy tubes, pacemaker leads, chest tubes, and sternal wires, along with other therapeutic interventions.

Appreciating where these lines and tubes should sit will require some practice. Of utmost importance is ETT placement. Consider the following case study to illustrate.

Case Study

Your patient was intubated this morning for acute respiratory failure. He has been agitated and difficult to sedate. The nurse comes to get you because peak pressure alarms have been going off and his saturations have dropped. You examine your patient and find diminished breath sounds to the left field. You determine you need a repeat CXR. Your primary differentials at this point include spontaneous pneumothorax, loss of volume, and mucous plugging. Do you have any other concerns?

Your CXR is obtained and you pull it up to review (Figure 4.5).

You see that you have a right internal jugular central line and an ETT. A common rule of thumb is to remember that you obtained this CXR for acute changes, so you should use your process to review and avoid jumping to any obvious conclusions as you may miss things. Your five Ps are as follows:

- Position: this is a portable film (AP), slightly rotated.
- Penetration: adequate, possibly slightly underpenetrated with reduced inspiratory effort.
- Pleura: evidence of lung markings to the periphery, no evidence of pneumothorax, hazy cost phrenic angles R > L.
- Parenchyma: perihilar congestion, evidence cephalization, L lung field seems hazier than R, and there is evidence of interstitial edema and diffuse consolidation L>R. There is evidence of volume loss on the Left.
- Plastics: This is an excellent example of right mainstem intubation. The ETT is coursing down in the right main bronchus when it should be 2 -4 cm above the carina. There is loss of volume on the left and the right lung may be overinflated.
- The ETT needs to be withdrawn at least 3 cm and CXR repeated.

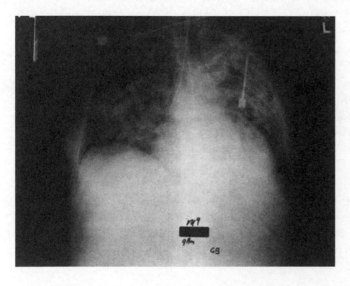

Figure 4.5 Plastics.

CONCLUSION

Your diagnostic process includes a systematic evaluation of the patient's history and physical examination, which will help you to develop a differential diagnosis and drive your choice of diagnostics. This process will include consideration for sensitivity, specificity, population, potential disease prevalence, pretest probability, cost, and benefit or risk to the patient. There are no perfect tests and your diagnostic process will require critical acumen, collaboration, testing, and oftentimes retesting based on findings. CDRs are evidence-based instruments that will assist you with your diagnosis. Along with various laboratory tests, other diagnostics that you must become familiar with include the 12-lead ECG, an echocardiogram, and radiographs. The CXR is a useful diagnostic tool and one of the most common tests you will order. As the provider ordering the film or examination, you need to be comfortable with basic interpretation of the tests you order and common findings. Establishing a systematic process and practicing it with a mentor will aid in your competence for interpretation of diagnostics. As demonstrated in this case, you cannot diagnose from a single test and need to align the findings of any data with your history, physical examination, and other diagnostic findings.

REVIEW QUESTIONS

1. Which of the following is true? Highly sensitive tests:
   a. Have a low percentage of false-negative results
   b. Have a low percentage of false-positive results
   c. Are used to confirm a diagnosis
   d. Provides an accurate true-negative rate

2. Interpretation of plain films includes technical as well as structural interpretation. If you cannot distinguish the vertebral bodies, then your film is
   a. Overexposed
   b. Rotated
   c. Over penetrated
   d. Underpenetrated

3. A meniscus sign is a common finding associated with
   a. Pneumonia
   b. Pleural effusion
   c. Pneumothorax
   d. Atelectasis

4. Volume loss, air bronchograms, and ipsilateral shift are commonly seen with
   a. Pneumonia
   b. Atelectasis
   c. Pleural effusion
   d. Emphysema

   Answers: 1, a; 2, d; 3, b; 4, b

REFERENCES

American Heart Association. (2020). *American heart association – about us*. https://www.heart.org/en/about-us
Carpenito-Moyet L. J. (2007). *Nursing diagnosis: Application to clinical practice* (14th ed.). Lippincott.
Chen, M., Pope, T., & Ott, D. (2011). *Basic Radiology*, (2nd ed.). McGraw-Hill.

Connolly, M. A. (2001). Black, white, and shades of gray: Common abnormalities in chest radiographs. *AACN Clinical Issues*, 12(2), 259–269, quiz 330–332.

Mettler, F. A. (2005). *Essentials of radiology*. Elsevier Saunders.

National Academies of Sciences, Engineering and Medicine. (2015). *Improving diagnosis in health care*. National Academies Press.

Pezzotti, W. (2014). Chest X-ray interpretation. *Nursing*, 44(1), 40–48.

Stern, S. C., Cifu, A. S., & Altkorn, D., (Eds.). Diagnostic process. In *Symptom to diagnosis: an evidence-based guide*(3rd ed.), McGraw-Hill, 2014. Retrieved July 31, 2019. http://accessmedicine.mhmedical.com/content.aspx?bookid=1088&sectionid=61696411.

Care of the Acutely Ill Patient and Prevention of Complications

Erin L. Hallinan

INTRODUCTION

Care of the critically ill patient is often complex and can often be a "rabbit hole" of discovery. As a critical care APRN, it is important to pay attention to the details and to provide comprehensive and holistic care to anticipate and prevent possible secondary complications. Thorough knowledge of disease processes, risk factors, and interventional risk is paramount in formulating a plan of care for the critically ill. In this chapter, we will focus on the immediate care of the critically ill and focus specifically on the prevention of secondary complications. Sepsis, respiratory failure, nutrition, and acute kidney injuries are covered in other chapters. This chapter will focus on hyperglycemia, GI bleeding and prevention of stress ulcers, VTE prophylaxis, toxic metabolic encephalopathy (TME), and post–intensive care syndrome (PICS), and ICU-acquired weakness.

Case Study

You are a critical care APRN intensivist working in a community-based hospital ICU, and you are called to the ED to evaluate Mrs. O, a 74-year-old Hispanic female for consideration for admission to the ICU. Mrs. O is a well-nourished ill-appearing female who appears her stated age who is lying on a stretcher in the ED after she had been intubated by EMS en route for a Glasgow Coma Scale (GCS) of 8. Mrs. O is unable to provide a review of systems; however, her daughter, who is at bedside, is able to provide her past medical history and her history of present illness. She had been feeling poorly for 6 days at home with a fever, chills, fatigue, shortness of breath, and a productive cough. Her daughter notes that she has not been eating well during this time and has been taking minimal oral fluid. Her daughter denies noting any vomiting or diarrhea during this time. Her daughter got scared and called 911 this morning when she found her mother "burning up" and minimally responsive in her bed with labored breathing.

According to her daughter, she has no known drug, food, or environmental allergies. Mrs. O does have a history of HTN, hyperlipidemia, or CAD; she had an MI in 1994 and carries a diagnosis of chronic diastolic congestive heart failure (CHF) and a history of asthma.

Her home medications include Lasix 20 mg orally daily, losartan 100 mg orally daily, amlodipine 10 mg daily, and albuterol metered-dose inhaler (MDI) p.r.n., and her daughter reports compliance with her medication regimen.

In the ED, you note the following physical examination: temperature, 102.7 °F; heart rate, 128 bpm; sinus tachycardia; respiratory rate, 32 set over 20 on the ventilator; and blood pressure, 76/42 mm Hg. Her SaO_2 is 89% on 70% FiO_2 and +5 positive end-expiratory pressure (PEEP). EMS communicates that they have had to go up on her FiO_2 multiple times to get her SaO_2 above 92%. She is poorly responsive, not on sedation, withdraws in all four extremities, and localizes to pain with her bilateral upper extremities. Her pupils are equal, round, and reactive to light and accommodation, and her pupil size is 4 mm. She has a positive gag and a positive cough reflex. Her lung sounds are diminished to both lower fields, and there are scattered rhonchi in her anterior fields. Her cardiovascular examination reveals regular rate and rhythm, normal S1 and S2, no murmurs, rubs, or gallops. Her abdomen is soft, obese, and nontender, with hypoactive bowel sounds and no palpable hepatosplenomegaly. Her skin is warm to the touch, dry and intact with poor turgor and tenting. It is noted that she has acanthosis nigricans at the back of her neck, in her armpits, and her groin. She has palpable +2 dorsalis pedis and posterior tibialis pulses in her bilateral lower extremities.

It is evident that Mrs. O is critically ill and will be admitted to the ICU for further clinical management and treatment. At this juncture, what do you see as your top clinical priorities? What are your main differential diagnoses? As a holistic and comprehensive critical care APRN, what do you anticipate at this point and what measures can you implement to prevent secondary complications?

Mrs. O is transported to the ICU, and her admission weight is 123 kg. As she is hypotensive and has not received any fluid in the ED, you quickly order a 30-cc/kg bolus of crystalloid, placement of an orogastric tube and Foley catheter for accurate intake and output, and broad-spectrum antibiotics (cefepime and vancomycin) after pan cultures are obtained (blood cultures × 2, sputum culture, and urinalysis) and a CXR. You order a CBC, comprehensive metabolic panel, lactic acid, Hgb A1c, prealbumin, LFTs, and coagulation studies. You also order an ECG and cardiac enzymes (creatine phosphokinase and troponin).

HYPERGLYCEMIA

It is well documented that there is an increased risk of cardiovascular disease and diabetes associated with obesity. More than one-third (35.7%) of adults are obese (World Health Organization, WHO, 2020), and 90% of type II diabetics are overweight or obese (American Society for Metabolic and Bariatric Surgery, 2018). The true prevalence of diabetes is difficult to quantify as it can go undiagnosed for a long period of time. In our case study, our patient is 5 ft 4 in tall and 270 lbs (123 kg). This gives her a BMI of 46.3 kg/m² and class III morbid obesity, a diagnosis not listed by her daughter in her past medical history. For this reason, her HbA1c was checked at time of admission, as diabetes is not listed in her history. However, our physical examination revealed acanthosis nigricans, which is often associated with diabetes. Untreated diabetes mellitus and poorly controlled blood glucose have been shown to increase morbidity and mortality (Egi et al., 2008), and in the critically ill population, the same is true regardless of reason for admission (Viana et al., 2014). Untreated diabetes can cause blindness/retinopathy, dental disease, strokes, heart attacks, HTN, surgical site infections, renal disease, limb ischemia, neuropathy, and pregnancy complications (American Society for Metabolic and Bariatric Surgery, 2018). Adults with diabetes have been shown to have a two- to threefold increased risk of stroke and myocardial infarction (Sarwal et al., 2010).

In the hospital setting, hyperglycemia is present in 40% of critically ill patients, with approximately 80% of patients without a prehospital diagnosis of diabetes (Farrokhi et al., 2011). Eighty percent of cardiac surgery patients are noted to have hyperglycemia, and in the critically ill population, 31% will have at least one blood glucose of 200 mg/dl recorded (Farrokhi et al., 2011). The American Diabetes Association and the American Association of Clinical Endocrinologists consensus of hospital-related or stress-related hyperglycemia is a blood glucose of >140 mg/dl or HbA1c > 6.5% without a prior diagnosis of diabetes and blood glucose 180–220 mg/dl in patients with diagnosed diabetes. It is important to differentiate between undiagnosed diabetes and stress-induced hyperglycemia to facilitate appropriate postillness care and follow-up. It is estimated that 30%–60% of new patients with hyperglycemia have confirmed diabetes or impaired carbohydrate intolerance at 1 year post illness (Greci et al., 2003). According to the American Diabetes Association, a diagnosis of diabetes can made if the patient's HbA1c is >6.5% or higher, fasting plasma glucose is 126 mg/dl or higher, oral glucose tolerance test is 200 mg/dl or higher, or random plasma glucose test is 200 mg/dl or higher on one isolated test and repeated testing. It is important to use the patient's HbA1c at time of admission to help identify potential undiagnosed diabetes if other risk factors are present.

Stress-Induced Hyperglycemia

Stress-induced hyperglycemia is an anticipated and frequent clinical manifestation of the acute metabolic and hormonal changes occurring during critical illness in response to trauma, injury, surgery, and stress.

Key Points

Hyperglycemia has been well documented in research as a marker of illness severity (Silva-Perez et al., 2017).

Stress-induced hyperglycemia often subsides as the causative underlying condition resolves. The pathophysiology is outlined in Figure 5.1 and is thought to be due to insufficient insulin secretion that cannot overcome the effects of the hyperglycemia from catecholamine stimulations (Silva-Perez et al., 2017).

It is important to note that for every 1-mmol/L or 18-mg/dl rise in admission fasting plasma glucose, there is approximately a 33% increase in mortality (Farrokhi et al., 2011). Poor glycemic control is also associated with more complications, wound infections, and increased LOS, which increases cost. Glycemic control in the ICU has been well studied and remains challenging, and treatment goals are controversial based on the population being discussed.

There is general consensus from the American Association of Clinical Endocrinologists and the American Diabetes Association (Moghissi et al., 2009) to maintain blood glucose

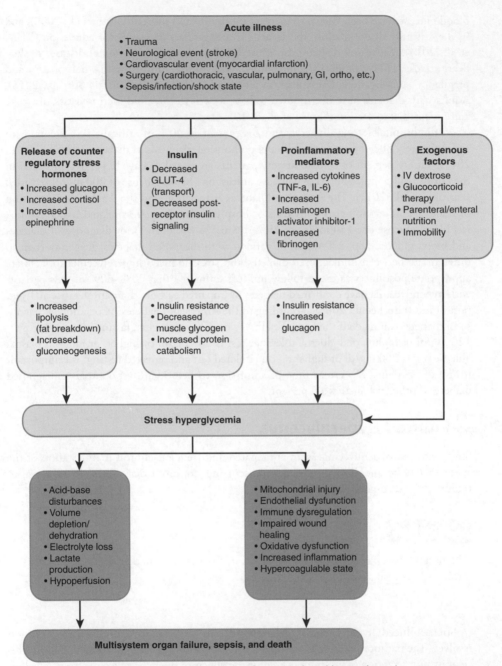

Figure 5.1 Pathophysiology of stress-induced hyperglycemia.

levels between 140 and 180 mg/dl for generalized ICU patients, and that the treatment for critically ill patients with blood glucose >180 mg/dl should be insulin (Silva-Perez et al., 2017). Intravenous insulin administration in both medical and surgical ICU patients demonstrated a reduction in systemic infections, reductions in incidence of multisystem organ failure, and a decrease in short- and long-term mortality (Van den Berghe et al., 2006). The Normoglycemia in Intensive Care Evaluation-Survival Using Glucose Algorithm Regulation (NICE-SUGAR) trial, the largest randomized controlled trial conducted to date, compared two different insulin-based control strategies. In a sample of 6104 ICU patients, the control group had a target blood glucose of <180 mg/dl and the intervention group had a blood glucose target of 81–108 mg/dl (Finfer et al., 2009). This trial discovered that there is a statistically significant increase in cardiovascular mortality associated with the intervention group and tighter glycemic control (Finfer et al., 2009). Further systematic review and meta-analysis discovered that strict glycemic control with blood glucose between 70 and 140 mg/dl had no clinical benefit but lead to higher risk and incidence of hypoglycemia (Silva-Perez et al., 2017).

Key Points

Hypoglycemia is an independent risk factor for death and is more associated with tighter glycemic control targets (Van den Berghe et al., 2001).

This is true for most studies in the neurologic, cardiovascular, cardiothoracic, and sepsis populations. For this reason, the current recommendations are to maintain blood glucose between 140 and 180 mg/dl, to avoid hypoglycemia, and in controlled settings (i.e., centers with experience, adequate nursing support, cardiac surgical patients, and patients without evidence of hypoglycemia), tighter targets of blood glucose between 110 and 140 mg/d/L can be considered.

Case Study

Mrs. O has responded nicely to the 30-cc/kg bolus of crystalloid, and her blood pressure is now 112/65 mm Hg. Her heart rate (HR) has come down to 82 bpm. Her fever has defervesced, and she is now 98.9 °F. Her SaO_2 is still 89% on 70% FiO_2 and +5 PEEP, and she is still tachypneic at 28/20 on the ventilator. She remains poorly responsive, not on sedation, with PERRLA 4. The admission CXR you ordered shows the ETT 3 cm above the carina, the orogastric tube with the tip in the gastric fundus, cardiomegaly, and a right lower lung (RLL) infiltrate. Her ECG does not reveal any ST segment abnormalities, and she is in a normal sinus rhythm. The Foley you placed shows dark amber urine, and the nurse reports to you that she is oliguric and making 22 ml/hr. Her first laboratory test results are as follows: WBC, 18.0/µl; Hgb, 8.2 g/dl; Hct, 24.6%; platelets, 132/µl, with 82% neutrophils; Na, 144 mEq/L; K, 3.2 mEq/L; CO_2, 31 mm Hg; Cl, 101 mEq/L; blood urea nitrogen (BUN), 45 mEq/L; Cr, 1.2 mEq/L; random glucose, 245 mg/dl; Mg, 1.2 mg/dl; Phos, 2.9 mg/dl; Ca, 7.8 mg/dl; international normalized ratio (INR), 1.25; prealbum, 10.4 mg/dl; HbA1c, 13.2%; troponin, 0.4 ng/ml; CK,94; LA, 3.1; ALT, 78 U/L; AST, 58 U/L; albumin, 2.8 g/dl; Alk Phos, 139 U/L; bilirubin total, 0.4 mg/dl; and total protein, 4.7 g/dl. Her arterial blood gas (ABG) is as follows: pH, 7.32; CO_2, 28 mm Hg; PaO_2, 54 mm Hg; oxygen saturation, 89%; and HCO_3, 20 mEq/L.

Based on the above information, you recognize that Mrs. O is likely an undiagnosed diabetic and you order glycemic control with insulin on a sliding scale per hospital protocol for someone who is NPO. You also recognize that she has protein calorie malnutrition at baseline and order a nutrition consult for tube feed recommendations (see Chapter 17). You replace her potassium, magnesium, and phosphorous and recognize her persistent metabolic and lactic acidosis in the setting of oliguria. You order an additional crystalloid fluid bolus and an echocardiogram to establish her baseline function and evaluate the cardiomegaly seen on CXR. You are concerned about her encephalopathy and the degree of hypoxemia she has, which seem disproportionate to the size of the infiltrate on CXR as she clearly has a pneumonia. You increase her PEEP to +8 and notice a decrease in her SBP to the 90s and no increase in her SaO_2. You place her on 100% FiO_2 and consider your next steps. What diagnostic tests should you consider next? When will you check laboratory test values again? What differential diagnoses are you considering?

While you are deliberating outside Mrs. O's room, the echo tech comes to you and tells you that Mrs. O's ejection fraction (EF) is 60% and that she appears to have a wall motion abnormality (akinesia) at the right ventricular mid-free wall and preserved function at the apex (consistent with McConnell sign). Upon hearing this, and in the setting of refractory hypoxemia, you are immediately concerned about a possible PE. As she is poorly responsive, you decide to obtain a noncontrast head computed tomography (NCHCT) angiography to rule out intracranial abnormality and to establish baseline. If she has a PE on the computed tomography angiography (CTA) of the chest you are simultaneously sending her down for, you will need to rule out a head bleed prior to initiation of anticoagulation regardless. As you consider possible systemic therapeutic anticoagulation vs. VTE prophylaxis, you also consider her for stress ulcer prophylaxis.

STRESS ULCER PROPHYLAXIS

Prophylaxis in the form of acid suppression is prescribed for 80%–90% of critically ill and injured patients (Cook & Guyatt, 2018). With the advent of the electronic medical record and predetermined ICU order sets, stress ulcer prophylaxis is often "prechecked" and prescribed without consideration for the clinical application or risk. The same can be true at the time of discharge, leading to an increase in prescriptions in the community after illness has passed (Cook & Guyatt, 2018). Understanding who is at risk and making a pragmatic clinical decision when prescribing stress ulcer prophylaxis is important as there is potential evidence that proton pump inhibitors (PPIs) and H_2 blockers are not without possible harm. The data on stress ulcer prophylaxis are nebulous, and the guidelines published are weak recommendations at best as the evidence for stress ulcer prophylaxis administration does not support a decrease in mortality or LOS (Zhikang et al., 2020).

Hospitalized and critically ill patients are widely considered to be at "high" risk for gastrointestinal bleeding. Perhaps this is based on basic knowledge of anatomy and physiology, wherein natural gastric defenses are depleted or altered during critical illness due to hypovolemia, shock states, blood loss, reduced splanchnic blood flow secondary to PEEP in ventilated patients, and vasopressor therapy administration. Normally, nitric oxide and prostaglandins help maintain a protective mucosal layer that sustains the gastric mucosa. Other factors such as alterations in neurohormonal control and the dysregulation of bicarbonate, phospholipids, and other peptides and proteins can cause alterations in pH while simultaneously causing vasoconstriction at the mucosal layer. Exogenous influence such as the direct trauma on the gastric mucosa caused by nasogastric tubes on suction also plays a role. This can all lead to mucosal damage and is the theoretical target end point for acid suppression therapy.

Research conducted over the last 50 years has demonstrated an evolution in schools of thought about gastrointestinal bleeding. In Cook and Guatt's (2018) review of the literature about gastrointestinal bleeding, endoscopies done 5 decades ago revealed stress-related gastric mucosal ulceration in over 75% of critically ill, injured, or burned patients. Their findings also revealed occult bleeding in 15%–50% of critically ill patients and overt bleeding in 5%–25% of critically ill patients who did not receive prophylaxis (Cook & Guyatt, 2018). As research has progressed and critical care medicine has advanced, we have learned that the evidence no longer supports those numbers. In a large study in 2015 by Krag et al., clinically significant bleeding was only found in 2.8% of patients, but the study yielded characteristics of patients at risk. Clinically significant bleeding is divided into two categories, primary and secondary. Primary bleeding is the predominant reason or cause of the patient being admitted to the hospital. Clinically significant secondary bleeding is theoretically what stress ulcer prophylaxis with acid suppression therapy is trying to prevent. Classifications of bleeding are defined in Table 5.1.

There are specific critically ill patient populations and characteristics that are considered to be higher risk for clinically significant secondary bleeding according to the literature. It is widely documented in the epidemiological data that patients with shock states, burns, neurologic trauma, and respiratory failure and those with underlying liver disease, renal impairment, known peptic ulcer disease, and coagulopathies are all at higher risk. In addition, patients who use nonsteroidal anti-inflammatory drugs (NSAIDs), antiplatelet therapy, anticoagulation, and high-dose glucocorticoids also have an amplified risk. Intensive care therapies such as patients requiring mechanical ventilation (>48 hr), renal replacement therapy (RRT), and extracorporeal membrane oxygenation therapy are also at a higher risk. Low-risk patients are those who are critically ill without risk factors, immunosuppression or use of corticosteroids, acute hepatic failure, use of anticoagulants, and cancer patients (Zhikang et al., 2020). Identifying and understanding those patients at risk is the first step in determining if your patient would require stress ulcer prophylaxis.

Key Points

Multiple randomized controlled trials and meta-analyses have revealed that the two general greatest risk factors for stress ulcer prophylaxis are mechanical ventilation without enteral nutrition for >48 hr and coagulopathy (Buendgens et al., 2016).

The highest risk patient population of all includes patients with chronic liver disease, on mechanical ventilation without enteral nutrition for >48 hr, and a coagulopathy. Current guidelines published in 2020 by Zhikang et al. examined the data from 12,660 critically ill patients in 72 trials, and the recent SUP-ICU randomized controlled trial from 2018. They found that prophylaxis provided approximately twice the absolute reduction of overt bleeding compared to clinically important bleeding (Zhikang et al.,

TABLE 5.1 DEFINITIONS OF BLEEDING AND RISK

CLASSIFICATION	DEFINITION	RISK
Clinically significant	Hematemesis/coffee grounds or frank bleeding/melena in addition to any of the following: • Decrease in BP > 20 mm Hg • Increase in HR > 20 bmp and decrease in SBP of 10 mm Hg • Decrease in Hgb of >2 g/dl over 24-hr period after bleeding • Administration of >2 units PRBCs pithing 24 hr after bleeding • Vasopressor initiation • Therapeutic endoscopy	3% of critically ill patients
Overt	Hematemesis/coffee grounds or frank bleeding/melena	5% of critically ill patients
Occult	Guaiac-positive fecal or gastric samples	15%–50% critically ill patients
Submucosal or mucosal alteration	Gastroduodenal mucosal or submucosal erosions and ulcerations document on endoscopy	Thought to be 75%–100% of critically ill patients in the past but no current data or evidence

Data from Krag, M., Marker, S., Perner, A., Wetterslev, J., Wise, M. P., Schefold, J. C., Keus, F., Guttormsen, A. B., Bendel, S., Borthwick, M., Lange, T., Rasmussen, B. S., Siegemund, M., Bundgaard, H., Elkmann, T., Jensen, V., Nielsen, R. D., Liboriussen, L., Bestle, M. H., …Møller, M. H., & SUP-ICU Trial Group. (2018). Pantoprazole in patients at risk for gastrointestinal bleeding in the ICU. *The New England Journal of Medicine, 379*, 2199–2208.

2020). The current guidelines make a weak recommendation for stress ulcer prophylaxis in patients considered to be moderate-high risk and a weak recommendation to not use stress ulcer prophylaxis in those considered to be at lower risk for clinically significant bleeding. The guidelines further recommend use of a PPI over a histamine-2 receptor antagonist (H2RA), although both are possible choices. When compared head to head, PPIs reduce the risk of overt bleeding over H2RAs, but the confidence interval in the data does not support the same when examining clinically important bleeding. Both can be administered intravenously or enterally, daily or twice daily, and both are low cost and generally well tolerated. There has been concern that PPIs and H2RAs are linked to higher incidence of pneumonia, *Clostridium difficile* infections, and increased LOS, but this was largely statistically insignificant in the research.

Key Points

There are also data to support that early enteral feeding may protect and restore the mucosa and may also protect patients from stress ulcers and gastrointestinal bleeding.

There is significant evidence to support the potential benefits of enteral nutrition. It can stimulate mucus and bicarbonate secretion by mucus glands and epithelial cells that maintains the mucus barrier and prevents translocation of bacteria. Enteral nutrition can also increase splanchnic blood flow, which may facilitate healing of any ulcerated mucosa (Rassameehiran et al., 2015). Other studies in critically ill burn and pancreatitis patients also support the same and have indicated that early enteral nutrition (EEN) significantly lowered the level of proinflammatory cytokines, aided in restoration of gastrointestinal function, decreased complications such as infection, and resulted in shorter LOS in patients with severe acute pancreatitis (Cui et al., 2013). In 2010, Marik et al. published a systematic review and meta-analysis that suggested that in patients with EEN, pharmacologic stress ulcer prophylaxis may not be needed at all. EEN has been shown in the literature in multiple studies to have a positive impact on mortality and shorter lengths of stay (Zhang et al., 2019). In addition, the European Society for Clinical Nutrition and Metabolism also strongly recommend early enteral feeding within 48 hr of admission for critically ill patients who would be considered to be high risk for stress ulcers based on the aforementioned patient populations with low-rate feeding and delayed feeding for specific conditions (Pironi et al., 2020). While stress ulcer prophylaxis risk reduction is not directly or specifically addressed in the guideline, the acuity and patient populations identified who would benefit from early nutrition are synonymous.

Key Points

A thoughtful and intentional approach to stress ulcer prophylaxis based on risk stratification, the patient's anticipated course, early administration of enteral feeding with aspiration risk reduction strategies, pharmacologic selection, and route administration should be considered at time of admission for critically ill patients.

Case Study

Mrs. O has returned to the ICU from her NCHCT and CTA chest. Her head CT did not reveal any acute intracranial abnormalities and demonstrated chronic microvascular white matter changes consistent with age. CTA of her chest was read as follows:

Impression: No evidence of pulmonary embolism in any of the pulmonary arteries. Bilateral extensive patchy consolidation and ground-glass opacities, consistent with extensive pneumonia, with likely aspiration pneumonia due to the dense airspace consolidation in the right lower lobe. ET tube at the level of carina. Retraction by 2–3 cm is recommended. Mediastinal and bilateral hilar lymphadenopathy. Indeterminate right adrenal mass. Further evaluation with noncontrast CT of the abdomen when the patient's clinical status improves is recommended.

The cardiologist has reviewed her echocardiogram and has read it as follows:

Echo Conclusions: Left ventricle: The cavity size is normal. Wall thickness is normal. Systolic function is normal. Estimated EF is 60%–65%. Right ventricle: wall motion abnormality (akinesia) at the right ventricular mid-free wall with preserved function at the apex. Left atrium: The atrium is dilated. No evidence of thrombus in the atrial cavity or appendage. Mitral valve: No evidence of vegetation. There is mild to moderate regurgitation.

As Mrs. O's echo was grossly normal and her CTA chest did not reveal a PE, but does show bilateral ground-glass opacities and an RLL infiltrate, in the setting of a PaO_2/FiO_2 ratio of 77, you diagnose her with acute hypoxemic respiratory failure 2/2 multilobar pneumonia. You increase her PEEP to +10, she does not have a decrease in her SBP this time, and her SaO_2 comes up to 97%. You titrate her FiO_2 down to 80% and maintain her SaO_2. You consider chemical paralysis and pronation therapy but decide against it, as her peak airway pressure (PAP) and plateau pressures are WNL and she is not overbreathing or bucking the ventilator, and her oxygenation is improving. You know that you may need to reconsider if her oxygenation gets worse. You add Pepcid for stress ulcer prophylaxis and follow up on the nutrition consult you placed earlier and start enteric tube feeds. You do not need to systemically anticoagulate her, but you do need to consider her for VTE prophylaxis. You also decide to recheck her laboratory work later this afternoon including an ABG and lactate as she was tachypneic and you assume her acidosis is resolving as she is no longer overbreathing the ventilator without sedation, although she appears quite comfortable.

VTE PROPHYLAXIS

Prescribing VTE prophylaxis to avoid DVT or pulmonary embolus is rooted in risk assessment. The literature reflects that patients have an increased for thromboembolism if they are elderly, are immobile, are admitted to the ICU with prior history of DVT/PE, have had a prior CVA with hemiparesis, are obese, are prescribed hormonal therapy, have active CHF, have active cancer, have thrombophilia, have acute respiratory failure, and have had recent surgery or trauma (Badireddy & Mudipalli, 2020).

Risk factors can be divided into two groups: genetic and acquired. Clotting disorders such as factor V Leiden or prothrombin mutations can increase risk of VTE, and any genetic condition that impacts coagulation function can either increase or decrease risk. Conversely, acquired risk factors can be further broken down to modifiable or nonmodifiable. Modifiable risk factors include smoking cessation, obesity reduction/weight loss, and avoiding long distance travel. Nonmodifiable risk factors include age, pregnancy, strokes, inflammatory conditions, cancers, and immobilization. Critically ill patients, and specifically those admitted to the ICU, have an independent risk factor for increased VTE due to the combination of immobility, mechanical ventilation, vasopressor use, organ failure (cardiac, respiratory, renal), and use of central venous access devices (CVADs). In fact, there is a threefold increase in risk for VTE in patients with a CVAD based on a 5-year retrospective review of the literature (Ejaz et al., 2018). In patients with sepsis and septic shock, the incidence of VTE is 37.2% (Kaplan et al., 2015), and the annual mortality rate for DVT and PE in the United States is 60,000 to 100,000 (Badireddy & Mudipalli, 2020).

Key Points

Research shows that half of all hospitalized patients are at risk for thromboembolism and that prevention of DVT/PE with prophylactic measures can decrease morbidity and mortality.

Risk Stratification

Risk stratification tools, such as the Pulmonary Embolism Rule Out Criteria (PERC), Geneva Score, or Wells Criteria are all reliable and validated (Guo et al., 2015). Each looks at specific factors such as immobility, age, heart rate, active malignancy, previous VTE, clinical signs of DVT, and more and assigns a numeric point score to stratify risk into clinical probability of DVT/PE. Other tools such as the HAS-BLED Score (**H**ypertension, **A**bnormal renal and liver function, **S**troke, **B**leeding, **L**abile INR, **E**lderly, and **D**rugs and alcohol) and the CHA_2DS_2-VASc Score (**C**ongestive heart failure, **H**ypertension, **A**ge ≥75 years, **D**iabetes mellitus, prior **S**troke, **V**ascular disease, **A**ge 65–74, **S**ex **c**ategory) are both acronym-based bleeding and thromboembolism prediction tools specifically for patients with atrial fibrillation. Tools such as these can be implemented in the clinical decision-making process when determining presence and risk of VTE for patients in the ICU.

> ### Key Points
>
> A careful history and physical examination should take precedence for decision-making, and these tools can be used to substantiate observations.

Physical examination noting signs and symptoms of DVT, including pain, edema, discoloration, and erythema, should prompt further investigation with venous duplex ultrasound, which is currently the best diagnostic tool for DVT (Theunissen et al., 2016). Signs and symptoms of PE include dizziness, tachycardia, sharp chest pain worse on inspiration, shortness of breath, and refractory hypoxemia. CTA of the chest is considered the gold standard of diagnostic therapies for PE (Ejaz et al., 2018).

> ### Key Points
>
> It is widely accepted that the roots of thrombogenesis for hospitalized patients lay in Virchow triad of venous stasis, hypercoagulability, and vessel (endothelial) damage.

Treatment

Mechanical Interventions

Mechanical interventions such as sequential compression devices (SCDs), intermittent pneumatic calf compression (IPCC) devices, venous foot pumps, or thrombo-embolus deterrent (TED) stockings were all developed to combat venous stasis. SCDs/IPCCs are designed to squeeze the muscles in a rhythmic, sequential manner, in an effort to stimulate blood flow through the deep veins, thus preventing stasis in patients with adequate blood supply and competent valves. The etiology of pump and cuff technology is rooted in the analysis of blood flow effect first studied in lymphedema patients (Morris and Woodcock, 2004). Research shows that regardless of the kind of device used, with compliance and appropriate application, even the gentlest systems work to prevent venous stasis and are effective (Morris and Woodcock, 2004). The literature and research also historically support the use of SCDs/IPCCs to decrease the incidence of VTE and are recommended as monointervention for patients at high risk of bleeding for whom pharmacologic prophylaxis is contraindicated (Ejaz et al., 2018).

Pharmacologic Prophylaxis

Pharmacologic prophylaxis has been well studied and is known to decrease mortality in the surgical patient population but is unfounded to decrease mortality in medical patients (Ejaz et al., 2018). Pharmacological prophylaxis includes low-molecular-weight heparin (LMWH), unfractionated heparin (UFH), fondaparinux, and direct oral anticoagulants (DOACs) such as rivaroxaban or warfarin. The Prophylaxis of Thromboembolism in Critical Care (PROTECT) Trial 2005 was a multicenter double-blinded prospective randomized controlled trial examining LMWH vs. UFH in reduction of incidence of VTE in general ICU patients with the primary end point of proximal lower extremity DVT and secondary end points including any DVT, PE, VTE, death, heparin-induced thrombocytopenia (HIT), or major bleeding (Przybysz & Huang, 2011). The study concluded that LMWH was comparable to UFH in reduction of risk of VTE but did not show a reduction in mortality and could be used as a safe alternative to UFH with no difference in major bleeding events between the two. The incidence of PE was also found to be lower in the LMWH group when compared to the UFH group.

Combination Therapy

Combination therapy is often routinely prescribed, aimed at mitigating both venous stasis and hypercoagulability. Mechanical VTE prophylaxis with IPCCs/SCDs is painless, non-invasive, and easy to prescribe, but is not always indicated in tandem with pharmacologic prophylaxis.

Other factors to consider when considering VTE prophylaxis are timing and frequency of medication administration, available route, renal function, platelet count, bleeding risk, monitoring of therapy efficacy (coagulation studies, factor Xa levels), duration of therapy, and compliance with interventions. LMWH is given once daily subcutaneously, UFH is given twice to three times daily subcutaneously, and DOACs are given once or twice daily orally if the patient is able to take PO or has an enteric feeding route. Frequency of medication administration can impact compliance, and other factors such as recent brain or gastrointestinal bleeding, upcoming surgery or procedures, or thrombocytopenia can all impact and interrupt prescriptive compliance with VTE prophylaxis, both mechanical and pharmacologic. In 2015, Manoucheri and Fallahi discovered that out of 472 patients examined, 54.9% were not being given appropriate VTE prophylaxis. Other studies in the literature revealed that 16%–45% of patients do not receive appropriate prophylaxis even when they have absolute indications for the reasons stated above (Ejaz et al., 2018). Prescriber education and electronic medical record reminders can theoretically help improve compliance.

Choosing which VTE prophylaxis to prescribe based on dynamic patient conditions can be challenging and requires critical thinking. Knowing your patient's clinical indication, mobility status, platelet count, and renal function and which pharmacologic agent to select while mitigating bleeding risk are important. For example, it is important to hold pharmacologic prophylaxis when a patient becomes thrombocytopenic and the platelet count drops to <50/μl; to use UFH in patients with decreased glomerular filtration rate (GFR), acute kidney injury (AKI), or end stage renal disease (ESRD), but doing so can be complicated and not straightforward; or to change pharmacologic agents to argatroban if HIT is suspected and prophylaxis is still indicated due to thrombosis risk (Ahmed et al., 2007). There have been multiple published guidelines and recommendations over the past several years. The most recent are the American Society of Hematology 2018 Guidelines for Management of Thromboembolism: Prophylaxis for Hospitalized and Nonhospitalized Medical Patients. The American Society of Hematology also came out with a 2019 guideline specifically for surgery patients. Box 5.1 summarizes selected recommendations from the American Society of Hematology.

BOX 5.1   VTE Prophylaxis

Select ASH Guideline Panel Recommendations and Suggestion for VTE Prophylaxis for Acutely Medically Ill Patients

- Use UFH, LMH, or fondaparinux over no parental anticoagulant
- Use LMWH or fondaparinux rather than UFH
- Anticoagulant choices are also recommended for patients with stroke who need VTE prophylaxis
- Use LMWH over UFH
- Use pharmacologic VTE prophylaxis over mechanical VTE prophylaxis
- In patients who cannot receive pharmacologic VTE prophylaxis, use mechanical VTE prophylaxis over no prophylaxis
- Use pharmacologic or mechanical VTE prophylaxis alone over combined prophylaxis
- When using mechanical prophylaxis, use pneumatic compression devices or graduated compression stockings
- Use LMWH over DOACs as VTE prophylaxis
- Use inpatient VTE prophylaxis with LMWH only over inpatient and extended duration outpatient with DOACs (unless on DOAC for other reasons)

Select ASH Guideline Panel Recommendations and Suggestions for Mechanical vs. Pharmacologic VTE Prophylaxis for Patients Undergoing Major Surgery, Major Trauma, or Neurosurgery

- Use pharmacologic or mechanical prophylaxis
- In patients who cannot receive pharmacologic VTE prophylaxis, use mechanical VTE prophylaxis over no prophylaxis
- Use intermittent pneumatic compression (IPC) devices over graduated compression stockings for patients receiving mechanical prophylaxis
- Use combined prophylaxis with mechanical and pharmacologic prophylaxis over pharmacologic prophylaxis alone
- Depending on risk of VTE and bleeding based on the patient and the surgery, use combined prophylaxis or mechanical prophylaxis alone
- Do not use inferior vena cava (IVC) filters for prophylaxis of VTE in patients undergoing surgery
- For patients undergoing major surgery, use extended pharmacologic VTE prophylaxis over short-term pharmacologic VTE prophylaxis
- Use early (less than 12 hrs post-op) pharmacologic prophylaxis
- Do not use pharmacology prophylaxis in neurosurgical patients
- For those neurosurgical patients for whom pharmacologic prophylaxis is necessary, use LMWH over UFH
- Use mechanical prophylaxis for all neurosurgical and major trauma patients
- For major trauma patients who are at a low to moderate risk of bleeding, use pharmacologic prophylaxis over no pharmacologic prophylaxis
- For major trauma patients who are at a high risk of bleeding, do not use pharmacologic prophylaxis
- For major trauma patients for whom pharmacologic prophylaxis is used, use LMWH or UFH

(continued)

BOX 5.1   VTE Prophylaxis (*continued*)

ASH, American Society of Hematology; DOAC, direct oral anticoagulant; LMWH, low-molecular-weight heparin; UFH, unfractionated heparin; VTE, venous thromboembolism.

Data from Schunemann, H. J., Cushman, M., Burnett, A. E., Kahn, S. R., Beyer-Westendorf, J., Spencer, F. A., Rezende, S. M., Zakai, N. A., Bauer, K. A., Dentali, F., Lansing, J., Balduzzi, S., Darzi, A., Morgano, G. P., Neumann, I., Nieuwlaat, R., Yepes-Nuñez, J. J., Zhang, Y., & Wiercioch, W. (2018). American Society of Hematology 2018 guidelines for management of venous thromboembolism: Prophylaxis for hospitalized and nonhospitalized medical patients. *Blood Advances*, 2, 3198–3225. and Anderson D., Morgano, G. P., Bennett, C., Dentali, F., Francis, C. W., Garcia, D. A., Kahn, S. R., Rahman, M. M., Rajasekhar, A., Rogers, F. B., Smythe, M. A., Tikkinen, K. A., Yates, A. J., Baldeh, T., Balduzzi, S., Brożek J. L., Ikobaltzeta, I. E., Johal, H., Neumann, I. D., …Dahm, P. (2019). American Society of Hematology 2019 guidelines for management of venous thromboembolism: Prevention of venous thromboembolism in surgical hospitalized patients. *Blood Advances*, 3(23), 3898–3944.

Case Study

Mrs. O is now making adequate urine, her FiO_2 is coming down on the ventilator, she is currently hemodynamically stable, and her repeat laboratory test results are as follows: WBC, 18.0/µl; Hgb, 7.8 g/dl; Hct, 23.4%; platelets 128/µl with 86 neutrophils; Na, 142 mEq/L; K, 4.1 mEq/L; CO_2, 27; Cl, 104 mEq/L; BUN, 40 mEq/L; Cr, 0.9 mEq/L; random glucose 142 mg/dl; Mg, 2.4 mg/dl; Phos 3.4 mg/dl; Ca, 8.2 mg/dl; INR, 1.11; and LA, 1.1. Her ABG is as follows: pH, 7.42; CO_2, 36 mm Hg; PaO_2, 89 mm Hg; O_2 saturation, 95%; and HCO_3, 23 mEq/L. Her laboratory test results, gas exchange, volume status, and hemodynamics are all markedly improved with the interventions you have placed thus far. You add Lovenox for VTE prophylaxis, and your nurse colleague asks you if it is okay that she already placed SCDs on her and asks you for an order. You reply that, based on the guidelines, they are not currently indicated, but you also praise her proactivity and patient advocacy and place an order anyway, as it will not harm the patient. Your nurse also tells you that the patient's daughter would like an update because she is concerned that her mother "isn't waking up" and would like the results of the CT scans. You ask the daughter to come with you to a quiet room at the end of the hall where you can sit and talk because you suspect that the patient has TME and you want to provide anticipatory guidance about the electroencephalogram (EEG), magnetic resonance imaging (MRI), and neurology consult you have ordered.

TME AND PICS AND ICU-ACQUIRED WEAKNESS

There is an old proverb that states, "An ounce of prevention is worth a pound of cure." The same can be true when discussing critically ill patients in the ICU, specifically when it comes to TME, PICS, and ICU-acquired weakness.

TME is a condition of global cerebral dysfunction in the absence of primary structural brain disease or direct central nervous system (CNS) infection that manifests as altered consciousness, behavior changes, or seizure as result of, or in response to, systemic dysfunction (Angel et al., 2008).

It is a common, complex, and multifactorial condition that requires the astute provider to proactively attempt to prevent in the critically ill population and to recognize and diagnose early. There are many conditions that mimic TME, and there are many possible causes and etiologies, which are listed in Box 5.2.

The etiologies most frequently seen in the ICU are hypoxemia, ischemia, organ dysfunction, medication effects, glycemic derangements, infection, and electrolyte abnormalities. It is thought that there is a correlation between advanced age and risk of encephalopathy (Berisavac et al., 2017). People who are older than 65 years or those who reside in a nursing home have a 60% chance of developing TME when ill (Berisavac et al., 2017). Hepatic encephalopathy is thought to have an incidence of 45%–80% in patients with liver cirrhosis depending on the severity of their underlying disease (Angel et al., 2008). In addition, emerging literature suggests that hyperglycemia in uncontrolled type II diabetics can be an independent risk factor for the development of delirium (Lopes & Pereira, 2018). Knowing the possible causes can help predict who is most at risk: the higher the age, compounded with more potential etiologies, the higher the risk.

Pathologic etiologies must be examined and ruled out prior to making a diagnosis of TME. Acute confusion and delirium are included in TME, and the clinical presentation is nonspecific and varies from patient to patient in severity and symptomology. The symptoms can be mild, spanning from inattention to severe agitation to psychosis and hallucinations to unresponsiveness and coma (Box 5.3).

The symptoms can also fluctuate, manifesting as hypoactive, hyperactive, or combined, focal or global, and can include both cognitive and motor deficits, altered pupillary responses, or respiratory and autonomic abnormalities. The most common symptom in TME is delirium (Krishnan et al., 2014). Hypoactive delirium is more frequent in the ICU and associated with a higher risk of mortality, as it results in a greater need for mechanical ventilation and prolonged LOS (Arumugam et al., 2017). In addition, the development of delirium and the duration of the delirium have also been linked to increased risks of prolonged critical illness, higher incidence of reintubation, poor global cognition, development of dementia, and long-term cognitive impairment (Park & Lee, 2019). According to Berisavac et al. (2017), mortality from TME depends on the quantitative disorder of consciousness as measured by the GCS wherein a GSC of 9–12 is associated with a 50% mortality rate, and the mortality rate of GCS < 8 is up to 63%.

The pathophysiology behind the development of TME is poorly understood, but there are multiple theories discussed in the literature. TME is thought to be caused by any systemic condition or illness causing alterations in blood flow, pH, osmolality, and temperature, which are all needed for normal brain function, leading to an imbalance in neurotransmitters and causing cytotoxic injury, neuroinflammation, and vasogenic edema. Alterations in neurotransmitters such as acetylcholine and proinflammatory mediators such as cytokines and chemokines all play a role in endothelial dysfunction, microvascular dysfunction, and thrombin formation, which can lead to delirium (Park & Lee, 2019).

BOX 5.2 Common Causes of TME

Pathologic Causes of Altered Mental Status

- Brain tumor/mass effect
- Intracranial hemorrhage (ICH) (epidural, subdural, subarachnoid, intraparenchymal)
- Hydrocephalus
- Cerebral venous thrombosis
- Seizures/postictal state
- Autoimmune/paraneoplastic encephalitis

TME

- Meningitis/encephalitis
- Hypoxemic-ischemic encephalopathy (anoxic brain injury)
- Sepsis/infection (due to systemic function, shock states/hypoperfusion)
- Hyper- or hyponatremia/osmotic demyelination syndrome (too rapid correction of hyponatremia)
- Myxedema coma (hypothyroidism)/thyroid storm (hyperthyroidism)
- Addison disease (adrenal insufficiency/crisis)
- Hypertensive encephalopathy/emergency
- Posterior reversible leukoencephalopathy (acute HTN causing vasogenic edema)
- Uremia (acute renal failure)
- Medications/drug/toxins/sedatives
- Hypocalcemia/hypomagnesemia/hypophosphatemia/hypercalcemia
- Salicylates/Reye syndrome
- Anticholinergics
- Immunosuppressants (steroids)
- Antibiotics (cephalosporins, quinolone, metronidazole)
- Sleep deprivation
- Delirium
- Ethanol or methanol intoxication
- Wernicke encephalopathy (thiamine deficiency/hepatic encephalopathy [hyperammonemia])
- Wilson disease (copper accumulation)
- Manganese accumulation (prolonged HD treatment/TPN)
- Heavy metal poisoning/organic phosphates

In addition, altered glucose metabolism, cellular membrane disruption from electrolyte alterations, and exogenous toxins or medications can all disrupt the blood-brain barrier leading to further interference with neuronal activity (Stokum et al., 2016). A recent study with human neuronal culture cells of the brain revealed hyperglycemia-induced inflammation and neurodegeneration secondary to oxidative stress, suggesting that chronic uncontrolled hyperglycemia can result in progressive structural abnormalities of the brain, leading to a lower cognitive reserve and increased risk of delirium when ill (Lopes & Pereira, 2018). Increased blood-brain barrier permeability can be found with an elevated protein level in the cerebral spinal fluid and is associated with neurologic injury (Schilde et al., 2018).

Recognizing the early signs of TME or delirium can often be challenging in the ICU, especially if the patient is on mechanical ventilation and is requiring sedation, or immediately post-op in a patient who has received anesthesia and pain medication. It is

BOX 5.3 Physical Clinical Symptoms of TME

- Attention deficit
- Disorientation
- Restlessness
- Impulsivity
- Agitation
- Irritability
- Confusion
- Delirium
- Hyperventilation
- Pupillary changes (mydriasis or miosis)
- Lethargy
- Hypoventilation
- Labile blood pressure/HTN
- Temperature instability
- Gastrointestinal dysmotility
- Obtundation
- Seizures
- Myoclonic jerking/fine tremors
- Decorticate or decerebrate posturing
- Coma

important to first assess the patient's level of sedation or consciousness before performing a cognitive evaluation. Tools that have been studied and proven valid can be used to assess sedation, including the Ramsay Sedation Scale, the Riker Sedation-Agitation Scale, or the Richmond Agitation-Sedation Scale (RASS) (Ely et al., 2003). Other predictive validated tools that can be used to identify delirium are the Intensive Care Delirium Screening Checklist (ICDSC) and the Confusion Assessment Method for the ICU (CAM-ICU) (Ely et al., 2001).

Key Points

The diagnosis of delirium and TME at time of admission or within 24 hr of admission with daily evaluation is important to improve outcomes.

Prevention is ideal but not always feasible in the critically ill. It is imperative to use predictive tools, validated assessment tools, comprehensive clinical laboratory tests and diagnostic data including head CT, brain MRI, EEG, and if necessary lumbar puncture for cerebrospinal fluid (CSF) analysis, as often the diagnosis of TME is made as a diagnosis of exclusion. Measuring procalcitonin, C-reactive protein (CRP), and ammonia levels and performing toxicology and virology screens can also be helpful in diagnosing TME (McGrane et al., 2011). Increased procalcitonin and CRP are associated with increased incidence and duration of delirium (Arumugam et al., 2017). Once all other organic differential diagnoses have been ruled out, focus should turn to immediate intervention and management to expedite recovery. Often, treating the underlying illness and maximizing all variables such as adequate nutrition, oxygenation, hemodynamic stability, volume status, and glycemic control can be enough to start the reversal of TME.

Critical illness and acute care hospital admission have been shown in the literature to demonstrate tangible consequences of long-term cognitive decline, PTSD, depression, and anxiety in the patients and their families. Critical illness polyneuromyopathy, dysphagia, cachexia, failure to thrive, chronic pain, sexual dysfunction, and chronic organ failure are all physical consequences of ICU stays (Mehlhorn et al., 2104). PICS was developed to describe the disability that has been identified in those surviving critical illness and the ICU and is comprised of impairment in cognition, psychological health, and physical function (Rawal et al., 2017). Emerging trends in research and literature are now focusing on ICU survivorship and reduction in incidence of PICS. One study demonstrated that, 12 months after critical illness, 25% of ICU patients had cognitive impairment similar to mild Alzheimer disease and moderate traumatic brain injury (TBI) (Pandharipande et al., 2013). Cognitive impairment and ICU-acquired muscle weakness are the two most common manifestations of PICS and are thought to occur in 25%–75% of ICU survivors. Delirium, deep sedation, dysregulation of the sleep-wake cycle, hypoxemia and prolonged mechanical ventilation, glucose dysregulation, hypotension and shock, use of RRT, immobility, and advanced age are the predominant contributing factors to developing PICS and neuromuscular weakness (Rawal et al., 2017).

Critical illness polyneuropathy and myopathy are seen in 25%–45% of admitted ICU patients and manifest as flaccid and symmetric paralysis (Zhou et al., 2014). The drivers of cognitive impairment and delirium are also the contributing factors for neuromuscular weakness.

Key Points

Proactive interventions to prevent delirium and mitigate PICS and neuromuscular weakness should begin at time of admission and be carried out consistently throughout hospitalization.

These two conditions are often concomitant, and polyneuropathy is thought to be characterized by axonal loss of motor and sensory fibers secondary to sepsis, whereas myopathy has been thought to be elicited from excessive doses of corticosteroids (Zhou et al., 2014). Two independent risk factors for these conditions have emerged in the literature: gram-negative bacteremia sepsis and hyperglycemia (Van den Berge et al., 2003). The diagnosis of critical illness polyneuropathy and myopathy is often included in the constellation of debilitation that is PICS. The gold standard for diagnosis is muscle biopsy, and there is no outright "cure" for this condition other than proactive prevention, supportive measures, tincture of time, and control of risk factors. Careful attention to treatment of causative factors, minimization of neuromuscular blockers, corticosteroids, glycemic management, early mobility, and aggressive physical therapy and rehabilitation are imperative. A study by Hermans et al., 2007 demonstrated that treatment of hyperglycemia with insulin lowered the risk of critical illness polyneuropathy and myopathy, and decreased ventilator days, ICU LOS, and overall mortality.

Key Points

Prolonged respiratory failure, immobility, and medications and infection are all linked to the development of critical illness polyneuropathy and myopathy.

In 2018, the SCCM, as part of their international ICU Liberation Initiative, released their Clinical Practice Guidelines for the Prevention and Management of Pain, Agitation/Sedation, Delirium, Immobility, and Sleep Disruption in Adult Patients in the ICU (PADIS) (Devlin et al., 2018). These guidelines incorporate a multimodal approach to the care of the critically ill to improve overall ICU outcomes and decrease ICU lengths of stay through the implementation of evidence-based, integrated, patient-centered care protocols. Evidence-based bundled care models have been shown to improve multidisciplinary collaboration, compliance with evidence-based protocoled care, and critical care outcomes and decrease mortality (Marra et al., 2017). One study published in 2015 by Kram et al. demonstrated that bundled care models decreased LOS by 26% and ventilator days by 29%, and delirium incidence was 19% with delirium prevention measures implemented and documented 89% of the time. The pragmatic implementation of an evidence-based care bundle is the ABCDEF bundle:

Assess, prevent, and manage pain and discomfort
Both sedation holidays and spontaneous breathing trials (SBTs)
Choice of multimodal analgesia therapies and pharmacologic sedation
Delirium: prevent, monitor, and manage
Early mobility and physical **E**xercise
Family participation, support, education, and empowerment (Marra et al., 2017)

A multidisciplinary team comprised of intensivist physicians and advanced practice providers (APPs), nurses, certified nursing assistants, pharmacists, respiratory therapists, nutritionists, physical and occupational therapists, and psychologists or psychiatrists is recommended to implement the ABCDEF bundle. Additional strategies to minimize PICS and the deleterious effects are maintaining glycemic control, avoiding hypoxemia, promoting normal sleep-wake cycles, ensuring adequate nutrition, aggressive physical therapy, and encouraging family participation. There is also emerging literature and research to support the development of post-ICU follow-up clinics to further study and manage PICS symptoms, but other interventions, such as maintaining an ICU diary, have not been proven to be effective in decreasing incidence of anxiety or PTSD in patients or their families (Barreto et al., 2019).

Case Study

Mrs. O is now on hospital day 11. She is hemodynamically stable, not on pressors, mildly volume overloaded, and being diuresed, on day 11 of her antibiotic course of Zosyn for her *Klebsiella pneumoniae* pneumonia and bacteremia. She had a repeat echocardiogram when her blood cultures came back positive, and she does not have evidence of vegetations on her valves. She has had a neurology consult, an EEG consistent with generalized slowing and no focal seizure activity, and an MRI that revealed normal age-related changes. She is opening her eyes, intermittently tracking, and moving around weakly with 3/5 strength in her extremities in the bed. She is failing her daily breathing trials with tachypnea, nasal flaring, and accessory muscle use. Her secretions burden is at a minimum, and her CXR shows resolution of her multilobar infiltrates. Her blood glucose has been difficult to control, and she is now on an insulin infusion per protocol. She is tolerating tube feeds at goal and moving her bowels. She requires intermittent potassium and phosphorous repletion based on the laboratory test results, and her family visits daily. She is out of bed to chair with a Hoyer lift daily, and the nursing staff is taking measures to open the shades during the day and promote a normal sleep-wake cycle.

Based on what you have read above, what do you think is currently happening? What are the next steps for Mrs. O?

You recognize that you have done all you can at this point to maximize Mrs. O's clinical condition, and you now have to be patient, assess her daily, attempt SBTs daily, and wait to see if she is going to improve and wean effectively. You must support her family during this difficult time, educate them, and provide anticipatory guidance.

On day 15, Mrs. O still has not improved from a pulmonary perspective and remains physically weak. You recommend tracheostomy and percutaneous gastrostomy tube placement and care management consult for disposition planning to a long-term acute care hospital (LTACH)/ventilator weaning facility.

CLINICAL PEARLS

- Check HbA1c at time of admission to differentiate between undiagnosed diabetes and stress-induced hyperglycemia.
- Maintain blood glucose between 140 and 180 mg/dl for the majority of generalized ICU patients.
- Avoid hypoglycemia.
- IV insulin administration is recommended.
- Evaluate who is at risk for stress ulcers and bleeding based on clinical conditions at time of admission.
- Consider and implement *early* enteral feeding (within 48 hr of admission).
- Discontinue GI prophylaxis when patients are taking an oral diet or transitioning out of the ICU (if no evidence of bleeding).
- Consider VTE prophylaxis for ALL patients being admitted to the ICU.
- Always check the renal function and for thrombocytopenia prior to prescribing pharmacologic VTE prophylaxis.
- Always know your patient's baseline mental status and cognitive functioning at time of admission.
- Always *first* rule out a pathologic etiology of altered mental status.
- Focus on mitigating contributing factors to TME at time of admission in your critically ill patients, as *prevention* is the key.
- Normalize sleep-wake cycles.
- Utilize assessment tools such as the CAM and implement the ABCDEF bundle at time of admission to help prevent TME.
- Early mechanical ventilation liberation, early physical mobility, conservative use of paralytics and corticosteroids, nutrition, and glycemic control all help mitigate critical illness myopathy.

REVIEW QUESTIONS

1. It is important to differentiate undiagnosed diabetes from stress-induced hyperglycemia. Which of the following can you use to identify undiagnosed diabetes in the hospitalized patient?
   a. Fasting glucose
   b. HbAlc
   c. Glucose tolerance test
   d. Blood glucose >200 mg/dl

2. An increase in mortality is associated with hyperglycemia; thus, glycemic control in the acute hospitalized patient is important. Tour range of blood glucose goal control for generalized ICU patients is
   a. 70–140 mg/dl
   b. 140–180 mg/dl
   c. 80–108 mg/dl
   d. Greater than 180 mg/dl

3. Patients at risk for secondary bleeding requiring stress ulcer prophylaxis include all of the following except
   a. Burns
   b. Shock states
   c. Neurologic trauma
   d. Use of anticoagulants

4. Stress ulcers may be prevented by
   a. PPIs
   b. H2RA
   c. Early enteral feeding
   d. All of the above

5. There is a threefold risk for VTE in patients with
   a. Sepsis
   b. Immobility
   c. Malignancy
   d. CVAD

6. Clinical decision-making for VTE risk is best implemented when based on
   a. PERC score
   b. Wells criteria
   c. History and physical
   d. Geneva score

7. Hold pharmacologic VTE prophylaxis when
   a. Platelet count drops below 100,000 u/L
   b. Hgb drops below normal limits
   c. Platelet count drops below 50,000 u/L
   d. Patient develops an AKI

8. TME has a constellation of symptoms, the most common being
   a. Seizures
   b. Delirium
   c. Weakness
   d. Hypoxemia

9. Recognizing early signs of TME is important as the ACNP caring for these patients. Which of the following is the most important step you can take in evaluating ICU patients?
   a. Careful choice of pharmacologic therapy for pain and sedation
   b. Recognize and address hypoxia
   c. Prevent hyperglycemia
   d. Assess the patient's baseline level of sedation before performing a cognitive evaluation

10. PICS requires an interdisciplinary approach. As the ACNP caring for these patients, you understand the importance of the ABCDE bundle and develop a strategy to implement the bundle in your unit. Your team should include
    a. Physicians
    b. Pharmacists
    c. Family members
    d. All of the above

Answers: 1, b; 2, b; 3, d; 4, d; 5, d; 6, c; 7, c; 8, b; 9, d; 10, d

REFERENCES

Ahmed, I., Majeed, A., & Powell, R. (2007). Heparin induced thrombocytopenia: Diagnosis and management update. *Postgraduate Medical Journal*, 83(983), 575–582.

American Diabetes Association. (2020). Classification and diagnosis of diabetes: Standards of medical care in diabetes—2020. *Diabetes Care*, 43(Suppl. 1), S14–S31.

American Society for Metabolic and Bariatric Surgery. (2020). *Type II diabetes and obesity: Twin epidemics*. https://asmbs.org/app/uploads/2009/03/Type-2-Diabetes-Fact-Sheet.pdf

Anderson, D., Morgano, G. P., Bennett, C., Dentali, F., Francis, C. W., Garcia, D. A., Kahn, S. R., Rahman, M. M., Rajasekhar, A., Rogers, F. B., Smythe, M. A., Tikkinen, K. A., Yates, A. J., Baldeh, T., Balduzzi, S., Brożek, J. L., Ikobaltzeta, I. E., Johal, H., Neumann, I. D., …Dahm, P. (2019). American Society of Hematology 2019 guidelines for management of venous thromboembolism: Prevention of venous thromboembolism in surgical hospitalized patients. *Blood Advances*, 3(23), 3898–3944.

Angel, M. J., Chein, R., & Young, G. B. (2008). Metabolic encephalopathies. *Handbook of Clinical Neurology*, 60, 115–166.

Arumugam, S., El-Menyar, A., Al-Hassani, A., Strandvik, G., Asim, M., Mekkodithal, A., Mudali, I., & Al-Thani, H. (2017). Delirium in the intensive care Unit. *Journal of Emergencies, Trauma, and Shock*, 10(1), 37–46.

Badireddy, M., & Mudipalli, V. R. (2020). *Deep venous thrombosis (DVT) prophylaxis*. In *StatPearls*. StatPearls Publishing.

Barreto, B. B., Luz, M., Rios, M. N., Lopes, A. A., & Gusmao-Flores, D. (2019). The impact of intensive care unit diaries on patients' and relatives' outcomes: A systematic review and meta-analysis. *Critical Care*, 23, 411.

Berisavac, I. I., Jovanović, D. R., Padjen, V. V., Ercegovac, M. D., Stanarčević, P. D., Budimkić-Stefanović, M. S., Radović, M. M., & Beslać-Bumbaširević, L. G. (2017). How to recognize and treat metabolic encephalopathy in Neurology intensive care unit. *Neurology India*, 65, 123–128.

Buendgens, L., Koch, A., & Tacke, F. (2016). Prevention of stress-related ulcer bleeding at the intensive care unit: Risks and benefits of stress ulcer prophylaxis. *World Journal of Critical Care Medicine*, 5(1), 57–64.

Cook, D., & Guyatt, G. (2018). Prophylaxis against upper gastrointestinal bleeding in hospitalized patients. *The New England Journal of Medicine*, 378, 2506–2516.

Cook, D. J., Rocker, G., Meade, M., Guyatt, G., Geerts, W., Anderson, D., Skrobik, Y., Hebert, P., Albert, M., Cooper, J., Bates, S., Caco, C., Finfer, S., Fowler, R., Freitag, A., Granton, J., Jones, G., Langevin, S., Mehta, S., ...Crowther, M., & PROTECT Investigators; Canadian Critical Care Trials Group (2005). Prophylaxis of Thromboembolism in Critical Care (PROTECT) Trial: A pilot study. *Journal of Critical Care.* 20(4), 364–372.

Cui, L. H., Wang, X. H., Peng, L. H., Yu, L., & Yang, Y. S. (2013). The effects of early enteral nutrition with addition of probiotics on the prognosis of patients suffering from severe acute pancreatitis. *Zhonghua Wei Zhong Bing Ji Jiu Yi Xue*, 25, 224–228.

Devlin, J. W., Skrobik, Y., Gélinas, C., Needham, D. M., Slooter, A. J., Pandharipande, P. P., Watson, P. L., Weinhouse, G. L., Nunnally, M. E., Rochwerg, B., Balas, M. C., van den Boogaard, M., Bosma, K. J., Brummel, N. E., Chanques, G., Denehy, L., Drouot, X., Fraser, G. L., Harris, J. E., ...Alhazzani, W. (2018). Clinical practice guidelines for the prevention and management of pain, agitation/sedation, delirium, immobility, and sleep disruption in adult patients in the ICU. *Critical Care Medicine*, 46, e825–e873.

Egi, M., Bellomo, R., Stachowski, E., French, C. J., Hart, G. K., Hegarty, C., & Bailey, M. (2008). Blood glucose concentration and outcome of critical illness: The impact of diabetes. *Critical Care Medicine*, 36(8), 2249–2255.

Ejaz, A., Ahmed, M. M., Tasleem, A., Rafay Khan Niazi, M., Ahsraf, M. F., Ahmad, I., Zakir, A., & Raza, A. (2018). Thromboprophylaxis in intensive care unit patients: A literature review. *Cureus*, 10(9), e3341.

Ely, E. W., Margolin, R., Francis, J., May, L., Truman, B., Dittus, R., Speroff, T., Gautam, S., Bernard, G. R., & Inouye, S. K. (2001). Evaluation of delirium in critically ill patients: Validation of the confusion assessment method for the intensive care unit (CAM-ICU). *Critical Care Medicine*, 29, 1370–1379.

Ely, E. W., Truman, B., Shintani, A., Thomason, J. W., Wheeler, A. P., Gordon, S., Francis, J., Speroff, T., Gautam, S., Margolin, R., Sessler, C. N., Dittus, R. S., & Bernard, G. R. (2003). Monitoring sedation status over time in ICU patients: Reliability and validity of the Richmond Agitation-Sedation Scale (RASS). *Journal of the American Medical Association*, 289, 2983–2991.

Farrokhi, F., Smiley, D., & Umpierrez, G. E. (2011). Glycemic control in non-diabetic critically ill patients. *Best Practice & Research. Clinical Endocrinology & Metabolism*, 25(5), 813–824.

Finfer, S., Chittock, D. R., Su, S. Y., Blair, D., Foster, D., Dhingra, V., Bellomo, R., Cook, D., Dodek, P., Henderson, W. R., Hébert, P. C., Heritier, S., Heyland, D. K., McArthur, C., McDonald, E., Mitchell, I., Myburgh, J. A., Norton, R., Potter, J., ...Ronco, J. J., & NICE-SUGAR Study Investigators. (2009). Intensive versus conventional glucose control in critically ill patients. *The New England Journal of Medicine*, 360(13), 1283–1297.

Greci, L. S., Kailasam, M., Malkani, S., Katz, D. L., Hulinsky, I., Ahmadi, R., & Nawaz, H. (2003). Utility of HbA(1c) levels for diabetes case finding in hospitalized patients with hyperglycemia. *Diabetes Care*, 26(4), 1064–1068.

Guo, D. J., Zhao, C., Zou, Y. D., Huang, X. H., Hu, J. M., & Guo, L. (2015). Values of the Wells and revised Geneva scores combined with D-dimer in diagnosing elderly pulmonary embolism patients. *Chinese Medical Journal*, 128(8), 1052–1057.

Hermans, G., Wilmer, A., Meersseman, W., Milants, I., Wouters, P. J., Bobbaers, H., Bruyninckx, F., & Van den Berghe, G. (2007). Impact of intensive insulin therapy on neuromuscular complications and ventilator dependency in the medical intensive care unit. *American Journal of Respiratory and Critical Care Medicine*, 175(5), 480–489.

Kaplan, D., Casper, T. C., Elliott, C. G., Men, S., Pendleton, R. C., Kraiss, L. W., Weyrich, A. S., Grissom, C. K., Zimmerman, G. A., & Rondina, M. T.. (2015). VTE incidence and risk factors in patients with severe sepsis and septic shock. *Chest*, 148(5), 1224–1230.

Krag, M., Perner, A., Wetterslev, J., Wise, M. P., Borthwick, M., Bendel, S., McArthur, C., Cook, D., Nielsen, N., Pelosi, P., Keus, F., Guttormsen, A. B., Moller, A. D., Møller, M. H., & SUP-ICU co-authors. (2015). Prevalence and outcome of gastrointestinal bleeding and use of acid suppressants in acutely ill adult intensive care patients. *Intensive Care Medicine*, 41, 833–845.

Krag, M., Marker, S., Perner, A., Wetterslev, J., Wise, M. P., Schefold, J. C., Keus, F., Guttormsen, A. B., Bendel, S., Borthwick, M., Lange, T., Rasmussen, B. S., Siegemund, M., Bundgaard, H., Elkmann, T., Jensen, V., Nielsen, R. D., Liboriussen, L., Bestle, M. H., ...Møller, M. H., & SUP-ICU Trial Group. (2018). Pantoprazole in patients at risk for gastrointestinal bleeding in the ICU. *The New England Journal of Medicine*, 379, 2199–2208.

Krishnan, V., Leung, L. Y., & Caplan, L. R. (2015). A neurologist's approach to delirium: Diagnosis and management of toxic metabolic encephalopathies. *European Journal of Internal Medicine*, 25, 112–116.

Lopes, R., & Pereira, B. D. (2018). Delirium and psychotic symptoms associated with hyperglycemia in a patient with poorly controlled type 2 diabetes mellitus. *Innovations in Clinical Neuroscience*, 15(5–6), 30–33.

Manoucheri, R., & Fallahi, M. J. (2015). Adherence to venous thromboprophylaxis guidelines for medical and surgical inpatients of teaching hospitals, Shiraz-Iran. *Tanaffos*, 14, 17–26.

Marik, P. E., Vasu, T., Hirani, A., & Pachinburavan, M. (2010). Stress ulcer prophylaxis in the new millennium: A systematic review and meta-analysis. *Critical Care Medicine*, 38, 2222–2228.

Marra, A., Ely, E. W., Pandharipande, P. P., & Patel, M. B. (2017). The ABCDEF bundle in critical care. *Critical Care Clinics*, 33(2), 225–243.

McGrane, S., Girard, T. D., Thompson, J. L., Shintani, A. K., Woodworth, A., Ely, E. W., & Pandharipande, P. P. (2011). Procalcitonin and C-reactive protein levels at admission as predictors of duration of acute brain dysfunction in critically ill patients. *Critical Care*, 15, R78.

Moghissi, E. S., Korytkowski, M. T., DiNardo, M., Einhorn, D., Hellman, R., Hirsch, I. B., Inzucchi, S. E., Ismail-Beigi, F., Kirkman, M. S., Umpierrez, G. E., & American Association of Clinical Endocrinologists; American Diabetes Association. (2009). American Association of Clinical Endocrinologists and American Diabetes Association consensus statement on inpatient glycemic control. *Endocrine Practice*, 15(4), 353–369.

Morris, R. J., & Woodcock, J. P. (2004). Evidence-based compression: Prevention of stasis and deep vein thrombosis. *Annals of Surgery*, 239(2), 162–171.

Pandharipande, P. P., Girard, T. D., Jackson, J. C., Morandi, A., Thompson, J. L., Pun, B. T., Brummel, N. E., Hughes, C. G., Vasilevskis, E. E., Shintani, A. K., Moons, K. G., Geevarghese, S. K., Canonico, A., Hopkins, R. O., Bernard, G. R., Dittus, R. S., Ely, E. W., & BRAIN-ICU Study Investigators. (2013). Long-term cognitive impairment after critical illness. *The New England Journal of Medicine*, 369(14), 1306–1316.

Park, S. Y., & Lee, H. B. (2019). Prevention and management of delirium in critically ill adult patients in the intensive care unit: A review based on the 2018 PADIS guidelines. *Acute and Critical Care*, 34(2), 117–125.

Pironi, L., Boeykens, K., Bozzetti, F., Joly, F., Klek, S., Lal, S., Lichota, M., Mühlebach, S., Van Gossum, A., Wanten, G., Wheatley, C., & Bischoff, S. C. (2020). ESPEN guideline on home parenteral nutrition, *Clinical Nutrition*, 39(6), 1645–1666. https://doi.org/10.1016/j.clnu.2020.03.005

Professional practice committee for the standards of medical care in diabetes-2016. (2016). *Diabetes Care*, 39(1), S107–S108.

Przybysz, T., & Huang, D. (2011). Does dalteparin PROTECT better than heparin? *Critical Care*, 15, 315.

Rassameehiran, S., Nugent, K., Rakvit, A. (2015). When should a patient with a nonvariceal upper gastrointestinal bleed be fed? *Southern Medical Journal*, 108, 419–424.

Rawal, G., Yadav, S., & Kumar, R. (2017). Post-intensive care syndrome: An Overview. *Journal of Translational Internal Medicine*, 5(2), 90–92.

Sarwar, N., Gao, P., Seshasai, S. R., Gobin, R., Kaptoge, S., Di Angelantonio, E., Ingelsson, E., Lawlor, D. A., Selvin, E., Stampfer, M., Stehouwer, C. D., Lewington, S., Pennells, L., Thompson, A., Sattar, N., White, I. R., Ray, K. K., Danesh, J., & Emerging Risk Factors Collaboration. (2010). Diabetes mellitus, fasting blood glucose concentration, and risk of vascular disease: A collaborative meta-analysis of 102 prospective studies. *Lancet*, 375, 2215–2222.

Schilde, L. M., Kösters, S., Steinbach, S., Schork, K., Eisenacher, M., Galozzi, S., Turewicz, M., Barkovits, K., Mollenhauer, B., Marcus, K., & May, C. (2018). Protein variability in cerebrospinal fluid and its possible implications for neurological protein biomarker research. *PloS One*, 13(11), e0206478.

Schunemann, H. J., Cushman, M., Burnett, A. E., Kahn, S. R., Beyer-Westendorf, J., Spencer, F. A., Rezende, S. M., Zakai, N. A., Bauer, K. A., Dentali, F., Lansing, J., Balduzzi, S., Darzi, A., Morgano, G. P., Neumann, I., Nieuwlaat, R., Yepes-Nuñez, J. J., Zhang, Y., & Wiercioch, W. (2018). American Society of Hematology 2018 guidelines for management of venous thromboembolism: Prophylaxis for hospitalized and nonhospitalized medical patients. *Blood Advances*, 2, 3198–3225.

Silva-Perez, L. J., Benitez-Lopez, M. A., Varon, J., & Surani, S. (2017). Management of critically ill patients with diabetes. *World Journal of Diabetes*, 8(3), 89–96.

Stokum, J. A., Gerzanich, V., & Simard, J. M. (2016). Molecular pathophysiology of cerebral edema. *Journal of Cerebral Blood Flow and Metabolism*, 36, 513.

Theunissen, J., Scholing, C., van Hasselt, W. E., van der Maten, J., & Ter Avest, E. (2016). A retrospective analysis of the combined use of PERC rule and Wells score to exclude pulmonary embolism in the Emergency Department. *Emergency Medicine Journal*, 33(10), 696–701.

Van den Berghe, G., Wouters, P., Weekers, F., Verwaest, C., Bruyninckx, F., Schetz, M., Vlasselaers, D., Ferdinande, P., Lauwers, P., & Bouillon, R. (2001). Intensive insulin therapy in critically ill patients. *The New England Journal of Medicine*, 345, 1359–1367.

Van den Berghe, G., Wouters, P. J., Bouillon, R., Weekers, F., Verwaest, C., Schetz, M., Vlasselaers, D., Ferdinande, P., & Lauwers, P. (2003). Outcome benefit of intensive insulin therapy in the critically ill: Insulin dose versus glycemic control. *Critical Care Medicine*, 31(2), 359–366.

Van den Berghe, G., Wilmer, A., Hermans, G., Meersseman, W., Wouters, P. J., Milants, I., Van Wijngaerden, E., Bobbaers, H., & Bouillon, R. (2006). Intensive insulin therapy in the medical ICU. *The New England Journal of Medicine*, 354(5), 449–461.

Viana, M. V., Moraes, R. B., Fabbrin, A. R., Santos, M. F., & Gerchman, F. (2014). Avaliação e tratamento da hiperglicemia em pacientes graves [Assessment and treatment of hyperglycemia in critically ill patients]. *Revista Brasileira de Terapia Intensiva*, 26(1), 71–76.

World Health Organization. (2020). *Obesity and overweight fact sheet*. https://www.who.int/news-room/fact-sheets/detail/diabetes

Zhang, H., Wang, Y., Sun, S., Huang, X., Tu, G., Wang, J., Lin, Y., Xia, H., Yuan, Y., & Yao, S.. (2019). Early enteral nutrition versus delayed enteral nutrition in patients with gastrointestinal bleeding: A PRISMA-compliant meta-analysis. *Medicine*, 98(11), e14864.

Zhikang, Y., Blaser, A. R., Lytvyn, L., Wang, Y., Guyatt, G. H, Mikita, J. S., Roberts, J., Agoritsas, T., Bertschy, S., Boroli, F, Camsooksai, J., Du, B., Heen, A. F., Lu, J., Mella, J. M., Vandvik, P. O., Wise, R., Zheng, Y., Liu, L., & Siemieniuk, R. A. C. (2020). Gastrointestinal bleeding prophylaxis for critically ill patients: A clinical practice guideline. *British Medical Journal*, 368, l6722.

Zhou, C., Wu, L., Ni, F., Ji, W., Wu, J., & Zhang, H. (2014). Critical illness polyneuropathy and myopathy: A systematic review. *Neural Regeneration Research*, 9(1), 101–110.

PART 3

Clinical Judgment

Psychosocial Health: Diagnosis and Management

Heather L. Spear • Anna M. Bourgault

SUBSTANCE ABUSE

Case Study

Mrs. R is a 70-year-old women admitted to the emergency room after she sustained a fall in her driveway while getting out of her car this evening. She is complaining of severe knee pain and has superficial abrasions and swelling around her right knee. A radiograph of the knee is ordered. While waiting for the result of the radiograph she develops tachycardia in the 170s. She states she feels her heart racing but otherwise she is asymptomatic. She is admitted to the cardiac step-down unit to stabilize her tachycardia episode and further work up her knee. You are the hospitalist APRN on call; you introduce yourself to the patient, take a chair, and sit by the patient's bed in an attempt to meet the patient at her eye level. You proceed to gain a detailed history and perform her physical assessment. In reviewing the patient's health history, it is identified that the patient lost her job 6 months ago. She has started drinking 3–4 glasses of wine at night with her husband. She finds the wine helps her fall asleep; the patient also admits she misses working and finds herself "bored" with nothing to occupy her time. As the APRN, you want to further explore the patient's substance use of alcohol.

Assessment of Substance Use and Abuse

The APRN will determine the level of intervention as a result of the Screening, Brief Intervention, and Referral to Treatment (SBIRT) assessment. Rosenthal et al. (2018) discuss SBIRT as an evidence-based instrument to assess for substance use and abuse. The SBIRT instruments identify if the patient is at low, moderate, or high risk for substance use of drugs and or alcohol (Table 6.1).

The patient-centered intervention is then developed to prevent further trajectory of abuse. APRNs may review billing guidance when assessing patients using the SBIRT assessment instrument (Department of Health and Human Services, 2011).

TABLE 6.1 EXAMPLES OF SBIRT ASSESSMENT INSTRUMENTS

INSTRUMENT	PURPOSE	LINK TO INSTRUMENT
Alcohol, Smoking, Substance Involvement, Screening Test (ASSIST)	Screening of substance use during the patient's lifetime	https://www.integration.samhsa.gov/clinical-practice/sbirt/Brief_Intervention-ASSIST.pdf
Alcohol Use Disorders Identification Test (AUDIT)	Screening of alcohol use	https://www.drugabuse.gov/sites/default/files/files/AUDIT.pdf
Drug Abuse Screening Test (DAST)	Screening for drug use	https://cde.drugabuse.gov/sites/nida_cde/files/DrugAbuseScreeningTest_2014Mar24.pdf
Cut Down, Annoyed, Guilty, Eye-Opener (CAGE)	Screening for alcohol use	https://pubs.niaaa.nih.gov/publications/arh28-2/78-79.htm

Key Points

The SBIRT instrument will assist the APRN to determine the amount of alcohol or other substances the patient is using and the level of dependency.

Take the time to sit with the patient when interviewing. Trust is essential in building rapport with your patient. Gerontology considerations for alcohol abuse include increased tolerance to alcohol with aging. Geriatric patients tend to have increased fatty tissue and less lean body tissue, which predisposes them to the risk of higher blood alcohol levels (BALs) in their system than a patient who is younger than 65 years. Their response to alcohol may cause memory loss and other cognitive deficits, including a risk for falls.

The Clinical Institute Withdrawal Assessment (CIWA-Ar) is an instrument to capture the severity of alcohol withdrawal symptoms (Figure 6.1). Symptoms measured by the CIWA scale include "tremors, anxiety, nausea or vomiting, transient and/or perceptual disturbances, diaphoresis, headache, and agitation and orientation" (Reoux & Oreskovich, 2006, p. 85). Alcohol withdrawal symptoms occur 24–48 hr after the last drink (Vacoralis & Halter, 2010).

Key Points

Consult a behavioral health (BH) professional, such as a BH APRN if available.

Differential Diagnosis

The differential diagnosis for substance use and abuse includes the following:

- Hypoglycemia
- Cerebral hemorrhage
- Benzodiazepine withdrawal
- Bacterial or viral meningitis

Case Study

According to the Alcohol Use Disorders Identification Test (AUDIT), Mrs. R is at high risk for alcohol use disorder. As the ARNP, you speak with her nurse about using the CIWA-Ar to ensure that she understands how to use it, and you write an order to complete the CIWA-Ar assessment every hour while Mrs. R is under observation.

Clinical Institute Withdrawal Assessment of Alcohol Scale, Revised (CIWA-Ar)

Patient: _____   Date: _____   Time: _____   (24 hour clock, midnight = 00:00)

Pulse or heart rate, taken for one minute: _____   Blood pressure: _____

NAUSEA AND VOMITING -- Ask "Do you feel sick to your stomach? Have you vomited?" Observation.
0 no nausea and no vomiting
1 mild nausea with no vomiting
2
3
4 intermittent nausea with dry heaves
5
6
7 constant nausea, frequent dry heaves and vomiting

TACTILE DISTURBANCES -- Ask "Have you any itching, pins and needles sensations, any burning, any numbness, or do you feel bugs crawling on or under your skin?" Observation.
0 none
1 very mild itching, pins and needles, burning or numbness
2 mild itching, pins and needles, burning or numbness
3 moderate itching, pins and needles, burning or numbness
4 moderately severe hallucinations
5 severe hallucinations
6 extremely severe hallucinations
7 continuous hallucinations

TREMOR -- Arms extended and fingers spread apart. Observation.
0 no tremor
1 not visible, but can be felt fingertip to fingertip
2
3
4 moderate, with patient's arms extended
5
6
7 severe, even with arms not extended

AUDITORY DISTURBANCES -- Ask "Are you more aware of sounds around you? Are they harsh? Do they frighten you? Are you hearing anything that is disturbing to you? Are you hearing things you know are not there?" Observation.
0 not present
1 very mild harshness or ability to frighten
2 mild harshness or ability to frighten
3 moderate harshness or ability to frighten
4 moderately severe hallucinations
5 severe hallucinations
6 extremely severe hallucinations
7 continuous hallucinations

PAROXYSMAL SWEATS -- Observation.
0 no sweat visible
1 barely perceptible sweating, palms moist
2
3
4 beads of sweat obvious on forehead
5
6
7 drenching sweats

VISUAL DISTURBANCES -- Ask "Does the light appear to be too bright? Is its color different? Does it hurt your eyes? Are you seeing anything that is disturbing to you? Are you seeing things you know are not there?" Observation.
0 not present
1 very mild sensitivity
2 mild sensitivity
3 moderate sensitivity
4 moderately severe hallucinations
5 severe hallucinations
6 extremely severe hallucinations
7 continuous hallucinations

ANXIETY -- Ask "Do you feel nervous?" Observation.
0 no anxiety, at ease
1 mild anxious
2
3
4 moderately anxious, or guarded, so anxiety is inferred
5
6
7 equivalent to acute panic states as seen in severe delirium or acute schizophrenic reactions

HEADACHE, FULLNESS IN HEAD -- Ask "Does your head feel different? Does it feel like there is a band around your head?" Do not rate for dizziness or lightheadedness. Otherwise, rate severity.
0 not present
1 very mild
2 mild
3 moderate
4 moderately severe
5 severe
6 very severe
7 extremely severe

Figure 6.1 Clinical Institute Withdrawal Assessment of Alcohol Scale, Revised (CIWA-Ar).

AGITATION -- Observation.
0 normal activity
1 somewhat more than normal activity
2
3
4 moderately fidgety and restless
5
6
7 paces back and forth during most of the interview, or constantly thrashes about

ORIENTATION AND CLOUDING OF SENSORIUM -- Ask "What day is this? Where are you? Who am I?"
0 oriented and can do serial additions
1 cannot do serial additions or is uncertain about date
2 disoriented for date by no more than 2 calendar days
3 disoriented for date by more than 2 calendar days
4 disoriented for place/or person

Total **CIWA-Ar** Score _____
Rater's Initials _____
Maximum Possible Score 67

*The **CIWA-Ar** is not copyrighted and may be reproduced freely. This assessment for monitoring withdrawal symptoms requires approximately 5 minutes to administer. The maximum score is 67 (see instrument). Patients scoring less than 10 do not usually need additional medication for withdrawal.*

Sullivan, J.T.; Sykora, K.; Schneiderman, J.; Naranjo, C.A.; and Sellers, E.M. Assessment of alcohol withdrawal: The revised Clinical Institute Withdrawal Assessment for Alcohol scale **(CIWA-Ar)**. *British Journal of Addiction* 84:1353-1357, 1989.

Figure 6.1 Cont'd

CLINICAL PEARLS

When substance use is suspected, the medical work-up must include the following:

- Substance, Brief Intervention, Referral to Treatment (SBIRT) assessment
- A BAL
- CIWA-Ar protocol initiated

Key Points

Care coordination is essential in the care of a geriatric patient with substance use disorder (SUD). Collateral information is important, such as genetic predisposition to alcoholism, a risk factor for SUD of alcohol.

Laboratory Analysis

Blood work should include a complete metabolic panel, hemoglobin (Hgb), hematocrit (Hct), folate, ferritin, magnesium, liver enzymes, and BAL. BAL is the amount of alcohol in 100 ml of blood, and it can be affected by body composition, medication, comorbidities, increased fatty tissue, and decreased lean tissue. A BAL of 20–50 mg/dl causes CNS depression, such as sedation (Merck Manual, 2019). A BAL of 50–100 mg/dl causes additional impairment of coordination, levels of 100–150 mg/dl may involve memory loss, levels of 150–300 mg/dl may involve delirium, levels of 300–400 mg/dl can cause unconsciousness, and a level over 400 mg/dl is fatal (Merck Manual, 2019).

Increased alanine aminotransferase (ALT) levels are indicative of liver disease (Leeuwen & Bladh, 2015, p. 20). Aspartate aminotransferase (AST) enzyme is tested in combination with ALT. An ALT/AST ratio of over 1.0 indicates alcoholic cirrhosis (Pagana & Pagana, 2007, p. 143). Gamma glutamyl transpeptidase (GGT) is an enzyme that can detect chronic alcohol intake. Patients who are alcoholic are prone to nutritional deficits (Leeuwen & Bladh, 2015, p. 471). Low folate levels indicate anemia, liver disease, and alcoholism. A low ferritin in combination with a low Hgb or Hct confirms iron deficiency anemia in a patient who has no other comorbidities that may impact the body's ability to store iron (Leeuwen & Bladh, 2015, p. 785). Decreased magnesium level seen in alcoholic patients is due to increased renal function and malnutrition (Leeuwen & Bladh, 2015, p. 1071).

CLINICAL PEARLS

- Assess for nutritional deficits including electrolyte imbalances
- Electrolyte imbalances increase the risk for a cardiac arrhythmia
- Monitor for seizure activity

Case Study

Mrs. R develops delirium tremens (DTs) 24 hr after being hospitalized. She exhibited signs of severe anxiety, elevated blood pressure, tachycardia, tremors, and periods of delirium. You are called to assess the patient. You review her vital signs and mental status, which includes orientation, level of consciousness, memory, thought process (coherent), thought content (delusion), mood, and speech. Your priority is to protect the airway and address cardiac symptoms. Standard measures also include IV administration of thiamine 100 mg, multivitamins, and magnesium. You give her a benzodiazepine to relieve her withdrawal symptoms in conjunction with the CIWA protocol. She remains on the intermediate unit for close monitoring. Over the next 48 hr, she improves, and her hemodynamics stabilize. She is lucid and cooperative. You work with case management, social services, and her family for discharge planning. She is discharged to short-term rehabilitation which includes a substance abuse, alcohol detoxification program.

Medications

Benzodiazepines, such as lorazepam, are given to relieve withdrawal symptoms; the hospital-based CIWA should be considered. Other medications used in a CIWA protocol are listed in Table 6.2.

TABLE 6.2 MEDICATIONS USED IN THE CLINICAL INSTITUTE WITHDRAWAL ASSESSMENT PROTOCOL

MEDICATION	ADULT DOSE	ACTION	CONTRAINDICATION
Disulfiram (Antabuse) Most effective in prescribing for a patient who is in their early sensation alcohol treatment; 12 hr after the patient's last intake of alcohol.	Initial dose is 500 mg orally once a day for 1–2 weeks, maintenance is 125–500 mg/day. Maximum dose is 500 mg/day.	The patient will exhibit disulfiram alcohol reaction when consuming any amount of alcohol. Disulfiram reaction includes headaches, nausea, and vomiting and compromises cardiac symptoms, such as tachycardia, dyspnea, diaphoresis, syncope, and confusion. Educate the patient to avoid alcohol or any alcohol containing products because they may exhibit a disulfiram reaction. Symptoms begin between 1 and 30 min and last for 2 hr (Varcarolis & Halter, 2010).	Metronidazole, paraldehyde, and patients with a history of coronary heart disease.
Acamprosate (Campral) Used for treating alcoholism and supporting the patient who has abstained from alcohol and wish to continue to abstain. Treatment may be initiated as soon as the patient withdraws from alcohol.	666 mg orally three times daily	Reduces craving for alcohol through its interaction with glutamate and GABA neurotransmitter (IBM Micromedex, 2019).	Hypersensitivity to acamprosate calcium and severe renal disease.
Naltrexone (Revia, Vivitrol) Treatment of alcohol and opioid dependence by blocking opiate receptors.	50 mg orally once daily, 380 mg IM gluteal injection every 4 weeks or once a month; prior to initiation of treatment patient must have stopped alcohol use.	Blocks opioid receptor interaction.	Use of opioid, hypersensitivity to naltrexone, polylactide-co-glycolide, and carboxymethylcellulose and other components of the diluent (IBM Micromedex, 2019, para. 1)
Benzodiazepines to treat withdrawl symptoms.	Lorazepam (Ativan) 1–2 mg IV or po. Diazepam 5–10 mg IV or po.		Use cautiously with older patients. Refer to the American Geriatric Society Beers Criteria.

DELIRIUM AND DEPRESSION

Case Study

Mrs. J is a 78-year-old widowed female who lives in independent senior living. Her daughter brings her to the emergency room and reports, "My mother is not herself! For the past 2 weeks, she hasn't answered her phone and her friends inform me she is not attending lunches at the senior center. When she visited me last Sunday, she was withdrawn and tearful, and slept all afternoon. Then in the past 2 days, she talked gibberish, was disoriented and was awake all night. She may have fallen. I'm afraid she may have had a stroke! When I went to pick her up to bring to the hospital, I found a note on her desk stating she wanted to die!"

On mental status examination, the patient is a frail, elderly female who is disoriented, inattentive, and irritable. She complains of chest and hip pain. She recognizes her daughter but does not understand where she is. Her speech varies from being inaudible to excessively loud. She frequently falls asleep during the interview but is easily aroused. She admits to feeling depressed and starts to cry. She denies suicidal thoughts but states, "I would be better off dead!" She is unable to describe her sleep patterns or recent appetite. Her thoughts are disorganized. She denies auditory or visual hallucinations. Her daughter reports that her mother's short-term memory has been worsening over the past 6 months, although her long-term memory is good. The patient lacks insight and judgment. As the AGACNP caring for the patient, you complete the history and physical examination of the patient, documenting and ordering the following:

- **Medical comorbidities:** HTN, hypercholesteremia, hypothyroidism, depression.
- **Medications:** Lisinopril 20 mg po qd, Lipitor 40 mg po qd, Synthroid 50 μg po qd, venlafaxine XR 37.5 mg po q am, nortriptyline (NTP) 100 mg po q hs.
- **Medical workup includes:** CBC w/diff, comprehensive metabolic panel, LFTs, thyroid panel, RPR, UA, toxicology screen (alcohol, acetaminophen, benzodiazepines, opioids), NTP level, vitamin B12, folate, vitamin D, ECG, head CT, CXR, hip XR, screen for cognitive impairment (Mini-Mental State Examination [MMSE] or Montreal Cognitive Assessment [MoCA]), screen for depression.

Key Points

Screening for baseline mental status and other mental disorders such as depression and anxiety is reliable ONLY following resolution of delirium.

CLINICAL PEARLS

Avoid polypharmacy and reduce medication risks:

- Familiarize yourself with the Beers Criteria designed for use in any clinical setting to identify potentially inappropriate medications (PIMs) that should be avoided in older adults (American Geriatrics Society, 2019).
- Notice most recent revisions are medications with strong anticholinergic effects, recategorized "nonbenzodiazepine" section for hypnotics and antidepressant history for falls and fractures (American Geriatrics Society, 2019 Beers Criteria update expert panel, 2019; Jacobs, 2019).
- Realize that "the Beers Criteria list has led to some unintended consequences and is meant to offer research-based guidance for the practitioner with a specific patient in a specific context" (American Geriatrics Society, 2019 Beers Criteria update expert panel, 2019).
- Know about Screening Tool of Older Persons Prescriptions (STOPP) and Screening Tool to Alert doctors to Right Treatment (START) criteria (Kok & Reynolds, 2017).

Case Study

While you are waiting for test results, medical treatment is ongoing and nursing care is attentive to Mrs. J's safety and elder sensitive needs. Staff ensures that the patient is safe on the stretcher at the lowest position to the floor, assesses for pain, administers essential home meds, offers toileting and hydration, determines when she ate last, and offers her food when appropriate. They also ensure that she has her eyeglasses and hearing aids, as appropriate, or offer an amplifier, which is available in many hospitals. Additionally, a large wall clock in the room offers orientation and a familiar comfort to the patient (Boltz et al., 2013; Doyle, 2017).

Key Points

Always examine the patient's body for any signs of abuse, failure to thrive, and neglect and observe any differences in the patient's communication and nonverbal behavior when the family is present. Any clinician who suspects elder abuse is mandated by state law to report it to the Department of Public Health. In addition, many hospitals coordinate this reporting with a licensed clinical social worker (Lachs & Pillemer, 2015).

CLINICAL PEARLS

Interviewing the family is essential with older adults.

- Obtain chronological history of patient's mood and memory.
- Review medications and identify who manages medications; confirm with home pharmacy.

- Ask about patient's participation in activities of daily living (ADLs) and with instrumental activities of daily living (IADLs) such as shopping, finances, and using phone and transportation.
- Inquire about family concerns and decisions about patient functioning that may require moving to a higher level of care. Evaluation of disposition starts in the emergency room; notify the case manager (Wolff et al., 2016).

It is crucial to be attentive to the family and to recognize that often the family members of an elderly patient are older adults themselves. Take notice of the older adult's sensory deficits, degree of caregiver strain, and level of fatigue. Inquire about medical illnesses, any medications they should be taking now, and last meal and hydration. Offer the family member a chair with arms. In the hospital, it is common to meet an older adult whose spouse was admitted overnight from the emergency room and the family member is without their home medication, such as insulin. Families need to be encouraged to go home, take their medications, eat, and have a nap before returning to the hospital (Doyle, 2017; Wolff et al., 2016).

Case Study

Your findings include the following: Head CT: No acute mass, midline shift, or hemorrhage; noted age-related atrophy of brain, white matter disease, and small vessel ischemic disease. Her CXR is normal. Her sodium is 125 mEq/l, and she is modestly anemic with an H/H of 9/27. Her NTP level is 160 (elevated). You search for a prior head CT or MRI for comparison and identify predisposing and precipitating factors for delirium. See Box 6.1. What is your differential?

Upon review of the patient's medical workup and results, you determine the patient has a delirium, mixed state (both hypoactive and hyperactive). While the patient has an altered mental status, you are unable to assess her depression. Before moving the patient to the medical floor, you slowly replace fluids and sodium so as not to cause a central pontine myelinolysis. You continue home medications except to hold the NTP and to order risperidone 0.25 mg po bid prn for agitation (Marcantonio, 2017).

Key Points

There are no medications to treat delirium. Antipsychotics such as haloperidol, olanzapine, and risperidone are administered only when the patient is severely agitated and presents as a safety risk. Recognize that antipsychotics in older adults have elevated risk for cardiac events and strokes (black box warning) and are known to cause QTc prolongation. Inform the family and discuss the risks and benefits of administering an antipsychotic prior to administration; document this discussion.

BOX 6.1   Conditions Frequently Associated With Delirium

The mnemonic I WATCH DEATH can be used to remember potential etiologies for delirium (Caplan, 2016).

- Infectious (e.g., Lyme disease)
- Withdrawal
- Acute metabolic
- Trauma
- CNS pathology (e.g., CVA)
- Hypoxia
- Deficiencies
- Endocrinopathies
- Acute vascular
- Toxins or drugs (e.g., polypharmacy)
- Heavy metals

CLINICAL PEARLS

Update and educate family about delirium, its course, and its treatment.

- Delirium is an acute neurocognitive, confusional state, often temporary, with inattention, disorganized thinking, possible hallucinations, misperceptions, and change in level of consciousness, either lethargy or agitation or both.
- The patient may or may not return to baseline cognitive status and is dependent on many factors: duration of delirium, previous episodes of delirium, comorbidities, and age. Should the patient have dementia, it is unlikely the patient will return to baseline function.
- Initial treatment is to treat all acute medical illnesses including withdrawal and to remove any agents that contribute to confusion, e.g., anticholinergics, hypnotics, and opioids.
- Ongoing treatment goals are to keep the patient safe, provide frequent reorientation, and strive to regulate the sleep/wake cycle.
- Encourage the family to engage the patient in conversation and reorient; provide familiar objects such as music, photos, and a blanket from home; share mealtimes; and be present, especially if patient is known to sundown.

Case Study

Once on the medical unit, the patient is settled into her room. Because the patient is impulsive and lacks awareness of safety risks, a 1:1 sitter is ordered but without restraints, as these exacerbate agitation. The assigned nurse greets the patient and her daughter and then takes a complete nursing history. The nurse evaluates the patient's mental status using the Confusion Assessment Method (CAM; Inouye et al., 1990).

She educates the daughter about this assessment and informs her of the results: her mother has a delirium. She meets the CAM criteria: (1) acute and fluctuating mental status, (2) inattention, and (3) change in level of consciousness (see Box 6.2). The nurse will monitor for evidence for hyperactive psychomotor activity with agitation, mood lability, and possible refusal of care (McKenzie, 2016; Inouye et al., 1990) as well as hypoactive psychomotor activity with lethargy and somnolence.

On day 2, Mrs. J is oriented to time, place, and person and is attentive but lethargic. She has poor safety awareness and occasional disorganized thinking. A physical therapy consult is ordered to promote mobility, prevent muscle atrophy and deconditioning, and facilitate wakefulness during the day. Her oral intake has improved, and her IV has been discontinued. Nurses recognize that the patient has not had a bowel movement since the day before admission and institute a bowel regimen with senna bisacodyl. The nurses work to establish good sleep hygiene, keeping the patient awake during the day, opening the blinds in the morning and closing the blinds at night, and at 9 p.m., offering the patient melatonin 3 mg to facilitate sleep.

A psychiatric consultation is ordered to evaluate the patient's depression and determine if she requires inpatient psychiatry level of treatment. The consultant administers the 9-question Patient Health Questionnaire (PHQ-9) now that the patient's delirium has resolved (Figure 6.2). The patient reports feeling hopeless and wanting to die; her PHQ-9 score is 25, and specifically, she scored 2 on the suicide item, further confirming her wish to die. The daughter has informed the psychiatrist/psych APRN that her mother had become more depressed over the past 3 weeks prior to developing delirium. She had been more socially isolated, had lost 10 pounds, and was waking up at 3 a.m. with an inability to return to sleep. With the medical issues resolved, the decision is made to admit the patient to inpatient psychiatry.

On day 3, Mrs. J is admitted to the psychiatric unit and is placed on q 15 min suicide checks. She ambulates independently, is eating and drinking without restriction, and has had a bowel movement. Her CAM is negative. Her mental status is depressed mood, flat affect, soft and slow speech, organized and goal-directed thoughts but with a paucity of thought, and psychomotor retardation. She is polite and cooperative and rarely makes eye contact. She shares a room with another patient, and she is often seen lying on her bed except when the staff arouse her for meals. She forgets to come to the medication room when her medications are due. She is neither exhibiting any bizarre behavior nor showing any signs of auditory or visual hallucinations. She sits quietly in group therapies offered on the unit and is the most engaged when the Recreational Therapist offers "Name That Tune" with songs from the patient's youth.

Your medical workup includes reordering the CBC, metabolic panel, and NTP level.

You meet with the patient to present the Geriatric Depression Scale (GDS). The original GDS is a 30-question scale; however, many acute care clinicians prefer to use the GDS-short form (Figure 6.3), with 15 questions. Any score 5 or greater is suggestive of depression. It is a self-administered scale. Mrs. J's GDS total score is 11.

Your assessment after reviewing all the medical history and interviewing the patient and daughter is that Mrs. J meets the criteria for major depressive disorder, recurrent, and severe.

BOX 6.2 Confusion Assessment Method (Inouye et al., 1990)

- Feature 1: Acute and fluctuating change in mental status AND
- Feature 2: Inattentive AND
- Feature 3: Disorganized thinking and perceptual disturbances OR
- Feature 4: Level of consciousness (LOC): refer to Richmond Agitation-Sedation Scale (RASS)

The Patient Health Questionnaire (PHQ-9)

Patient Name _____ Date of Visit _____

Over the past 2 weeks, how often have you been bothered by any of the following problems?	Not At all	Several Days	More Than Half the Days	Nearly Every Day
1. Little interest or pleasure in doing things	0	1	2	3
2. Feeling down, depressed or hopeless	0	1	2	3
3. Trouble falling asleep, staying asleep, or sleeping too much	0	1	2	3
4. Feeling tired or having little energy	0	1	2	3
5. Poor appetite or overeating	0	1	2	3
6. Feeling bad about yourself - or that you're a failure or have let yourself or your family down	0	1	2	3
7. Trouble concentrating on things, such as reading the newspaper or watching television	0	1	2	3
8. Moving or speaking so slowly that other people could have noticed. Or, the opposite - being so fidgety or restless that you have been moving around a lot more than usual	0	1	2	3
9. Thoughts that you would be better off dead or of hurting yourself in some way	0	1	2	3

Column Totals _____ + _____ + _____

Add Totals Together _____

10. If you checked off any problems, how difficult have those problems made it for you to
    Do your work, take care of things at home, or get along with other people?

☐ Not difficult at all   ☐ Somewhat difficult   ☐ Very difficult   ☐ Extremely difficult

Figure 6.2 The Patient Health Questionnaire. The PHQ-9 rating scale is 0–27: mild, 5–9; moderate, 10–14; moderately severe, 15–19; and severe, 20–27. Question 9 is a suicide screening question and, when positive, the patient needs further evaluation by a psychiatric expert. (From Kroenke, K., & Spitzer, R. L. (2002). The PHQ-9: a new depression diagnostic and severity measure. *Psychiatric Annals*, 32(9), 509–515.)

No.	Question	Answer	Score
	Geriatric Depression Scale (Short Form)		

Patient's Name: _____   Date: _____

Instructions: Choose the best answer for how you felt over the past week. Note: when asking the patient to complete the form, provide the self-rated form (included on the following page).

No.	Question	Answer	Score
1.	Are you basically satisfied with your life?	YES / *No*	
2.	Have you dropped many of your activities and interests?	*YES* / No	
3.	Do you feel that your life is empty?	*YES* / No	
4.	Do you often get bored?	*YES* / No	
5.	Are you in good spirits most of the time?	YES / *No*	
6.	Are you afraid that something bad is going to happen to you?	*YES* / No	
7.	Do you feel happy most of the time?	YES / *No*	
8.	Do you often feel helpless?	*YES* / No	
9.	Do you prefer to stay at home, rather than going out and doing new things?	*YES* / No	
10.	Do you feel you have more problems with memory than most people?	*YES* / No	
11.	Do you think it is wonderful to be alive?	YES / *No*	
12.	Do you feel pretty worthless the way you are now?	*YES* / No	
13.	Do you feel full of energy?	YES / *No*	
14.	Do you feel that your situation is hopeless?	*YES* / No	
15.	Do you think that most people are better off than you are?	*YES* / No	
		TOTAL	

(Sheikh & Yesavage, 1986)

Scoring:
Answers indicating depression are in bold and italicized; score one point for each one selected. A score of 0 to 5 is normal. A score greater than 5 suggests depression.

Sources:
- Sheikh JI, Yesavage JA. Geriatric Depression Scale (GDS): recent evidence and development of a shorter version. *Clin Gerontol*. 1986 June;5(1/2):165-173.
- Yesavage JA. Geriatric Depression Scale. *Psychopharmacol Bull*. 1988;24(4):709-711.
- Yesavage JA, Brink TL, Rose TL, et al. Development and validation of a geriatric depression screening scale: a preliminary report. *J Psychiatr Res*. 1982-83;17(1):37-49.

Figure 6.3 Geriatric Depression Scale-Short. (From Yesavage, J. B., Brink, T. L., Rose, T. L., Lum, O., Huang, V., Adey, M., & Leirer, V. O. (1983). Development and validation of a geriatric depression screening scale: A preliminary report. *Journal of Psychiatric Research*, 17(1), 37–49.)

Diagnosis

The diagnostic criteria for major depressive disorder, recurrent and severe, include depressed mood most of the day, nearly every day for 2 or more weeks, a change from previous functioning and/or loss of pleasure or interest, and five of nine symptoms listed in Box 6.3. Symptoms cause the patient to have significant distress or impairment (DSM-V, 2013). It is

---

BOX 6.3 Depression Symptoms Mnemonic: SIG: E Caps

- (S) Insomnia/hypersomnia
- (I) Reduced interest/pleasure
- (G) Excessive guilt or feelings of worthlessness
- (E) Reduced energy or fatigue
- (C) Diminished ability to concentrate or make decisions
- (A) Loss or increase of appetite/weight
- (P) Psychomotor agitation/retardation
- (S) Thoughts of suicide/death or an actual suicide attempt/plan

---

useful to familiarize yourself with the DSM-V specifically to review depressive disorders due to a medical condition. The mnemonic in Box 6.3 is a familiar and useful way to remember the symptoms of depression.

When older adults become depressed, they are more likely to describe their depression as lack of interest and pleasure, present with more somatic complaints, and explain their mood as a normal part of getting older. They may deny feeling depressed but will agree that they feel worthless and a burden to their family. However, depression in later life is quite serious. Twenty-five percent of older adults are affected by depression and cognitive impairment. The rate of suicide for the US population in adults 65 years of age and older is double that of the rate for the general US population; additionally, the highest suicide rates among any age group are highest in those 65 years of age and older (Box 6.4; Cremens, 2016). Late-life depression may follow acute illnesses such as stroke or hip fractures, and patients with dementia or Parkinson disease show increased risk for comorbid depression, the former up to 30% and the latter 50% (Cremens, 2016; Rackley, 2012). Patients with depression have poorer rehabilitation outcomes that affect their quality of life, thereby potentially necessitating a move to a higher level of care.

BOX 6.4 Suicide Risk Factors in Older Adults

- Widowhood
- Male > female
- Highest risk elders are 85 years of age and older
- Previous suicide attempts
- Affective disorder, e.g., major depressive disorder, increased risk with psychosis
- Active substance abuse
- New or chronic medical illness especially with chronic pain
- Access to lethal firearms
- Disruption in social relationships
- Exposure to suicidal behavior of others, e.g., relatives, peers, or media persons

Conwell and Caine (2002) and Cremens (2016).

Case Study

Mrs. J complains that she has been more forgetful for months and her daughter confirms this. She tells the APRN she is frightened that she may have Alzheimer disease. When pressed for time, administration of the mini-Cog is reasonable (Borson et al., 2000). For a more comprehensive screening, the APRN informs the patient and her daughter that she will begin cognitive screening using the MoCA instrument. Also, the APRN educates the patient and daughter that impaired concentration and memory are symptoms of depression. Once depression is treated, baseline cognitive status will be reevaluated and often is improved.

Cognitive Assessment

The MoCA is an easily administered brief screening instrument for mild cognitive dysfunction. The cognitive domains measured are attention and concentration, executive functions, memory, language, visuoconstructional skills, conceptual thinking, calculations, and orientation. The clinician will need about 10 min to administer (Nasreddine et al., 2005). Test scores 25 and above are considered normal, scores 21–24 are suggestive of mild cognitive impairment, and scores below 20 are suggestive of dementia. The MoCA (Figure 6.4) frequently identifies patient deficiencies that the MMSE misses (Folstein et al., 1975).

Case Study

The psychiatry treatment team holds an interdisciplinary meeting with the patient, family, nursing staff, medical staff, APRN/PA, hospital pharmacist, and community psychiatric provider to review the patient's record, course of hospitalization, and current medications (Wolff et al, 2016). Mrs. J's medication list is simplified and the hazards of polypharmacy are discussed. Her antidepressant NTP will be discontinued, and mirtazapine 7.5 mg po q hs will be started for sleep and appetite and to augment her venlafaxine XR. Mrs. J's venlafaxine XR will be increased to 75 mg qd and in the following week will be increased to 112.5 mg qd (Stahl, 2017). Ideally, a multimodal treatment plan for depression will be instituted (Box 6.5). The interdisciplinary treatment plan is as follows:

- Physical therapy evaluates patient for strength, endurance, and balance and makes recommendations to correct any acute problems and for outpatient follow-up.
- Occupational therapy reviews with the patient and family the safety concerns in her home and will make recommendations to improve safety. Also, OT will observe the patient organize a medication box, will assess patient's ability to meet her ADLs and IADLs, and will make recommendations post discharge. This is an opportune time to note if the patient needs long handle grabbers, a device to put on socks, a walker, new eyeglasses, hearing aids, modified utensils to facilitate eating, or other assistive devices.

- Social work reviews with the patient and family how well the home situation works for the patient and any prior visits to assisted living facilities (ALFs) or skilled nursing facilities (SNFs). The social worker will identify whether or not the patient has power of attorney (POA), healthcare agent, and end of living directive documents.
- Treatment team recommends the patient attend a Geriatric Intensive Outpatient Program (GIOP) 3 days a week following discharge. The patient's affect brightens when hearing about this. She admits she has been bored and lonely at home and has been unable to "get out of her rut."
- Nursing recommends a homecare nurse to make a home assessment and to observe the patient set up her medication box.
- The psychiatrist or APRN recommend neuropsychiatric testing, part of a dementia workup, to be completed as an outpatient once the patient's cognitive status and mood disorder have stabilized.

ANXIETY

Case Study

Mr. S is an 84-year-old married man who lives in an ALF and is admitted to medicine for a chronic obstructive pulmonary disease (COPD) exacerbation, increased anxiety, lethargy, and poor appetite. His medical conditions include COPD, CAD, HTN, hypothyroidism, hypercholesteremia, insulin-dependent diabetes mellitus, and generalized anxiety disorder (GAD). His surgical history includes coronary arterial bypass graft × 4 and cholecystectomy.

His current medications include the following: Lisinopril 20 mg qd, Lipitor 20 mg qd, Synthroid 75 μg qd, steroid inhaler, rescue inhaler, insulin meds, alprazolam 0.5 mg bid and 0.5 mg qd prn, NTP 75 mg q hs, vitamin B12, and vitamin D. He is allergic to penicillin.

His medical workup includes the following: CBC w/differential, comprehensive metabolic panel, liver functions, thyroid-stimulating hormone (TSH), urinalysis, O_2 saturation, serum toxicology screen, medication levels (NTP), CXR, and head CT.

You review the chief complaint and history of present illness, medical and surgical history, past psychiatric history, past and present substance abuse, family psychiatric and substance abuse history, and social and developmental history. Comprehensive assessment of the hospitalized older adult necessitates speaking with the nurse at the facility who is familiar with the patient, the closest family member, and the outpatient psychiatric provider who is managing the patient's psychiatric medications. It is important to be up-to-date with the patient's usual level of functioning relating to both ADLs and IADLs, acute illness symptoms leading up to admission, and the medications and behavioral approaches that are most effective for Mr. S's well-being.

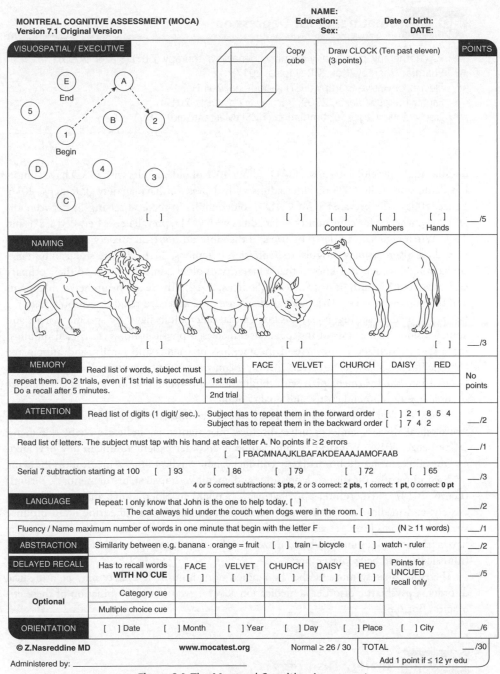

Figure 6.4 The Montreal Cognitive Assessment.

Introduction

All hospitalized patients experience situational anxiety. Patients usually demonstrate some behavioral regression in the new environment and when they are dependent on healthcare providers. However, patients may present with a preexisting anxiety disorder and these patients will need additional treatment to reduce anxiety symptoms. Approximately one-half

BOX 6.5 Treatments for Depression

- Psychotherapy, particularly cognitive behavioral therapy (CBT) (Blazer, 2009)
- Pharmacotherapy (Kok & Reynolds, 2017)
- Electroconvulsive therapy (ECT) (Goodman, 2011)
- Family therapy (Blazer, 2009; Rackley & Bostwick, 2012)
- Transcranial magnetic stimulation (TMS) (Marcantonio, 2017)

of older adults develop late-onset GAD. About 40% of older adults with GAD have comorbid depression while 60% of older adults with depression have anxiety (Cremens, 2016; Lenze, 2005). The prevalence for GAD in older adults in medical settings is between 1% and 28%, whereas for community older adults with GAD, prevalence is between 1.2% and 15%. When clinicians underrecognize and therefore do not treat anxiety and simple phobias, these disorders may progress to depression (Cremens, 2016). Depression can be a life-threatening disorder; it is known that a majority of older adults have visited their primary care physician 1 month prior to suicide (Steffens, 2014). The relationship between patients and their providers is key with older adults; more time is needed to address problems in the fast-paced medical setting. Next, it is known that older adults have age-specific worries and apprehensions such as loss of independence, increased physical illness, restricted mobility, more sensory deficits, reduced/fixed income, loss of friends and family, and anticipated changes in residence and caregivers. All these concerns must be taken seriously and incorporated into the treatment plan with implications for rehabilitation outcomes, adherence to discharge recommendations, and quality of life.

Many physical illnesses, such as heart disease, pulmonary disease, endocrine disease, neurological disease, and cognitive disorders like dementia, induce anxiety (Cremens, 2016; Lenze, 2014). Whenever a clinician hears an older patient complain of a new anxiety, the clinician should immediately consider a new medical illness, medication inducing or discontinued medications, depression, and cognitive impairment (dementia, delirium) (Lenze, 2014). Furthermore, polypharmacy, frequent in older adults, may contribute to anxiety, and medications such as steroids, bronchodilators, and ephedrine often produce anxiety symptoms (Stern et al., 2016). Some patients, especially those with dementia, may have a paradoxical response to benzodiazepines. Finally, anxiety is manifested in withdrawal from alcohol and benzodiazepines.

Therefore, anxiety must neither be ignored nor minimized; anxiety may be a medical disorder, a psychiatric disorder, a medication adverse event, or a combination of these etiologies (Box 6.6).

BOX 6.6 Anxiety Disorders

- Separation anxiety disorder
- Selective mutism
- Specific phobia
- Social anxiety disorder
- Panic disorder

(continued)

| BOX 6.6 | Anxiety Disorders (*continued*) |

- Agoraphobia
- Generalized anxiety disorder
- Substance-/medication-induced anxiety disorder
- Anxiety disorder due to another medical condition
- Other specified anxiety disorder
- Unspecified anxiety disorder

Data from American Psychiatric Association. (2013). Diagnostic and statistical manual of mental disorders, (5th ed.). American Psychiatric Association.

Case Study

On mental status examination, Mr. S is seated in the bedside chair. He is alert, oriented × 3, cooperative, and easily distracted. His affect is anxious and his mood is dysthymic. He demonstrates restlessness. He exhibits shortness of breath. His speech rate is slow and tone is soft. His thoughts are goal-directed and coherent. He denies paranoia, delusions, and auditory and visual hallucinations. His short-term memory is fair (recall 2/3 items after 5 min), and his long-term memory is intact. His insight is fair and his judgment is good. He asks you the same questions repeatedly and seeks your reassurance that he will get better to return to his wife who has her own health problems.

After determining that the patient is wearing his hearing aids and eyeglasses, you introduce yourself and sit down to be at the patient's eye level. You inquire what he is most concerned about and you share what you already know about him (Yager, 2011). You ask about his anxiety, although he may best relate to "concerns or stress" (Lenze, 2014). He describes uncontrollable worry, feeling restless, having trouble concentrating, and feeling muscle tension. Next, you ask him about his family living situation, work history, and present interests. This will serve to reduce his anxiety, build trust in your relationship, and facilitate review of his treatment plan. You also do a suicide screening, as elders with comorbid depression and anxiety are at higher risk for suicide (Lenze, 2014). While you are talking with him, you notice he is rearranging his personal items on the bedside table in a symmetrical pattern. He also requests that you write down your instructions. You recall the nurses informing you that he is very upset when they are late with his meds, insisting that they show him each individual medication before he is willing to swallow. You recognize his excessive anxiety, and in addition to his home medications, you order quetiapine 6.25 mg po bid prn anxiety; because the patient has COPD, it is preferable to treat his excessive anxiety with a nonbenzodiazepine.

The patient may or may not meet criteria for obsessive compulsive disorder (OCD), but you may be observing a personality disorder, in this example obsessive compulsive personality disorder (OCPD). More frequently, you will witness a personality trait, such as rigid, persistent, and exaggerated responses to interpersonal interactions that do not meet full criteria for a personality disorder.

Familiarize yourself with all the personality disorders in Box 6.7 to better prepare yourself for the behavioral nuances that will make you a more effective practitioner.

Later in the day after, the patient is medically stabilized, you return to speak with the patient and his wife. You reevaluate his anxiety symptoms: uncontrollable worry, restlessness, muscle tension, and poor concentration. You also ask about current life events as you know that there are other key stressors that can increase anxiety (Box 6.8). You learn from his wife that her husband has always been meticulous and focused on details and timeliness that confirms your thoughts that he has obsessive compulsive traits. You ask him if he is willing to complete an anxiety screening tool and he consents. The Hospital Anxiety and Depression Scale (HADS) is a valid instrument that measures emotional distress in patients with medical illnesses (Zigmond & Snaith, 1983). The most commonly used anxiety scale is the Hamilton Anxiety Rating Scale (HAM-A) (Hamilton, 1959; Porter, 2017; Stern et al., 2016). Or you may prefer to use anxiety scales specifically designed for older adults: the Geriatric Anxiety Inventory (GAI) (Pachana et al., 2007) or the Geriatric Anxiety Scale (GAS) (Segal et al., 2010; Mueller et al., 2015) (*Diagnostic and statistical manual of mental disorders*, DSM-5, 2013). The benefit of using an anxiety scale specific to older adults is that these scales account for physical illness symptoms that can erroneously increase anxiety scores. Other comorbid conditions that can exacerbate anxiety are shown in Box 6.9. Having the patient complete one of these scales periodically helps to identify the course of the patient's anxiety.

Key Points

Remember to send the rating scale results to the patient's primary care provider (PCP) and outpatient psychiatric provider.

Next you inquire about Mr. S's psychiatric medications: NTP and alprazolam. The patient is knowledgeable about his medications and informs you that NTP effectively reduces his anxiety and depressed mood and promotes a good night's sleep. He has been taking it for years and does not want it discontinued. You learned from his PCP that his annual ECG showed no changes in his cardiac rhythm. Fortunately at this dosage, he is

BOX 6.7   Personality Disorders

There are 10 personality disorders organized in three clusters:

Cluster A: paranoid, schizoid, schizotypal
Cluster B: antisocial, borderline, histrionic, narcissistic
Cluster C: avoidant, dependent, obsessive compulsive

Data from American Psychiatric Association. (2013). Diagnostic and statistical manual of mental disorders, (5th ed.). American Psychiatric Association.

BOX 6.8   Key Stressors Increasing Anxiety

- Aging with associated issues, e.g., loss of independence, loss of mobility, sensory deficits, loss of friends and relatives, change in residence, reduced finances
- Chronic illness and disability
- Caregiver status: unstable vs. stable, elder spouse, adult children who work or live long distance, and/or caregiver with chronic illness
- Bereavement

Data from Lenze (2014) and Stancu, I., & Von Gunten, A. (2014). Anxiety disorders in the elderly with an emphasis on generalized anxiety disorder. In R. Guglielmo, L. Janiri, & G. Pozzi (Eds.), *New perspectives on generalized anxiety disorder* (pp. 117–130, xiii). Hauppauge, NY, US: Nova Science Publishers, 215 anxiety disorder.

able to manage any side effects. In the older adult, it is more critical to remember that the tricyclic antidepressants (TCAs) have a side effect profile including anticholinergic effects, orthostasis, weight gain, and cardiac conduction delays and greater lethality in overdose (Bui, 2016).

Key Points

Remember to check a drug level and review side effect profiles and any medication interactions.

When Mr. S's anxiety worsened a few years ago, his PCP prescribed alprazolam and the patient reports it has been extremely helpful.

Treatment

Both alprazolam and NTP are on the Beers Criteria list (American Geriatrics Society, 2019). Revised in 2019, medical professionals identified high-risk medications for older adults and made recommendations regarding the level of risk as well as the strength of research evidence to support these risks. Recommendations are meant to highlight potential risks for older adults and to facilitate the clinician's decision-making whether or not to prescribe.

Disability is increased and quality of life is impaired in older adults with GAD. Because comorbid anxiety is extremely common in late-life depression, one needs to be attuned to higher suicide risk (Lenze, 2014). A majority of older adults visit their primary care physician within 1 month of suicide.

BOX 6.9   Conditions That Exacerbate or Cause Anxiety

- Dementia
- Hoarding syndrome
- Neurological disease, i.e., Parkinson disease, Huntington disease
- Heart disease, stroke, lung disease

There are limited evidence-based medication research studies in older adults. Benzodiazepines are commonly used in spite of serious side effects and are not recommended for long-term use (Lenze, 2014). The preferred medications to treat anxiety are the antidepressants serotonin selective reuptake inhibitors (SSRIs), primarily sertraline, and escitalopram in older patients. These medications are usually well tolerated and have low safety risks. When the patient does not respond to an SSRI, the selective nonspecific reuptake inhibitors (SNRIs) such as duloxetine and venlafaxine are recommended. Additional medications to reduce anxiety in older adults include mirtazapine, TCAs, buspirone, and low-dose trazodone (Bui, 2016). All of these medications require daily administration except trazodone and need to be prescribed at lower but therapeutic dosages. There is debate about using benzodiazepines in the elderly: many clinicians avoid them altogether, and others will prescribe a low dose for patients who are trustworthy, report efficacy, deny side effects, and do not receive adequate relief from an SSRI alone. Outpatient psychiatric providers are well trained in the nuances and treatment with all these medications and patients should be referred to them.

Elderly patients with anxiety may also report insomnia and the preferred medications are melatonin and trazodone. Hypnotics, on the Beers Criteria list (AGS, 2019; Noel et al., 2018), provide more risks than benefit and should be avoided. Box 6.10 lists other treatments for anxiety in older adults. A complete sleep evaluation may be necessary to first rule out any medical conditions and may be warranted as an outpatient procedure. Sleep hygiene including cognitive behavioral interventions for insomnia should be optimized (Segal et al., 2010).

Key Points

Consider consultation from a psychiatric APRN who may offer the evidence-based treatment interventions listed in Box 6.10 at the bedside and teaches skills that the patient may use post discharge.

Case Study

The following morning, the nurses inform you that Mr. S did not sleep last night and was confused and agitated. He attempted to punch the aide. Now he remains increasingly anxious, diaphoretic, and restless. You review his medical status. His blood pressure and heart rate are elevated. His laboratory test results are WNL. His UA is negative. On admission, his toxicology screen was positive for benzodiazepines, as alprazolam is one of his home meds. His NTP level is in the normal range at 70 (50–150 µg/L). He is oxygenating well; his O_2 saturation is above 90%; and his nasal O_2 has been decreased. You decide to review his administered medications. You discover that the patient's alprazolam was inadvertently discontinued in the ER and that the patient has not taken alprazolam in the past 36 hr. You recognize that although benzodiazepines are on the Beers Criteria list with risks in the elderly for falls, confusion, and sedation, Mr. S is now in benzodiazepine withdrawal. The mean half-life for alprazolam is 11.2 hr (6.3–26.9) in healthy adults and therefore longer in older adults. You therefore restart his home dose of alprazolam and give him his first dose now (Stahl, 2017).

BOX 6.10   Evidence-Based Treatment Interventions to Reduce Anxiety in Older Adults

- CBT, relaxation training, supportive therapy, and cognitive therapy (Segal et al., 2010)
- Psychoeducation, problem-solving training, and bibliotherapy (Thorp, 2009; van't Veer-Tazelarr, 2009)
- Interventions should be offered at a slower pace, supported with written or audio support, and may include a family member (Thorp, 2009, p. 180; Lenze, 2014)

Key Points

Successful management for an alprazolam taper is determined by the patient's dosage and number of years administered. For patients with long-term administration, especially alprazolam, it may take weeks to months to taper patient off and therefore will be managed as an outpatient.

Case Study

The next morning, Mr. S is medically and psychiatrically cleared for discharge to his ALF. The APRN meets with the patient and family and provides verbal and written discharge instructions and any helpful resources regarding anxiety management. Discharge documentation includes hospital course, most recent mental status examination, any changes in medical and psychiatric medications, results of his anxiety screening, and any additional recommendations. You send documentation to the patient's PCP, his MD/APRN at ALF, and his outpatient psychiatric provider.

CLINICAL PEARLS

- Medical disorders must be ruled out first before making a diagnosis of anxiety.
- Depression, delirium, and dementia may present with anxiety.
- Substance withdrawal (BZ, alcohol, cocaine, stimulants) must be a differential diagnosis.
- Conditions presenting as anxiety or agitation: UTIs, constipation, hypoxia, infection.
- An unfamiliar environment may be especially anxiety producing for older adults.
- Polypharmacy and medication side effects (e.g., akathisia) may induce anxiety.

(Cremens, 2016).

REVIEW QUESTIONS

1. What other risk factors should be assessed for SUD of alcohol?
   a. Genetics
   b. Age
   c. Profession
   d. Gender

2. When would you expect a patient to exhibit signs and symptoms of withdrawal from alcohol?
   a. 5–8 hr
   b. 24–48 hr
   c. 72–120 hr
   d. 121–168 hr

3. What medication is initially used for alcohol withdrawal symptoms?
   a. Acamprosate
   b. Excitalopram
   c. Lorazepam
   d. Fentanyl

4. Using the Beers Criteria, you are better able to assess an older adult's risk of:
   a. Mood disturbances and impulsivity
   b. Cognitive decline due to their diagnosis
   c. Medications with adverse effects
   d. Addiction to opioids and alcohol

5. Hypoactive delirium and depression may present similarly; select the best response to identify depression.
   a. Acute confusion, inattentive, somnolent, and apathetic
   b. Coherent thoughts, slow speech, somnolent, depressed mood
   c. Acute confusion, RASS "0," inattentive, perceptual disturbance
   d. Hyperactive state with delusions of grandeur, perceptual disturbance

6. Psychiatric medications upon discharge for Mrs. J are:
   a. Venlafaxine XR, mirtazapine, and risperidone
   b. Venlafaxine XR, mirtazapine, and NTP
   c. Venlafaxine XR, mirtazapine, and melatonin
   d. Venlafaxine XR and mirtazapine

7. What laboratory test will help identify conditions causing anxiety?
   a. LFTs
   b. Toxicology screen
   c. UA
   d. All of the above

8. What medications are recommended for older adult patients to reduce anxiety in the hospital?
   a. Clonazepam
   b. Buspirone
   c. Trazodone
   d. Sertraline

9. What therapeutic interventions may be offered at the bedside to reduce anxiety?
   a. Stand at bedside and educate patient
   b. Sit at bedside and teach breathing techniques
   c. Offer a printed relaxation exercise, in large print, after practicing with patient and answering patient's questions
   d. b and c

Answers: 1, a; 2, b; 3, c; 4, c; 5, b; 6, d; 7, d; 8, d; 9, d

REFERENCES

American Geriatrics Society. (2019). Beers Criteria update expert panel. American Geriatrics Society 2019 updated AGS beers criteria for potentially inappropriate medication use in older adults. *Journal of the American Geriatrics Society*, 67(4), 674–694.

American Psychiatric Association. (2013). *Diagnostic and statistical manual of mental disorders* (5th ed.). American Psychiatric Association.

Blazer, D. S. (2009). Mood disorders. In Blazer, D. S., & Steffens, D.C. (Eds.), *Textbook of geriatric psychiatry fourth edition* (pp. 275–299). American Psychiatric Publishing, Inc.

Boltz, D. S., Parke, B., Shuluk, B., Capezuti, E., & Galvin, J. E. (2013). Care of the older adult in the emergency department. *The Gerontologist*, 53(3), 441–453.

Borson, S., Scanlan, J., Brush, M., Vitaliano, P., & Dokmak, A. (2000). The mini-cog: A cognitive 'vital signs' measure for dementia screening in multi-lingual elderly. *International Journal of Geriatric Psychiatry*, 15(11), 1021–1027.

Bui, E. P. (2016). The pharmacotherapy of anxiety disorders. In Stern, T. F. (Ed.), *Massachusetts general hospital comprehensive clinical psychiatry* (pp. 464–474). Elsevier.

Caplan, J. C. (2016). Delirium. In Stern, T. F. (Ed.), *Massachusetts general hospital comprehensive clinical psychiatry* (2nd ed.,p. 176). Elsevier.

Conwell, Y., & Caine, E. D. (2002). Risk factors for suicide in later life. *Biological Psychiatry*, 52(3), 193–204.

Cremens, M. (2016). Geriatric psychiatry. In Stern, T. F. (Ed.), *Massachusetts general hospital comprehensive clinical psychiatry* (pp. 763–769). Elsevier.

Department of Health and Human Services. (2011). *Centers of medicare and medicaid services*. https://www.integration.samhsa.gov/sbirt/SBIRT_Factsheet_ICN904084.pdf

Doyle, A. (2017). *Mount Sinai's geriatric ED advances the patient experience for plder patients* (pp. 1–3). Industry Edge. A Press Ganey Publication.

Folstein, M.F., Folstein, S.E., & McHugh, P.R. (1975). Mini Mental State. A practical method for grading the cognitive state of patients for the clinician. *Journal of Psychiatric Research*, 12(3), 189–198.

Goodman, W.K. (2011). Electroconvulsive therapy in the spotlight. *New England Journal of Medicine*, 364, 1785–1787.

Hamilton, M. (1959). The assessment of anxiety states by rating. *British Journal of Medical Psychology*, 32, 50–55.

IBM Micromedex. (2019). *Search drug, disease toxicology, and more*. https://www.micromedexsolutions.com/micromedex2/librarian/CS/76FAE2/ND_PR/evidencexpert/ND_P/evidencexpert/DUPLICATIONSHIELDSYNC/CA41FA/ND_PG/evidencexpert/ND_B/evidencexpert/ND_AppProduct/evidencexpert/ND_T/evidencexpert/PFActionId/pf.HomePage?navitem=topHome&isToolPage=true

Inouye, S. K., van Dyck, C. H., Alessi, C. A., Balkin, S., Siegal, A.P., & Horwitz, R.I. (1990). Clarifying confusion: The confusion assessment method. A new method for detection of delirium. *Annals of Internal Medicine*, 113(12), 941–948.

Jacobs, L. G. (2019). For older people, medications are common; an updated AGS Beers Criteria' aims to ensure they are appropriate, too. *Geriatric Nursing*, 40(2), 230–231.

Kok, R. M., & Reynolds, C. F. (2017). Management of depression in older adults: A review. *Journal of the American Medical Association*, 317(20), 2114–2122.

Kroenke, K., Spitzer, R. L., & Williams, J. B. (2001). The PHQ-9: Validity of a brief depression severity measure. *Journal of General Internal Medicine*, 16(9), 606–613.

Lachs, M. S., & Pillemer, K. A. (2015). Elder abuse. *New England Journal of Medicine*, 373, 1947–1956.

Lee, H. H. (2013). Prevalence of depression in elderly patients with chronic physical illness. *European Neuropsychopharmacology*, S353.

Leeuwen, A. M., & Bladh, M. L. (2015). *Davis's comprehensive handbook of laboratory & diagnostic test with nursing implications* (6th ed.). F.A. Davis Company.

Lenze, E. W. (2014). Anxiety disorders. In Thakur, M. B. (Ed.), *Clinical manual of geriatric psychiatry* (pp. 175–192). American Psychiatric Publishing, Inc.

Marcantonio, E. R. (2017). Delirium in hospitalized older adults. *The New England Journal of Medicine, 377,* 1456–1466.

McKenzie, G. (2016). Late life depression, In M. Boltz , Capezuti, L., Fulmer, T. T., & Zwicker, D. A. (Eds.), *Evidence-based geriatric nursing protocols for best practice* (5th ed., pp. 211–232). Springer Publishing Company, LLC.

Merck Manual Professional Version. (2019). *Alcohol toxicity and withdrawal.* https://www.merckmanuals.com/professional/special-subjects/recreational-drugs-and-intoxicants/alcohol-toxicity-and-withdrawal?query=alcohol%20toxicity

Mueller, A. E., Segal, D. L., Gavett, B., Marty, M. A., Yochim, B., June, A., & Coolidge, F. L. (2015). Geriatric Anxiety Scale: Item response theory analysis, differential item functioning, and cretion of a ten-item short form (GAS-10). *International Psychogeriatrics, 27*(7), 1099–1111.

Nasreddine, Z. S, Phillips, N. A., Bédirian, V., Charbonneau, S., Whitehead, V., Collin, I., Cummings, J. L., & Chertkow, H. (2005). The montreal cognitive assessment: MoCA, a brief screening tool for cognitive assessment. *Journal of the American Geriatrics Society, 53*(4), 695–699.

Noel, O. P., Pifer, M., Mahoney, C., & Segal, D. (2018). The geriatric anxiety scale and the geriatric anxiety inventory: Relationships to anxiety risk factors. *Innovation in Aging, 2*(suppl 1), 283.

Pachana, N., Byrne, G. J., Siddle, H., Koloski, N., Harley, E., & Arnold, E. (2007). Development and validation of the geriatric anxiety inventory. *International Psychogeriatrics, 19*(1), 103–114.

Pagana, K. D., & Pagana, T. J. (2007). *Mosby's diagnostic and laboratory test reference* (8th ed.). Mosby Elsevier.

Porter, E., Chambless, D. L., McCarthy, K. S., DeRubeis, R. J., Sharpless, B. A., Barrett, M. S., Milrod, B., Hollon, S. D., & Barber, J. P. (2017). Psychometric properties of the reconstructed hamilton depression and anxiety scales. *The Journal of Nervous and Mental Disease, 205*(8), 656–664.

Rackley, S. B., & Bostwick, J. M. (2012). Depression in medically ill patients. *The Psychiatric Clinics of North America, 35*(1), 231–247.

Reoux, J. P., & Oreskovich, M. R. (2006). A comparison of two versions of the clinical institute withdrawal assessment for alcohol: The CIWA-Ar and CIWA-AD. *The American Journal on Addictions, 15,* 85–93. https://doi.org/10.1080/10550490500419136

Rosenthal, L. D., Barnes, C., Aagaard, L., Cook, P., & Weber, P. (2018). Initiating SBIRT, alcohol, and opioid training for nurses employed on an inpatient medical-surgical unit: A quality improvement project. *MEDSURG Nursing, 27*(4), 227–230.

Segal, D. L., June, A., Payne, M., Coolidge, F. L., & Yochim, B. (2010). Development and initial validation of a self-report assessment tool for anxiety among older adults: The geriatric anxiety scale. *Journal of Anxiety Disorders,* 709–714.

Stahl, S. (2017). *Stahl's essential psychopharmacology prescriber's guide.* Cambridge University Press.

Steffens, D. B. (2014). Mood disorders. In Thakur, M. B. (Ed.), *Clinical manual of geriatric psychiatry* (pp. 125–157). American Psychiatric Publishing, Inc.

Stern, T. F., Fava, M., Wilens, T. E., & Rosenbaum, J. F. (2016). *Massachusetts general hospital comprehensive clinical psychiatry.* Elsevier.

Thorp, S. R., Ayers, C. R., Nuevo, R., Stoddard, J. A., Sorrell, J. T., & Wetherell, J. L. (2009). Meta-analysis comparing different behavioral treatments for late-life anxiety. *The American Journal of Geriatric Psychiatry, 17,* 105–115.

van't Veer-Tazelaar, P. J., van Marwijk, H. W. J., van Oppen, P., van Hout, H. P., van der Horst, H. E., Cuijpers, P., Smit, F., Beekman, A. T. (2009). Stepped-care prevention of anxiety and depression in late life: a randomized controlled trial. *Archives of General Psychiatry, 66*(3), 297–304.

Varcarolis, E. M., & Halter, M. J. (2010). *Foundations of psychiatric mental health nursing: A clinical approach* (6th ed.). Mosby Elsevier.

Wetherell, J. L., Lenze, E.J., & Stanley, M. A. (2005). Evidence-based treatment of geriatric anxiety disorders. *Psychiatric Clinics, 28*(4), 871–896. https://doi.org/10.1016/j.psc.2005.09.006

Wolff, J. F., Feder, J., & Schulz, R. (2016). Supporting family caregivers of older Americans. *The New England Journal of Medicine, 375,* 2513–2515.

Yager, J. (1989). Specific components of bedside manners in the general hospital psychiatric consultation: 12 concrete suggestions. *Psychosomatics, 30,* 209–212.

Yesavage, J. B., Brink, T. L., Rose, T. L., Lum, O., Huang, V., Adey, M., & Leirer, V. O. (1983). Development and validation of a geriatric depression screening scale: A preliminary report. *Journal of Psychiatric Research*, 17(1), 37–49.

Zigmond, A. S., & Snaith, R. P. (1983). The hospital anxiety and depression scale. *Acta Psychiatrica Scandinavica*, 67(6), 361–370.

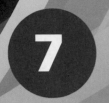

Hematologic and Oncologic Management

7

Laura Mulka

INTRODUCTION

ACNPs will encounter benign and malignant hematological and oncology patients on a daily basis. The following case studies are an overview of possible diagnoses which may be encountered. Hematology and especially oncology are rapidly transforming fields. According to Center Watch, between 2013 and 2018, there were 102 cancer fighting medications and/or new indications. As of August 2019, there were 22 new medications and/or indications approved by the FDA (CenterWatch, 2020). Some of this in part is due to the FDA's accelerated approval program. This allows for earlier approval of medications that meet a serious condition; however, they still require confirmatory studies to demonstrate the clinical benefit (Center for Drug Evaluation and Research, 2020).

MALIGNANT LESION

Case Study 1

Mr. G is a 57-year-old gentleman with past medical history of HTN who presents to the ED with increased DOE and fatigue that has been progressively worse over the last several days. He denies chest pain, cough, or recent exposure to infection. He drinks an occasional alcoholic beverage on the weekend and has no tobacco or illicit drug history.

His father had a history of CHF and stroke and died at age 74. His mother has a history of valvular heart disease and HTN. His siblings have histories of HTN and heart disease. There is no family history of blood disorders or cancer.

He reports increased fatigue over the past several months, which he attributes to "getting older." He has increased headaches and lightheadedness over the past few weeks. He noticed DOE a week ago while working outside, which has become progressively worse. He denies cough or chest pain, nausea, or vomiting; however, he has had a decreased appetite with a 10-pound weight loss over the last month. He denies dysphagia or reflux. He reports new onset of constipation over the last few days. He endorses complaints of lumbar back discomfort for the last few months which has not improved over time. He describes the pain as 4–5/10, achy in nature, with no precipitating event. Discomfort decreases with 600 mg ibuprofen.

His physical examination reveals the following: height, 67 inches; weight, 145 lbs; BP, 130/80; pulse, 140; respirations, 24; temperature, 99.2 °F; HEENT: normocephalic, sclera is anicteric; lymph: no cervical, supraclavicular, or inguinal adenopathy; CV: S1, S2 tachycardic, and no murmurs or gallops; lungs: clear throughout, with no crackles or rhonchi; abdomen: soft, nontender with positive bowel sounds, no hepatosplenomegaly; neuro: Pupil equal, round and reactive to light and accomidation (PERRLA), oriented to person, place, time, and situation, however lethargic; equal grasp strength 5/5 upper extremities; equal decreased strength of lower extremities 3/5; patellar reflexes decreased.

Based on Mr. G's history and physical examination, you make the following working list of problems:

1. Acute anemia
2. AKI
3. Hypercalcemia
4. Lytic lesion—concern for malignancy

Problem #1: Anemia

Anemia is the most common hematological diagnosis encountered in the acute care setting. To simplify anemia, one can approach it as increased destruction of red blood cells (RBCs) or decreased production (Table 7.1). Blood loss is not included in this chart but has a very high correlation with iron deficiency (Leung, 2019).

To further evaluate anemia, one must look at the RBC indices (Table 7.2). One can use RBC indices to help narrow down the causative factor for anemia. Many patients have multifactorial anemia, so this is only a guideline.

Microcytic causes of anemia include iron deficiency, thalassemic disorders, inflammation/chronic disease (early), sideroblasts, copper deficiency, lead poisoning, and hemolysis. Normocytic causes of anemia include acute blood loss, early iron deficiency, inflammation/

TABLE 7.1 CAUSES OF ANEMIA

INCREASED DESTRUCTION	DECREASED PRODUCTION
Aplastic anemia	B_{12} deficiency
Hemolytic anemia	Folate deficiency
Myelodysplasia	Iron deficiency
Tumor infiltration	Malabsorption
Hypersplenism	Dietary/alcohol
	Hypothyroid
	Renal insufficiency
	Chronic disease

TABLE 7.2 RBC INDICES

	LOW	HIGH
Mean corpuscular volume (MCV)	Microcytic	Macrocytic
Mean corpuscular hemoglobin (MCH)	Hypochromic	Hyperchromic
Mean corpuscular hemoglobin concentration (MCHC)	Low values correlate with low MCV and MCH	High values correlate with congenital or acquired spherocytosis or congenital hemolytic anemias (Leung, 2019)

chronic disease, bone marrow suppression, malignancy, chronic renal insufficiency, endocrine dysfunction, and hemolysis. Macrocytic causes of anemia include alcoholism, folate deficiency, B_{12} deficiency, myelodysplastic syndrome, acute myeloid leukemia, drugs, and liver disease (Leung, 2019).

The workup for anemia should include CBC with differential, iron, total iron binding capacity, ferritin, folate, B_{12}, reticulocyte count, TSH, creatinine, lactate dehydrogenase (LDH), indirect bilirubin, haptoglobin, and peripheral blood smear, along with stool for occult blood testing.

CLINICAL PEARLS

- Review the CBC and determine the indices to focus on causative factors.
- Order a general anemia workup.
- Remember: there may be more than one causative factor.

The American Association of Blood Banks (AABB) recommends an RBC transfusion for patients with Hgb less than 7 or with Hgb less than 8 if the patient is undergoing orthopedic or cardiac surgery or has preexisting cardiovascular disease (Carson et al., 2016). These recommendations do not apply to patients with ACS, oncologic patients, or patients with blood disorders and chronic transfusion–dependent anemia (Carson et al., 2016), as these patients often require transfusion at a higher Hgb level to avoid anemic hypoxia. Blood transfusions continue to have potential complications, including the risk of infection, allergic and immune transfusion reactions, volume overload, hyperkalemia, and iron overload (Carson & Kleinman, 2019). According to Kleinman et al. the risk of human immunodeficiency virus (HIV) infection from a blood transfusion is 1 in approximately 1.5–2 million. The risk of hepatitis B is 1 in 200,000–360,000, and the risk of hepatitis C is 1 in 1–2 million.

Problem #2: Acute Kidney Injury

The workup for acute renal failure (AKI) will be covered in Chapter 16. The differential diagnosis for AKI is vast and includes dehydration, hemorrhage, heart failure, liver disease, medications, obstruction, malignancy, and infection (Fatehi & Hsu, 2019).

Problem #3: Hypercalcemia

Hypercalcemia is a very common finding in acute and primary care settings. It is important to calculate the corrected calcium when you have a patient with a low albumin. A calcium value can be perceived as normal, when in fact it is elevated. The calculation to corrected calcium in a patient with low albumin is as follows (GlobalRxPh, 2017):

$$\text{Correct calcium} = \text{serum calcium} + 0.8\left(4 - \text{serum albumin}\right).$$

Hypercalcemia can be caused by many issues (Waltham, 2020). The first piece of the puzzle is to determine if it is a result of hyperparathyroidism. A parathyroid hormone (PTH) level should be ordered to rule this out. Once hyperparathyroidism is ruled out, the differential includes malignancy, vitamin D intoxication, chronic granulomatous disorders, medications, and other miscellaneous disorders such as hyperthyroidism and adrenal insufficiency (Shane, 2020). Signs and symptoms of hypercalcemia include nausea, vomiting, anorexia, abdominal pain, constipation, irritability, mental status changes, seizures, coma, fatigue, hyperreflexia, muscle weakness, orthostatic hypotension, cardiac arrhythmias, polyuria, polydipsia, dehydration, renal calculi, azotemia, and renal failure (Lewis, 2020).

CLINICAL PEARLS

- If serum calcium is high or high normal, assess patient's albumin level. If it is low, calculate a corrected calcium.
- If elevated serum calcium, or corrected calcium, check PTH level to rule out hyperparathyroidism.

Problem #4: Lytic Lesion

A lytic lesion is destruction of an area of bone caused by a disease process (National Cancer Institute, 2020). Many malignant and some nonmalignant diseases can cause lytic lesions. Included in the malignancies are breast, lung, prostate, renal cell, thyroid, and multiple myeloma. Nonmalignant causes include bone cysts and infections (Roodman, 2019).

Case Study

After a preliminary workup, Mr. G was found to have normocytic, normochromic anemia, with no vitamin deficiencies, source of bleeding, or hemolysis. The patient was transfused with two units of packed RBCs. AKI could be related to dehydration; however, no obstruction, medication, or other mechanical source was noted. The patient's corrected calcium was 13.52 and PTH was normal. The patient was treated with hydration and denosumab. Denosumab (Xgeva) is a RANK ligand inhibitor indicated for hypercalcemia of malignancy and prevention of skeletal-related events in patients with multiple myeloma and bone metastases from solid tumors (Xgeva package insert, 2019). The last concern was a lytic lesion. Differential diagnosis includes malignancy until proven otherwise. A computed tomography (CT) scan of the chest, abdomen, and pelvis without contrast (due to AKI) was ordered. The CT scan demonstrated no masses or organomegaly. Multiple areas of lytic lesions are noted in the spine, pelvis, and femur. The most likely culprit is multiple myeloma.

Multiple Myeloma

Multiple myeloma is a cancer of the immunoglobulin-producing plasma cells. Presenting symptoms of multiple myeloma include anemia, bone pain, elevated creatinine, fatigue, hypercalcemia, and weight loss (Laubach, 2019). Once the primary differential diagnosis is malignancy, a hematology/oncology consult should be requested. The hematologist/oncologist will order the following workup: serum protein electrophoresis, 24-hr urine protein electrophoresis, immunofixation of urine and serum, free light chains, beta-2 microglobulin, uric acid, and LDH (National Comprehensive Cancer Network, 2019c). The patient will need a bone marrow biopsy. A skeletal survey, not a bone scan, is the most appropriate test for multiple myeloma. The presentation of multiple myeloma lesions is primarily osteolytic associated with increased bone destruction and suppressed bone formation, which are often not detectable on bone scan as it relies on technetium uptake to identify areas of new bone formation (Roodman, 2019).

Treatments for myeloma have changed immensely in the past 5 years. New target agents including proteasome inhibitors, immunomodulating agents, and combinations of various agents have been exploding into clinical practice. The initial consideration for treatment is to determine if the patient is transplant eligible. Autologous hematopoietic cell transplantation has been proven to extend progression free and overall survival vs. chemotherapy alone. If the patient is determined to be transplant eligible, they will receive induction therapy, transplant, and then maintenance therapy. For patients who are not transplant eligible, they will receive single or combination therapy with a variety of medications (National Comprehensive Cancer Network, 2019c).

Case Study

Mr. G's diagnosis is immunoglobulin G myeloma. During the hospital stay, the patient started experiencing increased weakness of his lower extremities and new bowel incontinence. An MRI of his lumbar spine was performed and he was found to have a spinal cord compression.

Key Points

A spinal cord compression is an oncologic emergency. Spinal cord compression can lead to irreversible nerve damage that can cause paralysis or other losses of function depending on the level of the compression. Intervention includes steroids, potential surgery, or radiation therapy.

Transplant Eligibility

The next step is to determine if the patient is eligible for transplant. The provider then refers to the National Comprehensive Cancer Network (NCCN) guidelines for the most current recommendation for treatment. According to NCCN, category 1 recommendation is bortezomib/lenalidomide and dexamethasone (Laubach, 2019). Prophylaxis with Bactrim and acyclovir are added due to the high risk of infection. In addition, the patient will continue to receive denosumab monthly for osseous lesions. Potential side effects of treatment are dependent on the specific treatment used. The most common side effects of chemotherapy and targeted treatment include fatigue, nausea, diarrhea, immunosuppression, increased anemia and thrombocytopenia, neuropathy, and fertility issues/birth defects. Side effects of radiation include fatigue, skin irritation, and potential injury to structures radiated.

Case Study

Mr. G was treated initially in the hospital and released after day 1 of treatment. He received radiation therapy to L2 with high-dose steroids. He was also started on prophylaxis with Bactrim and acyclovir due to the high risk of infection. He was deemed eligible by transplant criteria. In addition, he will continue to receive denosumab monthly for osseous lesions.

He presented to the ED 10 days later with a fever of 101.6 °F and severe fatigue. On initial evaluation, a CBC revealed a WBC of 1.0, Hgb of 10.1, Hct of 30, platelets (Plts) of 403, and ANC of 200. Unfortunately, he had febrile neutropenia.

Neutropenia

Neutropenia is defined as an absolute neutrophil count (ANC) less than 1,500. The severity index for neutropenia classifies a count <1,500 as mild, <1,000 as moderate, and <500 as severe. Pan cultures, including blood, urine, and other sources (i.e., stool if having diarrhea), and CXR are the mainstay of practice (Wingard, 2019). Empirical coverage with IV antibiotics covering both gram-negative and gram-positive organisms should be started within 60 min of initial assessment (National Comprehensive Cancer Network, 2019a, 2019b, 2019c, 2019d). Febrile neutropenia is also considered and oncologic emergency.

Case Study

Mr. G has severe chemotherapy-induced neutropenia. He is treated with empiric antibiotics. He recovers from his unfortunate situation and completes his induction therapy, receives a transplant, and begins maintenance therapy with Revlimid and dexamethasone. He has been compliant with follow-up visits and transplant vaccines.

Survivorship

It is essential for all involved in the care of multiple myeloma patients, as for patients diagnosed with cancer, to understand that cancer is a chronic disease. One becomes a survivor the day they are diagnosed with cancer. Unfortunately, many cancers are not curable and treatment in this case is referred to as *palliative* or *control of disease*. The disease will be treated, go into remission, and then relapse. The cycle continues, but with each relapse, the remission time decreases. This leads to many issues that are not oncologic, such as depression, anxiety, and financial and social issues.

Key Points

Many side effects can have long-lasting effects which can alter quality of life. These include neuropathy, which may cause physical or sensory deficits and pain, increased risk for new malignancies, fertility issues, hypocalcemia, and osteonecrosis of the jaw.

LIVER DISEASE

Case Study 2

Mr. C is a 59-year-old male with a past medical history of diabetes, HTN, hyperlipidemia, colon cancer s/p colectomy in 2010, and alcohol dependence. He presents to the ED with DOE and progressive fatigue. He has not seen a physician in more than 5 years and has not been taking medications for diabetes, HTN or hyperlipidemia because of social issues. He has not had colon cancer follow-up. He has never used tobacco products. He drinks 3–4 glasses of liquor a day for more than 40 years. He denies illicit drug use. He is unemployed without insurance and divorced. He lives in a motel.

His father was diagnosed with breast cancer at age 56, rectal cancer at age 57, and renal cell carcinoma at age 88 and had a history of ETOH abuse. His mother has a history of Alzheimer disease, HTN, and hyperlipidemia. One sister was diagnosed with uterine cancer at age 49, and another sister was diagnosed with melanoma at age 65. Two paternal aunts have a history with breast cancer, one diagnosed at age 45 and the other at age 68. A paternal uncle was diagnosed with brain cancer at age 54.

Mr. C reports DOE and fatigue and lower extremity edema for the past few weeks. He denies chest pain, lightheadedness, palpations, melena, hematochezia, fever, night sweats, and cough. He has had no weight loss but has had increased abdominal discomfort and girth.

His physical examination reveals the following: height, 66 inches; weight, 210 lbs; B/P, 194/90; pulse, 102; respirations, 20; temp, 98.4 °F; HEENT: normocephalic, PEERLA, sclera is icteric; lymph: no cervical, supraclavicular, axillary, or inguinal adenopathy; coronary: S1, S2 with no murmurs or gallops; lungs: clear throughout; abdomen: distended, nontender with positive bowel sound; positive fluid wave and hepatomegaly, 4 fingerbreadths (FB) and splenomegaly 6 FB; neuro: alert and oriented × 4, equal and normal strength of upper and lower extremities, CN II–XII intact; skin: jaundice without petechiae or purpura.

His initial workup in the ED included CBC, chemistry profile, liver function test, CXR, and CT of the abdominal/pelvis. Results were as follows: WBC: 2.1 (**low**), Hgb: 5.9 (**low**), Hct 22.6 (**low**), Plts: 84,000 (**low**), BUN: 13; Cr: 0.9; T. Bili: 2.1 (**high**), Alk Phos: 72, ALT: 14, AST: 29. The CXR revealed no acute pulmonary pathology. His CT abdomen/pelvis revealed increased echogenicity of the liver with coarse nodular echotexture. The appearance is suggestive of hepatic cirrhosis. He also has moderate perihepatic ascites and splenomegaly.

Based on Mr. C's history and physical examination, you make the following working list of problems:

1. Pancytopenia
2. Uncontrolled HTN
3. Uncontrolled diabetes
4. Alcoholic cirrhosis
5. History of colon cancer

We will address the hematologic and oncologic issues here.

Problem #1: Pancytopenia

Pancytopenia is defined as a decrease in all peripheral blood cell lines. It can be caused by one source or multiple sources (Berliner, 2019). It is important that we refresh our knowledge of hematopoiesis to understand the possible sources of the problem.

Hematopoiesis

Hematopoiesis occurs in the bone marrow (Figure 7.1). The stem cell is the precursor cell. It is undifferentiated, which means that it does not have a specific function. It will differentiate into either a myeloid cell or lymphoid cell. Most disorders of the blood are either an excess or limitation in cell lines. Once the cells mature, they move into circulation and to the spleen. There is a careful balance and response of the bone marrow due to the needs of the body (Berliner, 2019). Thus, pancytopenia could be multiple problems that affect one or many cell lines or one problem that affects all cell lines. Table 7.3 outlines potential causes of pancytopenia.

CLINICAL PEARLS

- It is important to ascertain if the decrease of one or more cell lines is acute or chronic. If possible, obtain previous labs from months or a year ago.
- Assess for symptoms that may accompany pancytopenia, including frequent infections, shortness of breath, fatigue, and bleeding.
- Inquire about medications, both over the counter and prescription. Also ask about any treatments. The patient may forget to mention previous chemotherapy or treatment for various ailments such as eczema or psoriasis.

Diagnostics

Evaluation of pancytopenia should include the following: CBC with differential, reticulocyte count, folate, B_{12}, ferritin, iron, peripheral blood smear, prothrombin time (PT), partial thromboplastin time (PTT), fibrinogen, d-dimer, chemistry profile, liver function test, hepatic serology, HIV, LDH, and stool for occult blood (Berliner, 2019; Lipton, 2020). A hematologist referral may be required if the patient has unexplained pancytopenia, is unstable and symptomatic, or has blasts noted in peripheral smear.

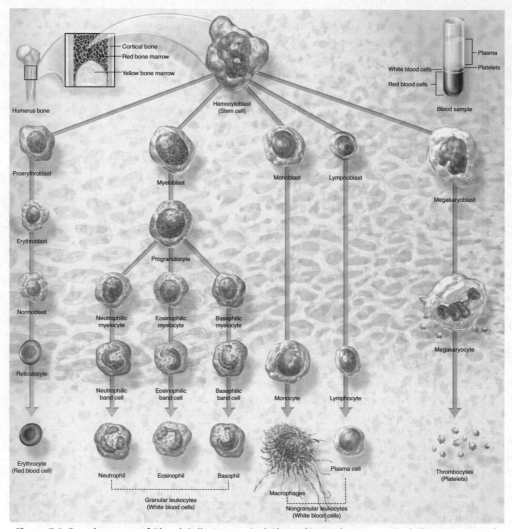

Figure 7.1 Development of Blood Cells Anatomical Chart. (From the Anatomical Chart Company.)

TABLE 7.3 CAUSES OF PANCYTOPENIA

PANCYTOPENIA SIGNS	POSSIBLE CAUSES
Decreased production of blood cells	B_{12} deficiency Folate deficiency Aplastic anemia Infectious disease (e.g., HIV, viral hepatitis) Medications
Bone marrow infiltration or replacement	Leukemia Lymphoma Myeloma Metastatic cancer Myelofibrosis
Increased destruction/sequestration	Disseminated intravascular coagulation Thrombotic thrombocytopenia purpura Myelodysplasia syndrome Hypersplenism (e.g., liver cirrhosis, autoimmune disease)

Adapted from Berliner, N. (2019). Approach to the adult with pancytopenia. In P. Newburger, & A. G. Rosmarin (Eds.), *UpToDate.*

Treatment

Treatment of pancytopenia is dependent on the cause. Treat the underlying issue, such as by discontinuing a medication that causes it, and it will improve. However, pancytopenia cannot improve if it is due to a chronic condition.

Case Study

Mr. C's results are as follows: reticulocyte count: 2.9 (**high**), reticulocyte absolute: 104.1 (**high**), ferritin: 6 (**low**), iron: 14 (**low**), Unsaturated iron binding capacity (UBIC): 366 (**high**), Total iron binding capacity (TIBC): 380, iron sat: 4 (**low**), vitamin B_{12}: 100 (**low**), folate: 1.2 (**low**), PT: 1.9 (**high**), PTT: 36 (**high**), LDH: 212, HIV and hepatic panel: negative; fibrinogen, d-dimer, uric acid, and calcium: normal, stool for occult blood: negative. His peripheral smear was normocytic, with microcytes, polychromasia, hypochromia, and ovalocytes present, with occasional macrocytes, target cells, and tear drop cells.

Mr. C has a decompensated liver disease, hypersplenism, and iron, folate, and B_{12} deficiency. Chronic alcohol abuse causes liver cirrhosis and leads to hypersplenism and iron, folate, and B_{12} deficiency.

Mr. C was treated for his vitamin deficiencies with folic acid 1 mg daily; B_{12} 1,000 μg injection weekly × 4 weeks, and then monthly; and iron infusions. The patient was severely anemic. Blood transfusion of three units of packed cells was prescribed. (Refer to case #1 for indications.) Should he receive platelets?

Transfusion Recommendations

For hospitalized adult patients, the recommendations from the AABB for platelets are as follows:

1. Prophylactic transfusion for platelet counts less than 10,000 (strong evidence)
2. Prophylactic transfusion for patients receiving central venous access placement if platelet count is less than 20,000 (weak evidence)
3. Prophylactic transfusion for lumbar puncture with platelet counts less than 50,000 (weak evidence)
4. Prophylactic transfusion for patients having major elective nonneurological surgery with platelet count less than 50,000 (weak evidence)
5. Recommends against routine prophylactic platelet transfusion for patients who are non-thrombocytopenic and have cardiac surgery with cardiopulmonary bypass (Kaufman et al., 2015)

Transfusion of fresh frozen plasma (FFP) is intended to correct deficiencies of clotting factors. Indications according to Liumbuno et al. (2015) are the following:

1. Ongoing bleeding with liver disease (Grade 1C recommendation)
2. Prevention of bleeding in the event of surgery or invasive procedure, in patients with liver disease (Grade 2C recommendation)
3. Patients being treated with vitamin K antagonist, in the presence of major hemorrhage or intracranial bleeding or in preparation of surgery that cannot be postponed (Grade 1C recommendation)

4. Patients with acute disseminated intravascular coagulation (DIC) and active bleeding in association with the correction of the underlying cause (Recommendation 1C)
5. Correction of microvascular bleeding in patients undergoing massive transfusion. If the PT and aPTT cannot be obtained within a reasonable period, FFP can be transfused in any case to attempt to stop the bleeding (Recommendation 1C)
6. Deficiencies of single clotting factors, in the absence of specific concentrate, in the presence of active bleeding, or in order to prevent bleeding in the case of surgery or invasive procedures (Recommendation 1C)
7. Apheretic treatment of thrombotic microangiopathies (thrombotic thrombocytopenia purpura, hemolytic uremic syndrome, hemolytic anemia with elevated liver enzymes and low platelets [HELLP] syndrome) as replacement of fluids (Grade 1A recommendation)
8. Reconstitution of whole blood for exchange transfusion (Grade 2C recommendation)
9. Hereditary angioedema due to deficiency of the esterase, in the absence of the inactivator of C_1 specific plasma derivative (Grade 2C recommendation)

Case Study

After receiving three units of packed cells, folic acid, B_{12}, and iron infusions, Mr. C's CBC is as follows: WBC: 1.2, Hgb: 8.9, Hct: 28.2, Plts: 88, ANC: 900. He continues to have pancytopenia. Unfortunately, this is a chronic condition due to his liver disease. His blood pressure and diabetes are now controlled with oral agents. He was started on a statin. Mr. C has not followed up with any provider in several years. You obtain a social worker consultation; she arranges for the patient to go to the clinic for primary care and assists with paperwork for insurance and options for more stable housing.

You provide the following discharge instructions for the patient:

- Good hand washing
- Report signs and symptoms of infection to clinic
- Continue folic acid daily
- Alcohol cessation
- Safety concerns, no contact sports
- Follow-up with clinic in 1 week for bloodwork
- Follow-up with gastroenterology for colonoscopy for colon cancer
- Obtain evaluation for potential genetic testing.

Problem #2: Colon Cancer

Cancer genetic testing is an essential component in prevention, early detection, and treatment planning. It is thought that 5%–10% of cancers are caused by a genetic mutation (National Cancer Institute, 2020). The remainder of cancer diagnoses is from either a familial or sporadic cause. The familial component could be due to environmental factors, common foods, or a genetic mutation that has not been identified at this time. Sporadic cancer occurs without a significant family history and is due to carcinogen exposure or unknown reasons. Each mutation carries a specific risk for certain cancers. A mutation does not mean the patient will be diagnosed with cancer or second cancer. It does increase the risk above the normal

---

BOX 7.1 NCCN Guidelines for Genetic Testing for Colon Cancer

- Family history with first- or second-degree relative with a genetic mutation
- Personal history of breast or high-grade prostate (Gleason score >7) cancer and Ashkenazi Jewish ancestry
- Personal or family history of a male with breast cancer at any age
- Personal history of triple-negative breast cancer diagnoses at age 60 years or younger
- Personal or family history of breast cancer diagnosed at age 45 years or younger
- Personal history of ovarian, pancreatic, metastatic breast, or metastatic prostate cancer
- Personal history of bilateral breast cancer
- Two relatives on the same side of the family with breast cancer, one under age 50 years
- Three or more of the following cancers on the same side of the family: breast, prostate, pancreatic, ovarian
- Family history of ovarian cancer
- Personal history of colon or uterine cancer before age 65 years
- Two relatives on the same side of the family with colon or uterine cancer, one diagnosed under age 50 years
- Three or more of the following cancers on the same side of the family: colon, uterine, ovarian, stomach, small bowel, kidney/urinary tract, pancreatic, or brain
- Ten or more cumulative polyps in the patient or a family member

Data from National Comprehensive Cancer Network. (2019). *NCCN clinical practice guideline in oncology for genetic/familial high-risk assessment: Colorectal* and National Comprehensive Cancer Network. (2019). *NCCN clinical practice guideline in oncology for genetic/familial high-risk assessment: Breast and ovarian.*

---

population. It is also important to note that if a person has a genetic mutation, each first-degree relative has a 50% risk of having that mutation and should be tested for that specific deleterious mutation. Once an individual is determined not to have a genetic risk, the next step is to determine a familial risk. There are several risk tools and models the genetic provider uses to determine this. These tools can demonstrate increased risk for family members, necessitating increased screening and hopefully prevention or early detection of a cancer. NCCN Guidelines are constantly updating screening criteria. The genetic counselor/provider will complete a pedigree and determine if the patient is appropriate for testing. It is essential for providers to have a basic awareness of high-risk patients who may need genetic testing. Box 7.1 provides a basic generalization of NCCN Guidelines. It is not an all-inclusive list.

Case Study

As an outpatient, Mr. C saw an oncology nurse practitioner and underwent cancer genetic counseling and testing. His pedigree is shown in Figure 7.2.

Genetic testing returns with a mutation in the *MSH6* gene. This is considered Lynch syndrome.

The *MSH6* gene increases the risk for colon, rectal, uterine, ovarian, stomach, small intestine, hepatobiliary system, renal and ureter, and brain cancers. Some people with *MSH6* mutation also can have skin tumors, including sebaceous adenomas and carcinomas (Win, 2019). Some very important interventions now need to be instituted. NCCN Guidelines dictate the required screening, including screenings listed in Table 7.4.

Mr. C's children and siblings will need to be tested for the specific mutation on the *MSH6* gene. The family has a very strong history of breast cancer. It is possible, but would be extremely rare for his father to have harbored a second mutation. It would be advisable for his sisters to have the full Lynch syndrome panel testing or whole genome sequencing performed and not just single mutation site testing. Referral to a genetic counselor can help the family make decisions on the ideal genetic testing plan and may recommend cascade genetic testing to identify all of the relatives who did or did not inherit the genetic mutation(s) of interest.

Key Points

A genetic counselor can be instrumental in guiding the patient and family through the process of genetic testing and the cascade genetic testing and screening that may follow.

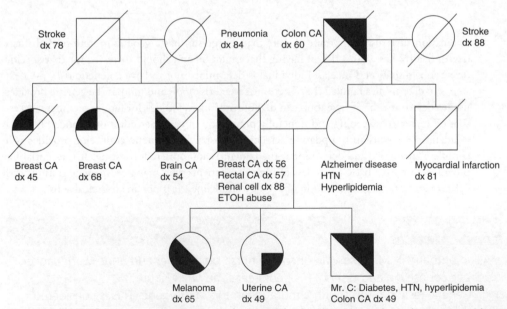

Figure 7.2 Lynch syndrome pedigree. Classic features of a family with Lynch syndrome are evident, including affected family members with colon, endometrial, and breast cancer, a young age at onset in some individuals, and incomplete penetrance (some individuals who carry the pathogenic variant express the associated trait while others do not).

TABLE 7.4 NCCN SCREENINGS REQUIRED FOR PATIENTS WITH SUSPECTED LYNCH SYNDROME

TYPE OF CANCER	SCREENINGS
Colon cancer	Colonoscopy screening every 1–2 years. There are data to suggest aspirin may decrease the risk of colon cancer in Lynch syndrome but the dose has not been established.
Gastric and small bowel cancers	There are no clear data to support surveillance for gastric, duodenal, and distal small bowel cancer. If surveillance is performed, upper endoscopy every 3–5 years.
Urothelial cancer	No clear evidence but surveillance options may include annual urinalysis.
Central nervous system cancer	Consider annual physical/neurological examinations
Pancreatic cancer	No recommendations at this time
Breast cancer	There have been suggestions that there is an increased risk for breast cancer in Lynch syndrome patients; however, there is not enough evidence.
Prostate cancer	There is insufficient evidence to recommend earlier or more frequent prostate screening among men with Lynch syndrome.

Data from Win, A. K. (2019). Lynch syndrome (hereditary nonpolyposis colorectal cancer): Clinical manifestations and diagnosis. In J. T. Lamont, & S. Grover (Eds.), UpToDate.

LUNG DISEASE

Case Study 3

Mr. B is a 76-year-old gentleman with past medical history of HTN and COPD. He presents to the ED with midsternal chest pain with no radiation that started today. He also reports increasing dyspnea and fatigue over the past several weeks.

He has a smoking history of 100 pack years (2 packs a day for a year × 50 years). He quit 8 years ago. He reports social alcohol use and no illicit drug use. His father has a history of CAD. His mother died of lung cancer (smoking history) and his brother of a stroke. He has no family history of thrombosis.

His review of systems reveals midsternal chest pain that started this morning after mowing the lawn on a tractor. There is no radiation of pain or nausea. He reports that he has had slight achiness of the chest for the last few days and noted increasing dyspnea over the last several weeks. He reports increasing fatigue and having a difficult time concentrating. Upon further discussion, he reveals decreased appetite and weight loss of 20 pounds over the last month. He has had no change of bowel or bladder habits and no bruising or bleeding. He also notes swelling in his left lower extremity for the past 2 days that is not painful.

His physical examination reveals the following: height, 72 inches; weight, 162 lbs; B/P, 162/88; pulse, 120; respirations, 32; pulse oximetry, 81% on ambient air; temperature, 97.7 °F; HEENT: normocephalic, PERRLA, oral mucosa intact; lymph: neck and right arm are edematous, 4-cm right supraclavicular lymphadenopathy and no cervical, axillary, or inguinal adenopathy; cor: S1, S2, tachycardic, and irregular; lungs: diminished throughout; abdomen: soft, nontender, no hepatosplenomegaly; extremities: right arm edema with positive pulses, left lower extremity edema with positive Holman sign, and positive pulses; skin: no petechiae or purpura.

Your initial workup revealed the following: CBC–WBC: 4.5, Hgb: 9.6 (**low**), Hct: 30 (**low**), Plts: 150, BUN: 12, Cr: 1.2, Na: 121 (**low**), K: 5.5 (**high**), CL: 92 (**low**), CO_2: 26, d-dimer: 350, CXR: large mediastinal mass, CTA: saddle pulmonary emboli: submassive, large mediastinal mass, supraclavicular adenopathy. The mass is compressing on the superior vena cava.

Based on Mr. C's history and physical examination, you make the following working list of problems:

1. Pulmonary emboli
2. Mediastinal mass
3. Hyponatremia

Problem #1: Pulmonary Emboli

A saddle pulmonary embolus is named for the location of the thrombus. It is located at the bifurcation of the main pulmonary artery, at times extending into the left and right pulmonary artery (Thompson & Kabrhel, 2019). More than 50% of patients with pulmonary emboli are found to have a DVT (Thompson & Kabrhel, 2019). Risk factors include immobility or decreased activity (travel or surgery), medications such as oral contraceptives or hormone replacement, pregnancy, malignancy, and family history (Bauer & Lip, 2019). If the practitioner identifies a family history of thrombus, a hematologist should be consulted for a hypercoagulable workup.

First, we need to review the coagulation cascade to understand the various risk factors and treatments (Figure 7.3).

The coagulation cascade is quite complicated; however, an excellent mnemonic to help remember the various components is shown in Box 7.2 (Shrestha, 2020).

Key Points

- The intrinsic pathway occurs from injury to a blood vessel. The extrinsic pathway is the tissue factor (only two of them to remember: factors III and VII), and then they join to the common pathway.

Factors II, VII, XI, and X require calcium and phospholipid for activation. These are vitamin K–dependent and are affected by warfarin and liver disease (Shrestha, 2020). The NOAC (novel oral anticoagulant) category mechanism of action is a selective inhibitor of

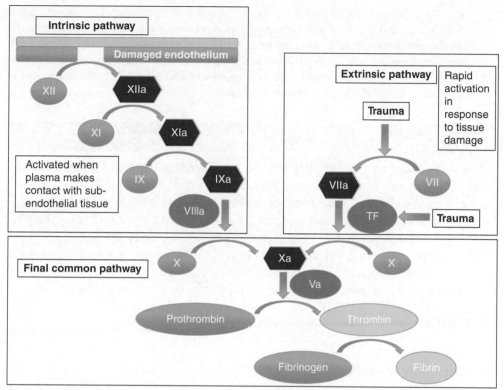

Figure 7.3 Classical clotting cascade. The classical clotting cascade is an in vitro representation; the cell-based model offers a more complete explanation of in vivo coagulation. The classical cascade is included here as it demonstrates which clotting factors are investigated with traditional coagulation tests (prothrombin and activated thromboplastin time). (From Bucklin, B. A., Baysinger, C. L., & Gambling, D. (2016). *A practical approach to obstetric anesthesia*. Wolters Kluwer Health.)

BOX 7.2 Mnemonic for the Components of the Coagulation Cascade

First person told cancer leads sickness, another chap said protein high fat

First	Factor I: Fibrinogen
Person	Factor II: Prothrombin
Told	Factor III: Tissue thromboplastin or tissue factor
Cancer	Factor IV: Calcium
Leads	Factor V: Labile factor, proaccelerin (factor VI no longer in coagulation cascade)
Sickness	Factor VII: Stable factor, proconvertin
Another	Factor VIII: Antihemophilic factor A
Chap	Factor IX: Christmas factor, antihemophilic factor B
Said	Factor X: Stuart power factor, autoprothrombin III
Protein	Factor XI: Plasma thromboplastin antecedent or PTA
High	Factor XII: Hageman factor, glass or contact factor
Fat	Factor XIII: Fibrin stabilizing factor or fibrinase

factor Xa and works by inhibiting free factor Xa and prothrombinase. It does not require a cofactor for activity. Although it has no direct effect on platelet aggregation, it indirectly inhibits platelet aggregation induced by thrombin, and because it inhibits factor Xa, it decreases thrombin generation (Rivaroxaban package insert, 2020). Heparin acts indirectly by binding to antithrombin (AT). AT is converted from a slow to a rapid inactivator of coagulation factors IIa and Xa (Hull et al., 2020).

Case Study

Mr. B was started on a heparin drip with an initial bolus of heparin. He was titrated according to a weight-based nomogram following either PTT or antifactor Xa levels. A duplex doppler was performed on his lower extremities and he was found to have an acute complete thrombosis of the perineal and common femoral veins on the left leg. Approximately 15% of patients with malignancy are diagnosed with thrombosis (Bauer & Lip, 2020). Patients with malignancies have an increased risk for thrombosis due to procoagulation activity that can promote clot formation. In addition, many patients have additional risk factors such as immobility, obesity, or surgery (Bauer & Lip, 2020).

Problem #2: Mediastinal Mass

The differential for a mediastinal mass is malignancy until proven otherwise.

Multiple types of malignancies can develop mediastinal masses, but the most common are aggressive lymphomas and lung cancers. The only way to diagnosis cancer is by biopsy. In addition to the biopsy, staging scans are ordered including a CT scan of the abdomen and pelvis and an MRI of the brain. These scans determine the metastasis of the cancer from the primary site. Staging in all types of cancer is graded from 1 to 4, with 4 being the most extensive spread of the disease.

Case Study

A biopsy of Mr. B's mass demonstrated small cell lung cancer. Staging studies demonstrate a large mediastinal mass, mass compressing superior vena cava (SVC), and supraclavicular adenopathy metastasis in the liver, and bilateral adrenal glands. There was no brain metastasis. Small cell lung cancer is an extremely aggressive disease with rapid doubling time, high growth fraction, and widespread metastasis. It is highly responsive to chemotherapy and radiotherapy but unfortunately relapses quickly (Gibson, Byers, and Gay, 2020). Small cell lung cancer can be staged in the typical I to IV staging system however at times it can be classified as limited or extensive stage. In the limited stage, the tumor is confined to the ipsilateral hemithorax and regional lymph nodes, which could be included in a single radiotherapy port. Extensive stage disease extends beyond the boundaries of limited disease (Glisson et al., 2020). This patient has stage IV or extensive stage disease.

Treatment

There are several treatment modalities for extensive stage small cell lung cancer including radiation therapy, chemotherapy, and immunotherapy. Care is directed according to NCCN Guidelines. The oncologist chooses first-line treatment with carboplatin, etoposide, and atezolizumab (Kelly, 2020; National Comprehensive Cancer Network, 2019d). Chemotherapy works by killing rapidly dividing cells during the process of cell division. Common side effects of chemotherapy include fatigue, myelosuppression with risk of infection, anemia, thrombocytopenia, nausea/vomiting, constipation, diarrhea, reduced kidney and liver function, hair loss, and neuropathy. Immunotherapy functions by enhancing the patient's own immune system to fight cancer. Side effects of immunotherapy include fatigue, peripheral edema, fever, diarrhea, nausea/vomiting, constipation, abdominal pain, decreased appetite, and infection. Unique side effects of immunotherapy include immune-mediated side effects such as pneumonitis, colitis, hepatitis, nephritis, and various endocrinopathies including hypothyroid or hyperthyroidism and diabetes (Tecentriq package insert, 2020).

Key Points

Some side effects of treatment can be long term and can interfere with the patient's quality of life. Some examples of these long-term effects include neuropathy and endocrine disorders such as hypothyroidism that can persist for the patient's lifetime.

Superior Vena Cava Syndrome

Superior vena cava syndrome (SVCS) is an oncologic emergency. SVCS results from an obstruction of blood through the superior vena cava by direct invasion or external compression (Drews & Rabkin, 2020). Presenting symptoms include facial, neck, and arm swelling. Dyspnea, stridor, cough, hoarseness, and dysphagia also can be symptoms.

Key Points

Assess the patient with an intrathoracic malignancy routinely for signs and symptoms of superior vena cava syndrome.

Treatment of SVCS is tumor directed, either chemotherapy or radiation therapy. In addition, endovenous recanalization with stent placement may be necessary. Radiation therapy can be delivered in a variety of ways. External beam radiation delivered by a linear accelerator is the most common method. Treatment planning occurs through a process of simulation, where CT scans and/or MRI is used to pinpoint the tumor and place "tattoo" marks on the skin. Side effects of radiation are dependent on the area radiated. Tissue swelling and irritation is the most common side effect. Other side effects include fatigue and skin irritation. In the case of small cell lung cancer, the heart may be in the radiation field, which could lead to cardiac toxicity. The lung is also in the radiation field, which can lead to a long-term side effect of radiation fibrosis (Mitin, 2020).

Problem #3: Hyponatremia

Hyponatremia can occur from an excess of water intake and impaired water excretion. One must determine the degree of hyponatremia and whether it is acute or chronic. Hyponatremia is considered severe when the serum sodium concentration is <120; it is considered moderate when the serum sodium concentration is 120–129, and it is considered mild when the serum sodium concentration is 130–134. Symptoms can include headache, fatigue, nausea, confusion, and muscle cramps and can progress to seizures, brain herniation, and death (Mitin, 2020). Syndrome of inappropriate antidiuretic hormone secretion (SIADH) is a disorder of impaired water secretion caused by inability to suppress the secretion on antidiuretic hormone, thereby causing reduced urinary output. If water intake exceeds the reduced urine output, the ensuing water retention leads to the development of hyponatremia. In SIADH, the serum sodium and the serum osmolality are low. The urine osmolality is above 100 mOsm/kg and urine sodium is usually above 40 mEq/L (Sterns, 2020a, 2020b).

Causative factors for hyponatremia could include malignancy, CNS disturbances such as stroke and hemorrhage, medications, HIV infection, surgery, pulmonary disease, hormone administration, and hormone deficiency such as hypopituitarism and hypothyroidism (Sterns, 2020a, 2020b).

Treatment of SIADH starts with managing the underlying disease such as by treating an infection or stopping an offending drug. Fluid restriction is the center of therapy with the goal of less than 800 ml/day. In severe symptomatic cases, intravenous hypertonic saline should be administered. Other interventions include salt tablets and vasopressin receptor antagonists (Sterns, 2019).

Case Study

On the second treatment day of radiation therapy, Mr. B developed an acute episode of tachycardia and hypotension. On further examination, you find that he has pulsus paradox, a significant decrease in systolic blood pressure on inspiration. On physical examination, you hear a pericardial rub. An ECG is performed and shows tachycardia. An echocardiogram demonstrates a large pericardial effusion (Hoit, 2020). Unfortunately, the patient has cardiac tamponade. This is an oncologic emergency.

You treat him by decreasing the pericardial fluid by percutaneous or surgical drainage. A pericardiocentesis or pericardiectomy (or pericardial window) can be performed; you treat him with a pericardiectomy. The advantage of the pericardiectomy in a pericardial biopsy can be performed and there is no concern for fluid reaccumulation (Hoit, 2020).

After the pericardial window, his heart rate returns to normal. The patient received the remainder of his radiation therapy and is preparing for his first dose of chemotherapy and immunotherapy. He was given allopurinol for prophylaxis of tumor lysis syndrome (TLS).

Tumor Lysis Syndrome

TLS is massive release of the waste products of the lysis of tumor cells along with uric acid and phosphate. This can lead to AKI. TLS occurs most frequently after initiation of cytotoxic therapy in patients with aggressive cancers with a high mitotic rate, such as highly aggressive lymphoma, T-cell acute lymphoblastic leukemia, and aggressive tumors with large tumor burden and high proliferative rate (Larson & Pui, 2020).

Case Study

After receiving cycle one of carboplatin, etoposide, and atezolizumab with aggressive hydration, Mr. B's uric acid is monitored closely. Unfortunately, on day 3, his uric acid is 8.9, his phosphorus is 6.0, his potassium is 7.0, his BUN is 37, and his Cr is 8.8. You give him hydration with normal saline at an increased rate of 150 ml/hr. One of the most dangerous issues with TLS is hyperkalemia and sudden death due to cardiac arrhythmias (Larson & Pui, 2020). You also order rasburicase, which can be given as a prophylactic medication for intermittent to high-risk patients or to assist in management of TLS. Rasburicase works differently than allopurinol by decreasing existing and newly created uric acid (Elitek package insert, 2020). The patient recovered from tumor lysis and completes four cycles of carboplatin, etoposide, and atezolizumab. His treatment will continue with maintenance atezolizumab until he has progression of the disease or unacceptable toxicity, such as myocarditis, pericarditis, arrhythmias, adrenal insufficiency, diarrhea or colitis, myositis, uveitis, or pneumonitis, which is not responsive to treatment.

CONCLUSION

The previous case studies are just a sample of possible scenarios one could encounter in the acute setting. Hematology and oncology are rapidly progressing fields. Estimates of new cancer cases and deaths in the United States for 2019 suggest an ongoing small decline in cancer mortality for both men and women and a 2% decline in annual incidence in men since 2006 and stable incidence in woman. Since 1991, the overall cancer death rate in the United States has dropped by 27% (Siegel et al., 2019). It is essential that practitioners keep themselves updated with the literature and use resources from specialty providers.

REVIEW QUESTIONS

1. Which of the following is a common cause of macrocytic anemia?
    a. Lead poisoning
    b. Acute blood loss
    c. Iron deficiency
    d. Alcoholism

2. Which of the following is a cause of pancytopenia involving bone marrow infiltration?
   a. Aplastic anemia
   b. Myelodysplasia syndrome
   c. Lymphoma
   d. Thrombotic thrombocytopenia purpura

3. TLS can lead to which of the following?
   a. Spinal cord compression
   b. AKI
   c. SVCS
   d. Microcytic anemia

Answers: 1, d; 2, c; 3, b

REFERENCES

Bauer, K. A., & Lip, G. Y. H. (2019). Evaluating adult patients with established venous thromboembolism for acquired and inherited risk factors. In L. L. K. Leung, J Mandel, & G Finlay (Eds.), *UpToDate*. Retrieved May 2, 2020. https://www.uptodate.com/contents/evaluating-adult-patients-with-established-venous-thromboembolism-for-acquired-and-inherited-risk-factors? Uptodate.com

Bauer, K. A., & Lip, G. Y. H. (2020). Overview of the causes of venous thrombosis. In L. L. K. Leung, J. Mandel, & G. Finlay (Eds.), *UpToDate*. Retrieved May 2, 2020. https://www.uptodate.com/contents/overview-of-the-causes-of-venous-thrombosis? Uptodate.com

Berliner, N. (2019). Approach to the adult with pancytopenia. In P. Newburger, & A. G. Rosmarin (Eds.), *UpToDate*. Retrieved May 2, 2020. https://www.uptodate.com/contents/approach-to-the-adult-with-pancytopenia? Uptodate.com

Carson, J. L., & Kleinman, S. (2019). Indications and hemoglobin thresholds for red blood cell transfusion in the adult. In A. J. Silverglied, & J. S. Timauer (Eds.), *UpToDate*. Retrieved May 2, 2020. https://www.uptodate.com/contents/indications-and-hemoglobin-thresholds-for-red-blood-cell-transfusion-in-the-adult.Uptodate.com

Carson, J. L., Guyatt, G., Heddle, N. M., Grossman, B. J., Cohn, C. S., Fung, M. K., Gernsheimer, T., Holcomb, J. B., Kaplan, L. J., Katz, L. M., Peterson, N., Ramsey, G., Rao, S. V., Roback, J. D., Shander, A., & Tobian, A. A. R. (2016). Clinical practice guidelines from the AABB. *The Journal of the American Medical Association*, 316(19), 2025. https://doi.org/10.1001/jama.2016.9185

Center for Drug Evaluation and Research. (2020). *Accelerated approval program, approach to the adult with anemia*. Retrieved May 2, 2020. https://www.fda.gov/drugs/information-healthcare-professionals-drugs/accelerated-approval-program

Drews, R. E., & Rabkin, D. J. (2020). Malignancy-related superior vena cava syndrome. In E Bruera, J. F. Eidt, J. L. Mills, & N. L. Muller (Eds.), *UpToDate*. Retrieved May 2, 2020. https://www.uptodate.com/contents/malignancy-related-superior-vena-cava-syndrome Uptodate.com

Elitek (rasburicase) [package insert] (2020). Sanofi-aventis U.S. LLC. Retrieved May 2, 2020. http://products.sanofi.us/elitek/Elitek.html

Fatehi, P., & Hsu, C. Y. (2019). Evaluation of acute kidney injury among hospitalized adult patients. In P. M. Palevsky, & J. P. Forman (Eds.), *UpToDate*. Retrieved May 2, 2020. https://www.uptodate.com/contents/evaluation-of-acute-kidney-injury-among-hospitalized-adult-patients. Uptodate.com.

Federal Drug Administration (FDA). (2019). *FDA approved drugs*. Retrieved May 2, 2020. https://www.centerwatch.com/directories/1067-fda-approved-drugs

Glisson, B. S., Byers, L. A., & Gay, C. M. (2020). Pathobiology and staging of small cell carcinoma of the lung. In R. C. Lilenbaum, A. Nicholson, & S. R. Vora (Eds.), *UpToDate*. Retrieved May 2, 2020. https://www.uptodate.com/contents/pathobiology-and-staging-of-small-cell-carcinoma-of-the-lung? Uptodate.com

GlobalRxPh. (2017). Corrected Calcium for serum albumin conc. GlobalRxPh.com. Retrieved May 2, 2020. https://globalrph.com/medcalcs/corrected-calcium-calculator-correction-for-serum-albumin-conc/

Hoit, B. D. (2020). Cardiac tamponade. In B. J. Gersh, J. Hoekstra, & B. C. Downey (Eds.), *UpToDate*. Retrieved May 2, 2020. https://www.uptodate.com/contents/cardiac-tamponade? Uptodate.com

Hull, R. D., Garcia, D. A., & Burnett, A. E. (2020). Heparin and LMW heparin: Dosing and adverse effects. In L. L. K. Leung, & J. S. Timauer (Eds.), *UpToDate*. Retrieved May 2, 2020. https://www.uptodate.com/contents/heparin-and-lmw-heparin-dosing-and-adverse-effects? Uptodate.com

Kaufman, R. M., Djulbegovic, B., Gernsheimer, T., Kleinman, S., Tinmouth, A. T., Capocelli, K. E., Cipolle, M. D., Cohn, C. S., Fung, M. K., Grossman, B. J., Mintz, P., Kleinman, S., Tinmouth, A. T., Capocelli, K. E., Cipolle, M. D., Cohn, C. S., Fung, M. K., Grossman, B. J., Mintz, P. D., …Tobian, A. A. R. (2015). Platelet transfusion: A clinical practice guideline from the AABB. *Annals of Internal Medicine*, 162(3), 205. https://doi.org/10.7326/m14-1589

Kelly, K. (2020). Extensive-stage small cell lung cancer: Initial management. In R. C. Lilenbaum, S. E. Schild, & S. R. Vora (Eds.), *UpToDate*. Retrieved May 2, 2020. https://www.uptodate.com/contents/extensive-stage-small-cell-lung-cancer-initial-management? Uptodate.com

Kleinman, S. (2019). Patient education: Blood donation and transfusion. Beyond the basics. In A. J. Silverglied, & J. S. Timauer (Eds.), *UpToDate*. Retrieved May 2, 2020. https://www.uptodate.com/contents/blood-donation-and-transfusion-beyond-the-basics. Uptodate.com

Larson, R. A., & Pui, C. H. (2020). Tumor lysis syndrome: Prevention and treatment. In R. E. Drews, A. S. Freedman, D. G. Poplack, & D. M. F. Saverese (Eds.). *UpToDate*. Retrieved May 2, 2020. https://www.uptodate.com/contents/tumor-lysis-syndrome-prevention-and-treatment? Uptodate.com

Laubach, J. P. (2019). Multiple myeloma: Clinical features, laboratory manifestations and diagnosis. In R. A. Kyle, S. V. Rajkumar, & R. F. Connor (Eds.), *UpToDate*. Retrieved May 2, 2020. https://www.uptodate.com/contents/multiple-myeloma-clinical-features-laboratory-manifestations-and-diagnosis? Uptodate.com

Leung, L. L. K. (2019). Approach to the adult with anemia. In W. C. Mentzer, J. S. Tirnauer, & L. Kunins (Eds.), *UpToDate*. Retrieved May 2, 2020. https://www.uptodate.com/contents/approach-to-the-adult-with-anemia. Uptodate.com

Lewis, J. L. (2020). *Hypercalcemia - Endocrine and metabolic disorders*. In *Merch manual*. Retrieved May 2, 2020. https://www.merckmanuals.com/professional/endocrine-and-metabolic-disorders/electrolyte-disorders/hypercalcemia

Lipton, J. M. (2020). *Evaluation of pancytopenia*. Epocrates. Retrieved May 2, 2020. https://online.epocrates.com/diseases/1024/Evaluation-of-pancytopenia

Liumbuno, G., Bennardello, F., Lattanzio, A., Piccoli, P., Rossetti, G., & Italian Society of Transfusion Medicine and Immunohaematology (SIMTI) Work Group. (2015). Recommendations for the transfusion of plasma and platelets. *Blood Transfusion*, 162(3), 132–150.

Mitin, T. (2020). Radiation therapy techniques in cancer treatment. In J. S. Loeffler, & S. R. Vora (Eds.), *UpToDate*. Retrieved May 2, 2020. https://www.uptodate.com/contents/radiation-therapy-techniques-in-cancer-treatment? Uptodate.com

National Cancer Institute. (2020). *Genetic testing fact sheet*. National Cancer Institute. Retrieved May 2, 2020. https://www.cancer.gov/about-cancer/causes-prevention/genetics/genetic-testing-fact-sheet

National Cancer Institute *Dictionary of cancer terms*. (2020). National Cancer Institute. cancer.gov. Retrieved May 2, 2020. https://www.cancer.gov/publications/dictionaries/cancer-terms/def/lytic-lesion

National Comprehensive Cancer Network. (2019a). *NCCN clinical practice guideline in oncology for genetic/familial high-risk assessment: Breast and ovarian*.

National Comprehensive Cancer Network. (2019b). *NCCN clinical practice guideline in oncology for genetic/familial high-risk assessment: Colorectal*.

National Comprehensive Cancer Network. (2019c). *NCCN clinical practice guidelines in oncology multiple myeloma*.

National Comprehensive Cancer Network. (2019d). *NCCN guidelines cell lung cancer*.

Xarelto (rivaroxaban) [package insert] (2020). Janssen Pharmaceuticals. Retrieved May 2, 2020. https://www.xareltohcp.com

Roodman, G. D. (2019). Mechanisms of bone metastasis. In R. E. Drews, D. M. F. Saverese (Eds.), *UpToDate*. Retrieved May 2, 2020. https://www.uptodate.com/contents/mechanisms-of-bone-metastases? Uptodate.com

Shane, E. (2020). Diagnostic approach to hypercalcemia. In C. J. Rosen, J. E. Mulder (Eds.), *UpToDate*.

Shrestha, S. K. (2020). *Simple coagulation cascade with mnemonics*. Epomedicine. Retrieved May 2, 2020. https://epomedicine.com/?s=simple+coagulation+cascade

Siegel, R. L., Miller, K. D., Jemal, A. (2019). Cancer statistics, 2019. *CA: Cancer Journal for Clinicians*, 69(1), 7–34.

Sterns, R. H. (2019). Treatment of Hyponatremia: Syndrome of inappropriate antidiuretic hormone secretion (SIADH) and reset osmostat. In M. Emmett, J. P. Forman (Eds.), *UpToDate*. Retrieved May 2, 2020. https://www.uptodate.com/contents/treatment-of-hyponatremia-syndrome-of-inappropriate-antidiuretic-hormone-secretion-siadh-and-reset-osmostat? Uptodate.com

Sterns, R. H. (2020a). Overview of hyponatremia in adults. In M. Emmett, Forman J. P. (Eds.), *UpToDate*. Retrieved May 2, 2020. https://www.uptodate.com/contents/overview-of-the-treatment-of-hyponatremia-in-adults? Uptodate.com

Sterns, R. H. (2020b) Pathophysiology and etiology of the syndrome of inappropriate antidiuretic hormone secretion (SIADH). In M Emmett, J. P. Forman (Eds.), *UpToDate*. Retrieved May 2, 2020. https://www.uptodate.com/contents/pathophysiology-and-etiology-of-the-syndrome-of-inappropriate-antidiuretic-hormone-secretion-siadh? Uptodate.com

Tecentriq (Atezolizumab) [package insert] (2020). Genentech. Retrieved May 2, 2020. https://www.gene.com/download/pdf/tecentriq_prescribing.pdf

Thompson, B. T., & Kabrhel, C. (2019). Overview of acute pulmonary embolism in adults. In J. Mandel, & G. Finlay (Eds.), *UpToDate*. Retrieved May 2, 2020. https://www.uptodate.com/contents/overview-of-acute-pulmonary-embolism-in-adults? Uptodate.com

Waltham, M. A. (2020). *UpToDate*. Retrieved May 2, 2020. https://www.uptodate.com/contents/diagnostic-approach-to-hypercalcemia. Uptodate.com

Win, A. K. (2019). Lynch syndrome (hereditary nonpolyposis colorectal cancer): Clinical manifestations and diagnosis. In J. T. Lamont, & S. Grover (Eds.), *UpToDate*. Retrieved May 2, 2020. https://www.uptodate.com/contents/lynch-syndrome-hereditary-nonpolyposis-colorectal-cancer-clinical-manifestations-and-diagnosis. Uptodate.com

Wingard, J. R. (2019). Treatment of neutropenic fever syndromes in adults with hematologic malignancies and hematopoietic cell transplant recipients. In E. Bow, & S. Bond (Eds.), *UpToDate*. https://www.uptodate.com/contents/treatment-of-neutropenic-fever-syndromes-in-adults-with-hematologic-malignancies-and-hematopoietic-cell-transplant-recipients-high-risk-patients? Uptodate.com

Xgeva (denosumab) [package insert] (2019). Amgen. Retrieved May 2, 2020. https://www.pi.amgen.com/~/media/amgen/repositorysites/pi-amgen-com/xgeva/xgeva_pi.pdf

8 Management of Endocrine Emergencies

Cheryl Wainwright Anderson

INTRODUCTION

This chapter will focus on medical emergencies associated with endocrine disorders: diabetic ketoacidosis (DKA), hyperosmolar hyperglycemic state (HHS), thyroid storm, and myxedema. As they represent some of the most serious endocrine complications, prompt identification of precipitating factors is critical and immediate treatment is essential.

Recall the questions to consider as you review each case study:

1. What is the likely diagnosis?
2. What are the precipitating factors?
3. What symptoms led you to the diagnosis?
4. What physical findings suggest the diagnosis?
5. What laboratory results support the diagnosis?
6. What additional laboratory tests would you order?
7. How would you treat this patient?
8. What are the possible differential diagnoses?

DIABETIC KETOACIDOSIS

Case Study

Ms. G is a 28-year-old female with history type 1 diabetes for 15 years. She has no other medical history. She uses an insulin pump and checks blood glucose four to seven times a day: before meals, 2 hr after meals, and at bedtime. Her most recent A1C was 6.8% and blood glucose had ranged from 65 to 235 mg/dl. She works full time as an administrative assistant and is pursuing a master's degree part time. She exercises 5 days a week at the gym. She eats three well-balanced meals a day and counts carbohydrates.

Due to increased stress at work and school, her normal routine was disrupted. She was working overtime to fill in for a colleague out on medical leave. As the semester was about to end, she was busy writing papers and studying for finals. She also had to travel out of state to attend a wedding as she was in the wedding party. She left for the wedding as soon as finals were over. As a result of these events, she had stopped exercising and regularly was skipping meals.

While away at the wedding, Ms. G realized that she had not packed enough insulin for her pump. She had to take a reduced amount until she could return home. She had also forgotten to bring her glucose meter and therefore was unable to check blood glucose. She indulged in food and drank more wine than usual. She was sleep deprived for several days. As she was preparing to return home, she began to experience symptoms of a UTI.

Upon returning home, Ms. G began to experience weakness, nausea, vomiting, and severe abdominal discomfort. As her symptoms persisted for more than 24 hr, she presented to the emergency room. You are the APRN assigned to her. Review of systems revealed polyuria, urinary frequency, burning upon urination, blurred vision, headache, and fatigue.

Upon physical examination, she was found to have the following: temperature 99.2°F, pulse 110 bpm, respiratory rate 30 breaths per minute, and blood pressure 90/50 mm Hg. Cardiovascular examination: fast regular rate, normal S_1 and S_2, and no murmurs, rubs, or gallops. Abdomen is guarded with decreased bowel sounds. Extremities: no edema, 2+ pedal pulses bilaterally, and no clubbing or cyanosis. Respiratory examination: labored breathing, clear lung sounds bilaterally, and fruity odor of the breath. Skin and mucous membranes are dry; skin turgor is poor. Neurological: lethargy noted.

You order a CBC with differential, complete metabolic panel, and blood and urine cultures. You also order a glucose point of care testing; result is 350 mg/dl. Based on this and her symptoms, you implement treatment before you receive laboratory results.

WBC count, Hgb, and Hct are elevated; glucose is greater than 250 mg/dl; sodium is mildly decreased, potassium is slightly elevated, serum bicarbonate is decreased, serum phosphate is normal, and BUN and creatinine are mildly increased.

You order ABG, Hgb A1C, serum osmolality, and urine for ketones. Arterial pH is less than 7, Hgb A1C is 12%, serum osmolality is greater than 320, and urine tested positive for moderate ketones. Results of blood and urine cultures are pending.

Overview of DKA

DKA and HHS are the most serious complications of diabetes requiring immediate intervention. Pathology, precipitating events, clinical presentation, diagnostic evaluation, differential diagnosis, and treatment will be reviewed. Although there are many similarities between DKA and HHS, there are significant differences. Hyperglycemia and ketonemia are indications of DKA, with metabolic acidosis being the major finding. HHS is characterized by more profound hyperglycemia and elevated plasma osmolality, but little or no ketoacidosis. Treatment for both states is similar.

DKA is a potentially life-threatening complication of diabetes. Onset of symptoms is usually rapid. It occurs more frequently with type 1 diabetes but can also develop with type 2 diabetes during periods of acute stress or illness. It may be the presenting symptom in individuals without a previous diagnosis of diabetes. It evolves rapidly because of fat breakdown, usually within 24 hr, and is diagnosed more often in younger patients (Kitabchi et al., 2009).

Pathology

Two major factors are responsible for the development of DKA: insulin deficiency and excess glucagon (Unger & Orci, 1981). Absolute insulin deficiency with little or no insulin production is characteristic of type 1 diabetes. Impaired glucose transport into peripheral tissue results in increasing hyperglycemia because of increased glycogenolysis (breakdown of glycogen to glucose) and gluconeogenesis (formation of glucose from amino acids and glycerol). Glucagon, a hormone secreted by the alpha cells of the pancreas, is normally suppressed by insulin. It stimulates glycogenolysis, breaking down glycogen in the liver to glucose, further contributing to hyperglycemia. This process is opposed by insulin and is switched off when an adequate amount of glucose has been transported into the cells. In addition, increasing stress promotes secretion of counterregulatory hormones, i.e., catecholamines, cortisol, and growth hormone (Kitabchi & Murphy, 2012). These hormones further stimulate hepatic glucose production resulting in more hyperglycemia (Kitabchi et al., 2009).

Oxidation of fatty acids occurs due to lipolysis of fat stores (breakdown of triglycerides to free fatty acids and glycerol). This occurs in an attempt to provide energy and can proceed to ketogenesis in the absence of insulin. Ketones provide an alternate source of energy when glucose cannot be metabolized properly. Fatty acids are transported to the liver where ketones are synthesized. One ketone, acetoacetic acid, is converted to acetone and is excreted through the lungs and has a fruity odor that can be detected on the breath. The most prevalent ketone, betahydroxybutyric acid, is excreted by the kidneys with glucose through osmotic diuresis. There is extensive loss of water leading to dehydration, concentrating glucose and resulting in more hyperglycemia. Water is pulled from the intracellular fluid (ICF) space to the extracellular fluid (ECF) space. Expansion of the ECF dilutes sodium, causing a decrease in its concentration. There is increased excretion of sodium and potassium, resulting in an electrolyte imbalance.

Key Points

Serum potassium levels may be normal in spite of total body potassium deficits, as it is primarily an ICF electrolyte. Acidosis occurs when ketones become excessive (Foster, 1984).

Hyperglycemia is not as severe in DKA as in HHS. Blood glucose is typically less than 800 mg/dl, often between 350 and 450 mg/dl. This is probably due to the fact that this population is younger and has a higher GFR, thus allowing for a greater capacity to excrete glucose than older patients with HHS (Delaney et al., 2000). Plasma osmolality is less elevated in DKA than in hyperosmolar, hyperglycemic, non-ketosis (Arieff & Carroll, 1972; Delaney et al., 2000).

Precipitating Factors

There are a number of common precipitating factors:

- Infection, especially involving pneumonia, UTIs, and sepsis, is the most common.
- Insufficient insulin therapy due to poor compliance, omission, malfunction of insulin pump, or discontinuation or too much food.
- Acute illnesses such as myocardial infarction, cerebral vascular accident, pancreatitis, gastrointestinal (GI) bleeding, and any major stress or trauma, physical or psychological, including surgery or pregnancy.
- Medications that impact carbohydrate metabolism, such as steroids, thiazide diuretics, sympathomimetic agents; other agents such as cocaine and certain antipsychotic drugs may precipitate onset (Kitabchi & Murphy, 2012; Newcomer, 2005).
- Sodium/glucose cotransporter 2 (SGLT2) inhibitors may trigger onset.

It may also be the declaration of new-onset type 1 diabetes related to any of these precipitating events.

Clinical Presentation

DKA usually evolves within 24 hr and is typically manifested by GI, respiratory, and neurologic abnormalities and dehydration.

- GI symptoms: patients usually present with nausea, vomiting, and abdominal pain. Abdominal pain is associated with the severity of acidosis and may be due to delayed gastric emptying and ileus caused by metabolic acidosis and electrolyte imbalance (Umpierrez & Freire, 2002). Pancreatitis should also be considered.
- Volume depletion: physical examination may reveal dry mucous membranes, poor skin turgor, dry skin, tachycardia, hypotension, and decreased jugular venous pressure.
- Neurologic symptoms: usually more profound with HHNK, but lethargy, headache, focal deficits, and obtunded mental status may develop and lead to coma.
- Other: polyuria, polyphagia, blurred vision, fruity odor of breath, Kussmaul respirations, and hypothermia.

Diagnostic Testing

Laboratory testing should include the following: glucose, electrolytes, BUN, creatinine, GFR, anion gap, bicarbonate, serum phosphate, CBC, plasma osmolality, Hgb A1C, ABG if bicarbonate is significantly reduced, routine urinalysis, urine ketones, serum ketones if urine ketones are present, urine culture if UTI is suspected, blood culture if sepsis is suspected, and sputum culture if upper respiratory infection is suspected.

Other diagnostic testing may include ECG and CXR.

Diagnostic Findings

Characteristics of DKA include hyperglycemia, hyperosmolality, osmotic diuresis, metabolic acidosis as reflected by the anion gap, and ketonemia. Blood glucose ranges from 350 to 500 mg/dl but DKA can occur with lower glucose values; it is typically less than 800 mg/dl but may exceed 900 mg/dl in patients who are comatose (Morris & Kitabchi, 1980).

Glucosuria results, producing osmotic diuresis and promoting excretion of sodium, potassium, and water, thus increasing plasma osmolality. Most patients with DKA have mild hyponatremia, but serum sodium may be normal or elevated depending on the extent of hyperglycemia and osmolality, as these factors influence the shift of water and electrolytes from ICF to ECF Total body potassium depletion occurs as potassium moves from the ICF to ECF due to osmotic diuresis (Adrogue et al., 1986). Serum potassium can be normal or elevated initially due to this shift (Defronzo et al., 1994).

Serum creatinine and BUN can be significantly elevated secondary to polyuria from uncontrolled hyperglycemia. Dehydration and hypovolemia are reflected by the decrease in GFR (Molitch et al., 1980). DKA results in the elevation of the anion gap, typically >20 mEq (reference range 3–10 mEq), caused by the accumulation of beta-hydroxybutyric and acetoacetic acids. Serum bicarbonate levels are usually markedly decreased, <16 mEq/L (Porter et al., 1997). Serum phosphate tends to be normal or high due to phosphate shift out of the cells (Kebler et al., 1985). Arterial pH will be less than 7.0 if DKA is severe.

CBC with differential may show elevated Hgb and Hct levels due to volume depletion. It often reveals leukocytosis in patients with DKA. This is due to counterregulatory hormones (catecholamines, cortisol) in the absence of infection (Nematollahi et al., 2007).

Key Points

Serum osmolality is more elevated in HHS than in DKA due to extreme dehydration. Serum ketones should be performed if urine is positive for ketones. Nitroprusside test is used to detect urine ketones.

Treatment Goals

Treatment goals for DKA include correction of dehydration, repletion of electrolytes, administration of insulin, and prevention of complications.

1. Correct dehydration. Replace fluids with 0.45% or 0.9% saline to restore volume and decrease osmolality. On average, fluid should be replaced at 1,000 ml/hr for 1–2 hr in patients with hypovolemia, but without shock or heart failure. Infusion after 2 hr is dependent upon fluid volume, urine output, hyperglycemia, and electrolytes (25, Kit). Volume overload is to be avoided. Rate generally should be decreased to 250–500 ml/hr as patient becomes rehydrated.
2. Provide sufficient insulin to restore normal glucose metabolism. Low-dose regular or rapid-acting insulin (0.1 units/kg body weight per hour) should be administered intravenously if serum potassium ≥ 3.3 mEq. If serum potassium <3.3 mEq, insulin administration should be delayed until potassium replacement has been begun and the level has increased. Insulin administration causes potassium to shift from ECF to the cells. This can significantly decrease extracellular potassium levels depending on how quickly the shift occurs. Arrhythmias and death can occur (Nyenwe & Kitabchi, 2011).
3. Restore electrolyte balance. 20–30 mEq potassium should be infused per each liter of intravenous fluid if serum potassium is between 3.3 and 5.3 mEq/L and once urine output is established. Monitoring of serum potassium should be done hourly until stable.
4. Provide glucose when needed.

To prevent hypoglycemia, 5% dextrose should be added to intravenous when blood glucose is 200–250 mg/dl.

5. Prevent complications. Hypoglycemia, hypokalemia, hyperglycemia, and hyperkalemia are potential complications of treatment. Therefore, monitoring is essential. Serum glucose and potassium should be checked hourly until stable. Sodium, chloride, bicarbonate, BUN, creatinine, venous pH, and ketones should be checked every 2–4 hr. Ketosis is usually reversed in 12–24 hr.
6. Consider indications for bicarbonate replacement. Use of sodium bicarbonate is controversial because of potential harmful effects. It is not indicated if arterial pH is greater than 7.0 as hydration and insulin will reverse acidosis (Defronzo et al., 1994).

Case Study

You implemented treatment prior to receiving all laboratory results. You did a POCT glucose which indicated DKA. When results were available, you confirmed presence of acidosis based on arterial pH and serum bicarbonate. Hgb and Hct as well as BUN and creatinine were elevated resulting from dehydration. Ketosis was confirmed by presence of ketones in the urine. Serum osmolality was increased, sodium was decreased, and potassium was slightly elevated as a result of osmotic diuresis. Elevation in glucose promoted osmotic diuresis, causing dehydration, increased excretion of sodium, and movement of potassium from intracellular to ECF. Urine culture was positive for *Escherichia coli*.

You identified the precipitating factors as increased stress, which contributed to excess secretion of counterregulatory hormones; noncompliance with insulin dose; departure from healthy eating habits; and UTI.

You started an IV of normal saline at 1,000 ml/hr. The patient had urine output, so you added regular insulin 0.1 unit/kg/hr. You checked electrolytes. Potassium was 3.5 mEq/L, so you administered potassium and monitored blood levels hourly. After 2 hr, glucose was 190 mg/dl. Potassium further decreased to 3.2 mEq/L as insulin decreased hyperglycemia and potassium moved back from ECF to ICF. You added additional potassium and 5% dextrose to the IV. You also decreased the amount of insulin. You treated the UTI with the appropriate antibiotics.

Twenty-four hours later, electrolytes were normal and urinary ketones were small. You discussed the precipitating factors with the patient and reviewed prevention strategies.

Differential Diagnosis

The differential diagnosis for DKA includes the following:

- HHS
- Gastroenteritis
- Metabolic encephalopathy, usually from systemic illness
- Fasting ketoacidosis, from low-carbohydrate diets, anorexia
- Alcoholic acidosis
- Lactic acidosis
- Uremia
- Pancreatitis
- Aspirin or acetaminophen toxicity

Conclusion

It is important to recognize the early signs and symptoms of DKA to begin prompt treatment. Initial evaluation should include identification of precipitating factors so that they can be resolved or minimized. Assessment of cardiopulmonary, neurologic, and volume status is a priority. DKA evolves rapidly and morbidity and mortality remain high. Therefore, treatment should be initiated, even before laboratory results are available.

HYPEROSMOLAR HYPERGLYCEMIC STATE

Case Study 2

Mr. FG is an 82-year-old male with history of type 2 diabetes for over 20 years, CAD status post myocardial infarction, HTN, hyperlipidemia, atrial fibrillation, and angina, who is status post hip replacement surgery. He was discharged to an SNF for short-term rehabilitation and remained there for 3 weeks. Prior to his surgery his diabetes was controlled with diet and metformin; his A1C was 6.3%. His other medications included aspirin 81 mg, metoprolol succinate 50 mg, atorvastatin 80 mg, Eliquis 5 mg bid, and lisinopril 5 mg. He was quite active prior to surgery, exercising in cardiac rehab three times a week.

Following surgery, his recovery was slow even though he had physical therapy. He was experiencing hip pain, which impacted on his ability to regain strength and mobility. His fasting blood glucose was checked daily while in the S. It ranged from 130 to 250, and he was started on lantus 10 units daily. He was discharged to home with minimal improvement in his blood glucose. Therefore, lantus was increased to 12 units and he was instructed to check blood glucose before meals and at bedtime. Due to the cost of the test strips and lantus, which were only minimally covered by his insurance, Mr. FG did not test blood glucose and decreased his lantus dose to 5 units. A week after discharge, he developed a productive cough and was experiencing increasing shortness of breath. His appetite decreased, and he was not drinking much fluid.

Mr. FG's wife noticed that he appeared weak and lethargic. He was losing weight. He complained of thirst and polyuria. His skin became extremely dry. He began to experience dizziness and confusion. His lethargy and weakness continued to increase. Several days later, he had a seizure and collapsed on the floor. His wife called 911, and he was rushed to the hospital.

Upon presentation in the emergency room, you are called to evaluate him. Review of systems revealed polyuria, extreme thirst, weakness, leg cramps, and blurred vision. Upon physical examination, you note that his skin turgor is poor, his mucous membranes are extremely dry, his eyes appear sunken, and he has mild confusion. His temperature is 100.2°F, blood pressure is 100/50, and respiratory rate is 26 breaths per minute. Cardiovascular examination reveals heart rate of 110 beats per minute, irregular rhythm of 2/6 SEM, and no rubs or gallops. Abdomen is flat, no tenderness, with normal bowel sounds. Extremities show no edema and weak pedal pulses bilaterally. Respiratory examination reveals decreased breath sounds, inspiratory rales, and expiratory wheezes bilateral bases. Fruity odor of breath is absent. His skin shows extreme dryness, flakiness, poor turgor, and dry mucous membranes. Neurological examination reveals lethargy and mild confusion.

You check POCT glucose; it is greater than 600 mg/dl. You order a CBC with differential, complete metabolic panel, ABG, serum osmolality, urine for ketones, blood and urine cultures, and Hgb A1C. You begin treatment before laboratory results are received.

Serum glucose is 1,100 mg/dl; WBC count, Hgb, and Hct are elevated; sodium is elevated; potassium is decreased; BUN and creatinine are elevated; serum phosphate is elevated; serum bicarbonate and arterial pH are normal; serum osmolality is elevated.

You order a blood culture, CXR, and ECG. CXR reveals bilateral infiltrates. The blood culture is positive for *Streptococcus pneumoniae*, and the ECG shows flattened T waves.

Overview of HHS

HHS is characterized by hyperglycemia greater than 600 mg/dl (frequently exceeds 1,000 mg/dl), but with little or no ketoacidosis (Kitabchi et al., 2009). Blood glucose gradually escalates over a long period of time (average 12 days) before it becomes a serious problem.

Key Points

As DKA occurs in patients with type 1 diabetes with absolute insulin deficiency, HHS is most often seen in undiagnosed or older adults (older than 65 years) with type 2 diabetes who have decreased, but not absent, insulin production.

It infrequently occurs in children and in those with type 1 diabetes (Khardori & Soler, 1984). Symptoms of polyuria, polydipsia, and weight loss can persist for several days without GI symptoms of DKA; therefore, medical attention is often not sought or the condition is misdiagnosed. Extreme dehydration, electrolyte imbalance, and hyperosmolarity contribute to the severity of illness. Mortality rate for HHS is between 10% and 20%, approximately 10 times higher than for DKA (Pasquel & Umpierrez, 2014). This is primarily due to the fact that patients with symptoms of DKA seek medical attention sooner.

Pathology

HHS is similar to DKA, with several differentiating factors. As with DKA, there is impaired peripheral glucose utilization and increased glycogenolysis and gluconeogenesis (Kitabchi et al., 2009). However, insulin is not totally absent, blood glucose is significantly more elevated, and dehydration is more profound. Lipolysis is absent or minimal as there is some circulating insulin. Insulin concentration required to prevent lipolysis and ketoacidosis is approximately one-tenth of that required to promote glucose transport into cells (Zierler & Rabinowitz, 1964). However, insulin secretion is not sufficient to suppress gluconeogenesis, thus resulting in severe hyperglycemia (Kitabchi & Fisher, 1981). Glucosuria results when blood glucose exceeds 180 mg/dl, and there is excessive loss of water via the kidneys because of osmotic diuresis. Hyperglycemia, osmolality, and renal water loss become more extensive, further contributing to dehydration. As there is little or no ketosis, symptoms of DKA (abdominal discomfort and hyperventilation) do not develop and the correct diagnosis is often overlooked. Neurologic symptoms, including lethargy, focal deficits, alterations in mental status, and coma, are more common with HHS because of extreme hyperosmolality (Lorber, 1995).

Precipitating Factors

Precipitating factors for HHS are related to insufficient insulin production and include similar causes of DKA.

- Undiagnosed or new-onset type 2 diabetes
- Insufficient insulin
- Infection (factor in 60% of cases) (Nugent, 2005)
- Surgery
- Acute illnesses such as myocardial infarction, cerebrovascular accident, GI bleeding, uremia, pancreatitis, pulmonary embolism, and arterial thrombosis
- Medications that affect carbohydrate metabolism such as steroids, thiazides, beta blockers, and phenytoin
- Dehydration resulting from osmotic diuresis, fever, burns, diarrhea, diuretics, dialysis, and impaired thirst mechanism

Clinical Presentation

The clinical presentation of HHS is similar to DKA, with several exceptions.

- Gradual development over a period of days
- Severe hyperglycemia
- Extreme dehydration including dry mucous membranes, poor skin turgor, and sunken eyes

- Neurologic changes including lethargy, confusion, aphasia, focal deficits, seizures, and coma are more common with HHS; decreases in mentation correlate with serum osmolality (Nugent, 2005)
- Absence of ketosis and GI symptoms
- Other: polyuria, polydipsia, blurred vision, weakness, leg cramps, anorexia, and dizziness (Nugent, 2005).

Diagnostic Testing

Laboratory testing should include the same tests as DKA: glucose, electrolytes, BUN, creatinine, GFR, anion gap, bicarbonate, serum phosphate, CBC, plasma osmolality, Hgb A1C, ABG if bicarbonate is significantly reduced, routine urinalysis, urine ketones and serum ketones if urine ketones should be absent, and cultures of urine, sputum, and blood if infection is suspected.

Other diagnostic testing may include ECG and CXR.

Diagnostic Findings

Key Points

HHS is characterized by hyperglycemia that is more extreme than DKA (frequently greater than 1,000 mg/dl and sometimes as great as 3,000 mg/dl) (Daugirdas et al., 1989) and dehydration, but no ketoacidosis.

As with DKA, patients with HHS usually have mild hyponatremia (Adrogue et al., 1986); however, with severe osmotic diuresis, these patients may present with normal or elevated sodium because of marked sodium concentration (Khardori & Soler, 1984). Serum osmolality tends to be markedly elevated and can lead to neurologic symptoms such as seizures and coma. Potassium deficit exists in both DKA and HHS because of osmotic diuresis. This results in potassium loss through renal excretion. However, serum potassium is usually normal or elevated because of shift from ICF to ECF (Aurora et al., 2012). As with DKA, creatinine and BUN are often acutely elevated indicating a decrease in GFR due to hypovolemia (Rumbak et al., 1991). Serum phosphate tends to be normal or high due to phosphate shift out of the cells (Kebler et al., 1985). Serum bicarbonate and arterial pH are typically normal, but serum osmolality is greater than 320 (Kitabchi et al., 2009). CBC with differential may show elevated Hgb and Hct levels due to volume depletion. Serum osmolality is more elevated in HHS than in DKA due to extreme dehydration. ECG abnormalities can indicate hyperkalemia or hypokalemia.

Treatment Goals

Treatment goals are similar for DKA and HHS:

1. Aggressively replace fluids. Restore intravascular volume with 1 L of normal saline per hour. Fluid deficit is typically more severe with HHS. Blood glucose may decrease significantly with restoration of fluid balance alone. Proceed with caution with elderly patients, especially those with a history of myocardial infarction, CHF, or renal failure. Cardiovascular status needs to be carefully monitored.

2. Replace electrolytes. Total body potassium deficit is often unknown as serum level may be normal or high. Potassium depletion tends to be more severe with HHS. Insulin administration may cause a severe decrease in serum potassium. Monitor hourly until stable.

3. Administer insulin. Low-dose insulin should be administered intravenously. As hydration can effectively lower blood glucose in HHS, insulin requirements are typically less. Insulin administration should be delayed until potassium replacement is implemented if serum potassium is less than 3.3 mEq/L. As insulin causes potassium to shift back into the cells, hypokalemia is a potential threat. Add 5% dextrose to intravenous fluids and decrease insulin when blood glucose is 200–250 mg/dl.

4. Identify and treat underlying medical condition.

5. Prevent complications.

Case Study

You suspected HHS, as POCT glucose was greater than 600 mg/dl, and therefore initiated treatment before testing results were back. You identified the several precipitating factors, including stress associated with surgery, increasing hyperglycemia, lack of appetite, increasing dehydration, and pulmonary infection.

You started intravenous fluids, initially at 1,000 ml/hr, and monitored the patient on telemetry. Blood glucose, which was greater than 1,000 mg/dl, decreased to 699 after an hour. Potassium was less than 3.3 mEq, and this was reflected by the flattened T waves on the ECG. You therefore delayed administration of intravenous insulin. Potassium eventually increased to 3.6 mEq, and insulin was started intravenously. Within 24 hr, blood glucose decreased to less than 200 mg/dl, and electrolytes were normal. Intravenous was discontinued, and insulin was switched to subcutaneous. You discussed the precipitating events with the patient and family and helped the patient to realize the importance of prevention.

Differential Diagnosis

The differential diagnosis for HHS includes the following:

- DKA
- CNS infection
- Sepsis
- Severe dehydration
- Uremia
- Intoxication (ethanol, narcotics)
- Excessive diuretic use

Conclusion

HHS is often misdiagnosed as patients often do not seek prompt medical attention. This is due to the fact that onset of symptoms is gradual; symptoms therefore are attributed to other causes. The seriousness of this condition, resulting from pronounced hyperglycemia, severe dehydration, and significant electrolyte imbalance, requires immediate treatment in order to prevent mortality.

Features and treatment for DKA and HHS have many similarities but specific differences that guide your differential diagnoses. Table 8.1 distinguishes the specific features of each state.

TABLE 8.1 FEATURES OF DKA AND HHS

DKA	HHS
Usually with type 1 diabetes	Usually with type 2 diabetes
Younger age	Older age, >65 years
Blood glucose <800 mg/dl	Blood glucose frequently >1,000 mg/dl
Evolves over 24 hr	Evolves over days, weeks
pH <7.3	pH >7.3
Bicarbonate <18	Bicarbonate >18
Positive urine ketones	Usually no urine ketones
Serum osmolality variable	Serum osmolality >320
	Greater mortality

CLINICAL PEARLS

Common treatment guidelines for DKA and HHS include the following:

1. Rehydrate
2. Replace electrolytes
3. Administer insulin
4. Provide glucose as appropriate
5. Identify and treat underlying cause
6. Prevent complications
7. Provide education for prevention

THYROID STORM

Case Study

Ms. BT is a 44-year-old female with history of HTN and Graves disease. She presented to the emergency room with abdominal bloating, diarrhea, tachycardia, agitation, exertional dyspnea, increasing fatigue, and edema, which she had been experiencing for a week. She had nausea and vomiting 24 hr prior to admission. Her medications included losartan 50 mg daily and levothyroxine 75 μg daily. She had surgery for hernia repair 2 weeks prior to her admission.

Upon examination, she was found to have an enlarged thyroid gland, exophthalmos, warm moist skin, and tremors; temperature 104.2°F, blood pressure 160/98 mm Hg, pulse 140 beats per minute, and respirations 28. Cardiovascular examination revealed fast irregular rate, normal S_1 and S_2, low-grade systolic murmur, and no rubs or gallops. ECG revealed rapid atrial fibrillation. Extremities revealed 1+ pitting edema bilaterally. Abdomen showed ascites and decreased bowel sounds. Respiratory examination revealed late inspiratory crackles bilateral bases. A CXR was consistent with pulmonary edema.

You order a TSH test due to new-onset atrial fibrillation. You also order a CBC with differential, complete metabolic panel, lactate, pro BNP, blood culture, and urine culture. Her TSH is 0.04 mIU/L, and her lactate is 8.8 mmol/L. Thus, you order free T4 as TSH is extremely low, but you initiate treatment before this laboratory result is obtained. You also order thyrotropin receptor antibodies (TRAb). Glucose is 145 mg/dl, calcium is 11.0 mg/dl, total cholesterol is 140 mg/dl, pro BNP is 1,500 pg/ml, and WBC count is elevated. Free T4 was 6.8 mg/dl. TRAb and blood and urine cultures are pending.

Overview of Thyroid Storm

Thyroid storm is a rare but serious and life-threatening condition. Most episodes occur in individuals with known hyperthyroidism; therefore, characteristics of hyperthyroidism are evident in thyroid storm. Thyroid storm is often fatal without prompt and aggressive treatment (Sarlis & Gourgiotis, 2003).

Pathology

Hyperthyroidism is due to excessive production of thyroid hormone. Thyrotoxicosis refers to any cause of excessive thyroid hormone; thus, it includes hyperthyroidism.

Key Points

Thyroid storm, also known as thyrotoxic crisis, is a severe form of thyrotoxicosis with excessive release of thyroid hormones.

In overt hyperthyroidism (as compared with mild hyperthyroidism), symptoms are usually more apparent than in mild hyperthyroidism. Patients can present with anxiety, agitation, tremor, weakness, palpitations, weight loss, increased appetite, and heat intolerance (Trzepacz et al., 1989). Weight gain may occur in some patients, especially younger people, due to excessive increase in appetite (Nordyke et al., 1988). Other symptoms include hyperdefecation, urinary frequency, amenorrhea, gynecomastia, and erectile dysfunction (Krassas et al., 1994). Heart failure and myocardial infarction are potential outcomes. New-onset atrial fibrillation, myopathy, osteoporosis, hypercalcemia, dyspnea, and poor glycemic control can also indicate presence of hyperthyroidism, especially in older patients (Boelaert et al., 2010).

| BOX 8.1 | Precipitating Factors in Thyroid Storm |

Undertreated hyperthyroidism
Infection
Trauma
Thyroid or other surgery
Acute iodine load
Pregnancy
Antithyroid medication

Precipitating Factors

Thyroid storm can occur in patients with undertreated hyperthyroidism (as in Graves disease, also known as toxic diffuse goiter) and with solitary toxic thyroid nodule, but it is often triggered by an acute event such as thyroid or other surgery, damage to the thyroid gland, acute iodine load, infection, trauma, pregnancy, or misuse of antithyroid medication (Swee du et al., 2015). Risk factors include trauma, stroke, DKA, and pulmonary embolus. Although the exact causes are not known, it has been hypothesized that catecholamines and rapid increase in thyroid hormone contribute (Sarlis & Gourgiotis, 2003). However, elevation of thyroxine (T4) and triiodothyronine (T3) levels and reduction of TSH were not more pronounced than in patients with uncomplicated thyrotoxicosis (Nayak & Burman, 2006).

Box 8.1 summarizes common precipitating factors for thyroid storm.

Clinical Presentation

Symptoms of hyperthyroidism typically appear exaggerated or accelerated in thyroid storm (Angell et al., 2015) and have been associated with mortality (Swee du et al., 2015).

- Cardiovascular symptoms: extreme tachycardia (greater than 130 beats per minute), atrial fibrillation or other arrhythmias, HTN with widened pulse pressure, heart failure, myocardial infarction, and sudden cardiac death
- Neurologic symptoms: alterations in mental status—anxiety, agitation, delirium, psychosis, and coma
- GI symptoms: abdominal pain, nausea, vomiting, diarrhea, or jaundice from hepatic failure
- Other symptoms: fever (up to 106°F); may also be prothrombotic.

Diagnostic Testing

Laboratory testing should include TSH, T4, T3, TRAb, glucose, CBC, and calcium and liver function tests. ECG should be checked for arrhythmia. Table 8.2 lists laboratory findings in thyroid storm.

Diagnostic Findings

TSH is decreased, and free T3 and/or T4 is elevated, but usually not more elevated than in uncomplicated hyperthyroidism. TRAb can be positive if hyperthyroidism is a result of

TABLE 8.2 LABORATORY FINDINGS IN THYROID STORM

TEST	FINDING
TSH	Decreased
Free T3, T4	Elevated
Glucose	Mildly elevated
Calcium	Mildly elevated
Total cholesterol	Decreased
Liver function tests	Elevated alkaline phosphatase and bilirubin
RBCs	Elevated
WBCs	Elevated or decreased

autoimmunity. Mild hyperglycemia is typical due to increased glycogenolysis, secondary to catecholamine release. Mild hypercalcemia may be seen due to hemoconcentration and increased bone reabsorption. Other findings include low total cholesterol, abnormal liver function tests, elevated red blood cells (RBCs), and leukocytosis or leukopenia (Nayak & Burman, 2006).

A scoring system developed by Burch and Wartofsky may be utilized to guide care. It grades diagnostic criteria for thyroid storm. A score of 45 or higher strongly suggests presence of thyroid storm, whereas a score below 25 indicates that thyroid storm is not likely. Although this system is believed to be sensitive, it is not specific (Burch & Wartofsky, 1993).

Treatment

Radioiodine therapy, medications, and thyroid surgery are options.

Treatment guidelines for thyroid storm are often expanded from those used in treating patients with uncomplicated hyperthyroidism who do not meet criteria for thyroid storm. Medications are given in higher doses and are administered more frequently, and additional medications may be given for thyroid storm (Angell et al., 2015). Treatment involves use of several medications, as different mechanisms of action are required (Chiha et al., 2015). Guidelines (Ross et al., 2016) include the following medications:

- Beta blockers: immediate treatment, usually with propranolol, to decrease heart rate. A cardioselective beta blocker such as metoprolol or atenolol should be considered in patients with asthma. Calcium channel blockers can be used if beta blockers are contraindicated or cannot be tolerated (Milner et al., 1990). Can be discontinued when thyroid function tests are normal and cardiovascular symptoms resolve.
- Thionamide: immediate treatment of life-threatening thyroid storm with propylthiouracil (PTU) in an intensive care setting. It blocks conversion of T4 to T3 with a significant decrease in T3 within 24 hr. Patients treated with PTU should be transitioned to methimazole prior to discharge. Methimazole can be administered for severe but not life-threatening hyperthyroidism. It decreases synthesis of T3 and T4 and has a longer duration of action than PTU. Maximum effect is usually achieved in a month. Higher doses of thionamides are typically given in thyroid storm due to increased risk of mortality and potential for poor absorption secondary to GI dysfunction (Isozaki et al., 2016).

Once stable, the dose should be titrated to maintain euthyroidism. If thionamides are contraindicated due to side effects (agranulocytosis or hepatic toxicity) or cannot be tolerated, thyroidectomy is the treatment of choice (Panzer et al., 2004).

- Iodine solution: should be delayed 1 hr after first dose of thionamide. It blocks release of T3 and T4 from the thyroid gland (Nayak & Burman, 2006). Can be discontinued after mental status symptoms subside.
- Glucocorticoids: used in thyroid storm, but not routinely used with severe but not life-threatening hyperthyroidism. They decrease conversion of T4 to T3 (Tsatsoulis et al., 2000).
- Bile acid sequestrants: decrease levels of thyroid hormone by interfering with hepatic circulation, where thyroid hormone is metabolized (Kaykhaei et al., 2008). They can be useful in patients who are unable to tolerate thionamides.
- Plasmapheresis: has been used when routine therapy has been ineffective. It extracts thyroid hormone from plasma (Muller et al., 2011).
- Radioactive iodine: should be administered as a preventive measure if thyroid storm was precipitated by Graves disease. Thyroidectomy can also be considered.
- Thyroidectomy: Preoperative preparation.

Case Study

You noted multiple organ failure seemed to be occurring. You implemented treatment prior to receiving all laboratory results. You ordered antibiotics, as severe sepsis was initially suspected due to lactate elevation. The extremely low TSH, as well as recent history of surgery and findings from the physical examination, caused you to suspect thyroid storm. This was further supported by the elevated free T4 and positive TRAb. You ordered PTU and radioactive iodine and had the patient transferred to intensive care. She was started on a beta blocker to control heart rate and a diuretic for CHF. You would have considered plasmapheresis if the treatment had been unsuccessful, but as a result of your prompt treatment, the patient's prognosis greatly improved.

Differential Diagnosis

Differential diagnosis for thyroid storm includes the following:

- Sepsis, septic shock
- CNS infection
- Malignant hyperthermia
- Acute mania with catatonia
- Pheochromocytoma
- Neuroleptic malignant syndrome
- Hypertensive encephalopathy

Conclusion

Early recognition of life-threatening symptoms and immediate treatment of thyroid storm is critical as the mortality rate for thyroid storm is high.

CLINICAL PEARLS

TSH should be evaluated whenever thyroid storm is suspected (fever, alterations in mental status, goiter, atrial fibrillation, abnormal cardiac function, recent thyroid or other surgery, antithyroid drug therapy, or recent exposure to contrast containing iodine).

If TSH is decreased, free T3 and T4 should be assessed.

TRAb can also be measured, but treatment should not be delayed in patients with symptoms.

Thyroidectomy should be considered if thyrotoxicosis remains uncontrolled (Swee du et al., 2015).

MYXEDEMA COMA

Case Study

Mrs. PG is a 65-year-old female who was brought to the emergency room by her husband for alterations in mental status and extreme weakness. The patient has a history of hypothyroidism, HTN, COPD, hyperlipidemia, peripheral vascular disease, and atrial fibrillation. She is status post thyroidectomy 10 years ago for hyperthyroidism. She was recently started on amiodarone 200 mg bid after she developed atrial fibrillation with a rapid ventricular response. Other medications include metoprolol succinate 75 mg, levothyroxine 100 μg, losartan 50 mg, atorvastatin 40 mg, Breo Ellipta 100–25 μg, and warfarin. She had recently been diagnosed with bacterial pneumonia and was treated with antibiotics. She experienced nausea/vomiting and diarrhea from taking antibiotics and therefore stopped her medications. She had previously been noncompliant with her medications since and had often missed doses. When she takes her levothyroxine, she does not take it appropriately, but takes it with food and with her other medications. She denied abnormal vision, fever, chest pain, abdominal pain, diarrhea, numbness, and tingling. She does have fatigue, occasional palpitations, dyspnea with exertion, cough, and constipation. She has gained 10 lbs in the past month and has been experiencing hoarseness. She is also complaining of feeling cold. She has been experiencing mild confusion.

Her temperature is 97.1°F, blood pressure is 98/50 mm Hg, pulse is 52 beats per minute and irregular, and pulse ox is 90%. Cardiovascular examination reveals slow rate, irregular rhythm, and no murmurs, rubs, or gallops. ECG reveals bradycardia and atrial fibrillation. Respiratory examination reveals hypoventilation, decreased breath sounds, and rhonchi bilaterally. CXR reveals small bilateral pleural effusions. Her abdomen is obese with decreased bowel sounds. Eye, ears, nose and throat examination shows periorbital edema and macroglossia. Neurologic examination revels that she is lethargic with mild confusion. Her extremities show puffiness in hands; 2+ pitting edema bilateral lower extremities. Her skin shows a thyroidectomy scar present on the neck and extreme dryness.

You order a stat TSH and free T4 based on the patient's presentation. You also order CBC, complete metabolic panel, lipid panel, ABGs, and cortisol level. You initiate treatment with a combination of T3 and T4. You also order hydrocortisone. The TSH is extremely high and the free T4 is severely decreased at 0.23 ng/dl, indicating primary hypothyroidism. Cortisol level is normal, ruling out concomitant adrenal insufficiency; hydrocortisone is therefore not administered. Laboratory results reveal leukocytosis, hyponatremia, and hypoglycemia. Creatinine is 2.0, and lipids are elevated.

Overview

Myxedema coma is severe hypothyroidism and is an endocrine emergency. It is more common in women than in men (Ono et al., 2017). Typical symptoms of hypothyroidism include weight gain, dry skin, fatigue, constipation, cold intolerance, and menstrual abnormalities; they depend on the duration and severity of hormone deficiency (McDermott, 2009).

Key Points

Myxedema coma is more extreme and can be manifested by multisystem organ failure due to significant decrease in organ function. Alterations in mental status and hypothermia are classic indicators, but renal insufficiency, respiratory failure, and depressed cardiac function may occur. Prompt recognition and aggressive treatment are critical. Mortality remains a risk even if treatment is initiated.

Diagnosis is based on history, physical examination, and laboratory testing. Fortunately, as testing of TSH is readily available, diagnosis can be made immediately. This has been beneficial in reducing the severity of hypothyroidism. However, if suspected, treatment should be initiated before laboratory results are obtained.

Pathology

Myxedema is a state of severely decompensated hypothyroidism which increases progressively in severity. It can develop as a result of ongoing poorly controlled hypothyroidism and can be precipitated by factors such as illness or certain substances. There is a severe lack of thyroid hormone which results in a significant decrease in metabolism. It can occur in patients with primary or central hypothyroidism and in those with chronic autoimmune thyroiditis.

Key Points

Primary hypothyroidism is characterized by an elevated TSH and low free T4, whereas a low T4 and nonelevated TSH indicate central hypothyroidism.

Primary hypothyroidism results from previous treatment for hyperthyroidism, i.e., thyroidectomy, radioiodine, or antithyroid drugs. There is insufficient TSH stimulation of the thyroid gland in central hypothyroidism, caused by disease of the pituitary gland or hypothalamus (Samuels & Ridgway, 1992).

Precipitating Factors

Infection, surgery, exposure to cold, trauma, acute illness, and myocardial infarction are events that can trigger myxedema coma. Myxedema coma has been diagnosed in patients taking sedatives, opioids, and lithium (Waldman & Park, 1989). It has also been seen in patients taking amiodarone (Hawatmeh et al., 2018).

Clinical Presentation

Symptoms of hypothyroidism are typically present. Classic symptoms of myxedema coma include hypothermia (decrease in thermogenesis) and alterations in mental status. A decrease in function of multiple organ systems, as in the following list, may be noted:

- Neurologic: lethargy, confusion, seizures, and obtunded mental status due to hypoxia and decreased cerebral blood flow; can progress to myxedema madness and coma if untreated
- Cardiovascular: bradycardia, hypotension, decreased cardiac output, narrow pulse pressure, decreased contractility, pericardial effusion
- Pulmonary: hypoventilation, hypercapnia, hypoxia due to CNS depression; mechanical ventilation may be necessary
- GI: anorexia, malabsorption, reduced intestinal motility, paralytic ileus
- Renal: decreased GFR due to decreased cardiac output
- Other: weight gain, fatigue, and dry skin
- Physical examination: nonpitting edema from abnormal deposits of albumin, enlarged tongue from mucopolysaccharide edema, hypoventilation from respiratory acidosis, muscle weakness, puffiness in hands and face, periorbital edema, presence of thyroidectomy scar

Diagnostic Findings

Diagnostic findings of myxedema coma include decreased T4, elevated TSH if primary hypothyroidism, and mildly elevated, normal, or low if central hypothyroidism. Hypoglycemia due to decreased gluconeogenesis and hyponatremia results from impaired excretion of free water. A decreased cortisol level may be seen secondary to adrenal insufficiency. Hyperlipidemia may be found.

Treatment Goals

Treatment should be immediate, without waiting for laboratory results. Patients should be treated in the ICU depending on the severity of the condition and mechanical ventilation implemented as required. Improvement in clinical status does not usually occur for several days. Treatment should include the following steps:

1. Replace thyroid hormone. Thyroid hormone should be administered intravenously to rapidly correct low thyroid hormone level. Administration of oral thyroid hormone will not achieve normal blood level for several days. Choice of treatment has been

controversial as there have been no clinical trials evaluating different regimens. Some experts advise that either levothyroxine (T4) or liothyronine (T3) be given; others recommend that both be administered. Conversion of T4 to T3 is impaired in hypothyroidism. Onset of action is more rapid with T3; its activity is greater.

Key Points

Thyroid hormones should initially be administered intravenously.

2. Administer intravenous fluids and electrolytes.
3. Rule out adrenal insufficiency. Glucocorticoids should be given unless cortisol levels are normal.
4. Reverse hypothermia. Use of a warming blanket is recommended.
5. Monitor for respiratory failure. Mechanical ventilation may be indicated.
6. Treat infection.

Differential Diagnosis

The differential diagnosis for myxedema coma includes the following:

- Septic shock
- CHF
- COPD exacerbation
- Hypothermia
- Hepatic encephalopathy
- Hypothyroidism
- Pneumonia

Case Study

The patient continues to deteriorate rapidly with further reduction in mental status and increasing respiratory failure. The patient is transferred to intensive care where she is intubated. T3 and T4 are administered intravenously. TSH and T4 levels are monitored daily. Her mental status begins to improve when the TSH approaches normal. Renal insufficiency resolves when cardiac output returned to normal. You order a cardiology consult to evaluate amiodarone. The importance of recognizing precipitating events was discussed with the patient. In this case, noncompliance with thyroid medication, amiodarone, infection, and history of thyroidectomy were all factors.

Conclusion

Early recognition of myxedema coma and immediate treatment are essential due to the high mortality rate (Beynon et al., 2008). Diagnosis is based on history, physical examination, and exclusion of other causes.

CLINICAL PEARLS

Myxedema coma should be suspected if the patient presents with hypothermia, hypercapnia, hyponatremia, depressed mentation, presence of thyroidectomy scar, or coma.

Blood should be drawn if myxedema is suspected, but treatment should not be delayed.

Death is usually attributed to respiratory failure.

Mortality is still as high as 50% even with prompt treatment (Ono et al., 2017). The severity of the hypothermia impacts on mortality. Most abnormalities can be reversed with thyroid hormone replacement, but improvement is often not seen for several days.

REVIEW QUESTIONS

1. Which of the following is not true?
   a. HHS has a higher mortality rate than DKA.
   b. Lethargy and confusion are more common in DKA than in HHS.
   c. Onset of DKA usually occurs rapidly.
   d. Dehydration is typically more profound in HHS.

2. One major difference between DKA and HHS is:
   a. Hyperglycemia is typically more profound in DKA.
   b. Onset of HHS occurs rapidly whereas blood glucose gradually increases over a period of days in DKA.
   c. Serum osmolality is more elevated in HHS.
   d. Lipolysis usually occurs in both HHS and DKA.

3. Thyroid storm can occur in undertreated hyperthyroidism, but is often triggered by:
   a. Surgery
   b. Pregnancy
   c. Acute iodine load
   d. All of the above

4. Which of the following are symptoms of myxedema coma?
   a. Tachycardia, lethargy, and dry skin
   b. Confusion, weight loss, and edema
   c. Weight gain, bradycardia, and hypothermia
   d. Hyperventilation, HTN, and seizures

   Answers: 1, b; 2, c; 3, d; 4, c

REFERENCES

Adrogue, H. J., Lederer, E. D., Suki, W. N., & Eknoyan, G. (1986). Determinants of plasma potassium levels in diabetic ketoacidosis. *Medicine (Baltimore)*, 65(3), 163–172.

Angell, T. E., Lechner, M. G., Nguyen, C. T., Salvato, V. L., Nicoloff, J. T., & LoPresti, J. S. (2015). Clinical features and hospital outcomes in thyroid storm: A retrospective cohort study. *The Journal of Clinical Endocrinology and Metabolism*, 100(2), 451–459.

Arieff, A. I., & Carroll, H. J. (1972). Nonketotic hyperosmolar coma with hyperglycemia. *Medicine*, 51(2), 73–94.

Aurora, S., Cheng, D., Wyler, B., & Menchine, M. (2012). Prevalence of hypokalemia in ED patients with diabetic ketoacidosis. *The American Journal of Emergency Medicine*, 30(3), 481–484.

Beynon, J., Akhtar, S., & Kearney, T. (2008). Predictors of outcome in myxedema coma. *Critical Care*, 12(1), 111.

Boelaert, K., Torlinska, B., Holder, R. L., & Franklyn, J. A. (2010). Older subjects with hyperthyroidism present with a paucity of symptoms and signs: A large cross-sectional study. *The Journal of Clinical Endocrinology and Metabolism*, 95(6), 2715–2726.

Burch, H. B., & Wartofsky, L. (1993). Life-threatening thyrotoxicosis: Thyroid storm. *Endocrinology and Metabolism Clinics of North America*, 22(2):263–277.

Chiha, M., Samarasinghe, S., & Kabaker, A. S. (2015). Thyroid storm: An updated review. *Journal of Intensive Care Medicine*, 30(3), 131–140.

Daugirdas, J. T., Tzamaloukas, A. H., & Ing, T. S. (1989). Hyperosmolar coma: Cellular dehydration and serum sodium concentration. *Annals of Internal Medicine*, 110(11), 855–857.

Defronzo, R. A., Matzuda, M., & Barret, E. (1994). Diabetic ketoacidosis: A combined metabolic-nephrologic approach to therapy. *Diabetes Review*, 2, 209.

Delaney, M. F., Zisman, A., & Kettyle, W. M. (2000). Diabetic ketoacidosis and hyperglycemic hyperosmolar nonketotic syndrome. *Endocrinology and Metabolism Clinics of North America*, 29(4), 683–705.

Foster, D. W. (1984). From glycogen to ketones and back. *Diabetes*, 33(12), 1188–1199.

Hawatmeh, A., Thawabi, M., Abuarqoub, A., & Shamoon, F. (2018). Amiodarone induced myxedema coma: Two case reports and literature review. *Heart and Lung*, 47(4), 429–431.

Isozaki, O., Satoh, T., Wakino, S., Suzuki, A., Iburi, T., Tsuboi, K., Kanamoto, N., Otani, H., Furukawa, Y., Teramukai, S., & Akamizu, T. (2016). Treatment and management of thyroid storm: Analysis of the nation-wide surveys. *Clinical Endocrinology*, 84(6), 912–918.

Kaykhaei, M. A., Shams, M., Sadegholvad, A., Dabbaghmanesh, M. H., & Omrani, G. R. (2008). Low doses of cholestyramine in the treatment of hyperthyroidism. *Endocrine*, 34, 52–55.

Kebler, R., McDonald, F. D., & Cadnapaphomchai, P. (1985). Dynamic changes in serum phosphorus levels in diabetic ketoacidosis. *The American Journal of Medicine*, 79(5), 571–576.

Khardori, R., & Soler, N. G. (1984). Hyperosmolar hyperglycemic nonketotic syndrome. Report of 22 cases and brief review. *The American Journal of Medicine*, 77(5), 899–904.

Kitabchi, A. E., & Fisher, J. N. (1981). Insulin therapy of diabetic ketoacidosis: Physiologic versus pharmacologic doses of insulin and their routes of administration. In M. Brownlee (Ed.), *Handbook of diabetes mellitus* (p. 95). Garland STPM Press.

Kitabchi, A. E., & Murphy, M. B. (2012). Consequences of insulin deficiency. In Skyler J. (Ed.), *Atlas of diabetes* (pp. 39–63). Springer.

Kitabchi, A. E., Umpierrez, G. E., Miles, J. M., & Fisher, J. N. (2009). Hyperglycemic crises in adult patients with diabetes. *Diabetes Care*, 32(7), 1335–1343.

Krassas, G. E., Pontikides, N., Kaltsas, T., Papadopoulou, P., & Batrinos, M. (1994). Menstrual disturbances in thyrotoxicosis. *Clinical Endocrinology*, 40(5), 641.

Lorber, D. (1995). Nonketotic hypertonicity in diabetes mellitus. *Medical Clinics of North America*, 79(1), 39–52.

McDermott, M. T. (2009). Hypothyroidism. *Annals of Internal Medicine*, 151, ITC61.

Milner, M. R., Gelman, K. M., Phillips, R. A., Fuster, V., Davies, T. F., & Goldman, M. E. (1990). Double-blind crossover trial of diltiazem versus propranolol in the management of thyrotoxic symptoms. *Pharmacotherapy*, 10(2), 100–106.

Molitch, M. E., Rodman, E., Hirsch, C. A., Dubinsky, E. (1980). Spurious serum creatinine elevations in ketoacidosis. *Annals of Internal Medicine*, 93(2), 280–281.

Morris, L. R., & Kitabchi, A. E. (1980). Efficacy of low-dose insulin therapy for severely obtunded patients in diabetic ketoacidosis. *Diabetes Care*, 3(1), 53–56.

Muller, C, Perrin, P., Faller, B., Richter, S., & Chantrel, F. (2011). Role of plasma exchange in thyroid storm. *Therapeutic Apheresis and Dialysis*, 15(6), 522–531.

Nayak, B., & Burman, K. (2006). Thyrotoxicosis and thyroid storm. *Endocrinology and Metabolism Clinics of North America*, 35(4), 663–686.

Nematollahi, L. R., Taheri, E, Larijani, B., Mohajeri, M., Gozashti, M., Wan, J. Y., & Kitabchi, A. E. (2007). Catecholamine-induced leukocytosis in acute hypoglycemic stress. *Journal of Investigative Medicine*, 55(1), S262.

Newcomer, J. W. (2005). Second generation antipsychotics and metabolic effects: A comprehensive literature review. *CNS Drugs*, 19(suppl 1), 1–93.

Nordyke, R. A., Gilbert, F. I. Jr., & Harada, A. S. (1988). Graves' disease: Influence of age on clinical findings. *Archives of Internal Medicine*, 148(3), 626–631.

Nugent, B. W. (2005). Hyperosmolar hyperglycemic state. *Emergency Medical Clinics of North America*, 23(3), 629–648.

Nyenwe, E. A., & Kitabchi, A. E. (2011). Evidence-based management of hyperglycemic emergencies in diabetes mellitus. *Diabetes Research and Clinical Practice*, 94(3), 340–351.

Ono, Y., Ono, S., Yasunaga, H., Matsui, H., Fushimi, K., & Tanaka, Y. (2017). Clinical characteristics and outcomes of myxedema coma: Analysis of a national inpatient database in Japan. *Journal of Epidemiology*, 27(3), 117–122.

Panzer, C., Beazley, R., & Braverman, L. (2004). Rapid preoperative preparation for severe hyperthyroid Grave's disease. *Journal of Clinical Endocrinology and Metabolism*, 89(5), 2142–2144.

Pasquel, F. J., & Umpierrez, G. E. (2014). Hyperosmolar hyperglycemic state: Historic review of the clinical presentation, diagnosis and treatment. *Diabetes Care*, 37(11):3124–3131.

Porter, W. H., Yao, H. H., & Karounos, D. G. (1997). Laboratory and clinical evaluation of assays for beta-hydroxybutyrate. *American Journal of Clinical Pathology*, 107(3), 353–358.

Ross, D. S., Burch, H. B., Cooper, D. S., Greenlee, M. C., Laurberg, P., Maia, A. L., Rivkees, S. A., Samuels, V., Sosa, J. A., Stan, M. N., & Walter, M. A. (2016). 2016 American thyroid association guidelines for diagnosis and management of hyperthyroidism and other causes of thyrotoxicosis. *Thyroid*, 26(10), 1343–1421.

Rumbak, M. J., Hughes, T. A., & Kitabchi, A. E. (1991). Pseudonormoglycemia in diabetic ketoacidosis with elevated triglycerides. *American Journal of Emergency Medicine*, 9(1), 61–63.

Samuels, M. H., & Ridgway, E. C. (1992). Central hypothyroidism. *Endocrinology and Metabolism Clinics of North America*, 21(4), 903–919.

Sarlis, N. J., & Gourgiotis, L. (2003). Thyroid emergencies. *Reviews in Endocrine and Metabolic Disorders*, 4(2), 129–136.

Swee du, S., Chng, C. L., & Lim, A. (2015). Clinical characteristics and outcome of thyroid storm: A case series and review of neuropsychiatric derangements in thyrotoxicosis. *Endocrine Practice*, 21(2), 182–189.

Trzepacz, P. T., Klein, I., Roberts, M., Greenhouse, J., & Levey, G. S. (1989). Graves' disease: An analysis of thyroid hormone levels and hyperthyroid signs and symptoms. *American Journal of Medicine*, 87(5), 558–561.

Tsatsoulis, A., Johnson, E. O., Kalogera, C. H., Seferiadis, K., & Tsolas, O. (2000). Effect of thyrotoxicosis on adrenocortical reserve. *European Journal of Endocrinology*, 142(3), 231–235.

Umpierrez, G, & Freire, A. X. (2002). Abdominal pain in patients with hyperglycemic crises. *Journal of Critical Care*, 17(1), 63–67.

Unger, R. H., & Orci, L. (1981). Glucagon and the A cell: Physiology and pathophysiology. *The New England Journal of Medicine*, 304(25), 1518–1524.

Waldman, S. A., & Park, D. (1989). Myxedema coma associated with lithium therapy. *American Journal of Medicine*, 87(3), 355–356.

Zierler, K. L., & Rabinowitz, D. (1964). Effect of very small concentrations of insulin on forearm metabolism. *Journal of Clinical Investigation*, 43(5), 950–962.

9 Dermatology and Ophthalmology

Bettina Magliato

FUNDAMENTALS OF SKIN ASSESSMENT

Case Study

You are the APRN working in the critical care unit of an acute care community hospital. You are managing 10 patients this Saturday evening. Ms. G has just arrived to the unit. You received report from the ED with the following information: 72-year-old female with new altered mental status. According to the patient's daughter, she presented with a 5-day history of increasing somnolence and confusion and a new skin rash. Two weeks ago, she was started on a new medication to help with migraine prophylaxis.

Her past medical history includes HTN, mild renal insufficiency, migraines, and a mood disorder. She has no past surgical history. Her current medications include Depakote, clonazepam, Paxil, hydrochlorothiazide (HCTZ), and lisinopril. Topiramate was recently added for her migraines. She has no known drug allergies. Her vaccination history is unknown.

Her review of systems was difficult to obtain because of her altered mental status. According to her daughter, the patient has been very fatigued and sleepier than usual. She has been sleeping on the couch almost all day, every day, for the past week. Her appetite is poor, and she is not drinking enough fluids. According to the daughter, she did not seem to be short of breath or have any chest pain or palpitations. The daughter states the rash over the right eye developed yesterday. The daughter denies any other skin issues.

Your physical examination reveals the following:

- **Constitutional:** Temperature, 99.8°F; pulse, 94 bpm; respirations, 18 breaths/min; blood pressure, 110/70 mmHg. She can be roused by voice but does not respond coherently.
- **HEENT:**
  - Head: Normocephalic
  - Eyes: R eye: Mild periorbital edema, vesicular rash along inner aspect of lid and lower forehead, extending down to the tip of the nose; hyperemic conjunctivitis; EOM not evaluated due to lethargy; pupils are equal and reactive to light and accommodation

- Neck: Full range of motion (ROM), trachea is midline, no carotid bruit, JVD (jugular venous distention), Brudzinski or Kernig sign
- **Cardio**: Regular rhythm; normal rate; nondisplaced PMI (point of maximum impulse); normal heart sounds; normal S1, S2; no S3, S4; no friction rub or murmur; carotid, radial, femoral, dorsal, pedal, and posterior tibial pulses 2+ bilaterally
- **Pulmonary**: Effort normal, no respiratory distress, no accessory muscle use; breath sounds normal, no wheezes, rales, or rhonchi
- **Abdomen:** Soft, flat, normoactive bowel sounds; no tenderness when palpated; no CVA (costovertebral angle tenderness) tenderness; no hepatosplenomegaly
- **Lymph:** No adenopathy
- **Neurological**: She is lethargic and confused to place and time; her speech is slow but clear. She is unable to assess motor or sensory state; she responds to noxious stimuli by pushing you away. She moves all four extremities with normal strength. She has no facial droop. You are unable to evaluate her cranial nerves as she will not cooperate with the examination.
- **Skin**:
  - Warm and dry. Capillary refill <2 s. No clubbing or cyanosis of nails.
  - Right eye: Unilateral distribution of vesicular lesions along inner aspect of the right eye lid, lower forehead, extending down to the tip of the nose. There is mild erythema of the surrounding skin, without induration, fluctuance, or crepitus. There is periorbital edema.
  - On her coccyx/right and left inner buttock, there is a deep maroon/purple, nonblanchable skin lesion measuring 4 × 8 cm. The central area is a deflated purple blister; it is not black eschar. There is some partial thickness skin loss. No drainage, induration, fluctuance, crepitus, or warmth.

Figure 9.1 shows her facial lesions, and Figure 9.2 shows her coccyx wound.

In the ED, a workup was started for altered mental status. Labs were drawn and the results were as follows: Her urine drug screen and alcohol detection tests were negative. Her urinalysis was negative for leukocyte esterase, bacteria, and nitrates; the culture is pending. Her hepatic and renal functions are normal, but her ammonia level is elevated at 145 µmol/L (20–70). Her valproic acid level is therapeutic at 110 µg/ml (50–150).

Ms. G was admitted with a diagnosis of encephalopathy with elevated ammonia thought to be due to the concomitant use of topiramate and valproate. A treatment plan has been initiated to deal with the elevated ammonia, but what about the alterations in skin integrity? Based on the given information, what are your top three differentials? There are two areas of concern: the right eye and the coccygeal/buttock area. It is 11 p.m. on a weekend. The wound APRN is not in house. Where do you start?

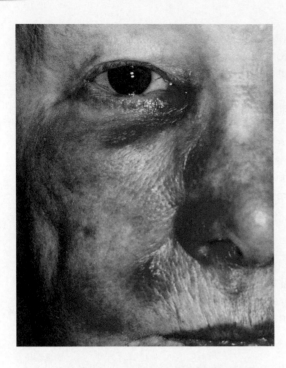

Figure 9.1 Ms. G's facial rash. (From Rapuano, C. (2018). *Cornea* (3rd ed.). Lippincott Williams & Wilkins.)

Systematic Skin Assessment

A systematic skin assessment and an accurate description of any skin lesions or abnormalities are essential to capture a reasonable list of differential diagnoses. Additional diagnostic tests and assessments can be performed to further refine the most likely diagnosis.

Key Points

Developing a systematic skin and wound assessment process and using available web-based resources that are integrated into the electronic medical record are key to ensuring that you make an accurate diagnosis and initiate an effective treatment plan for your patient.

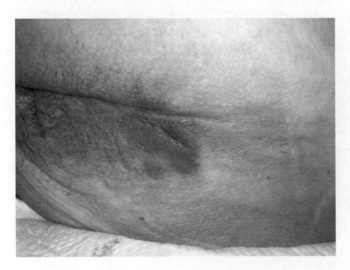

Figure 9.2 Ms. G's coccygeal wound.

Skin lesions have specific morphologic characteristics and should be described by five parameters: distribution, shape, border and margins, changes within the lesion, and pigmentation (Bryant & Nix, 2016). The underlying cause of the skin condition must be determined before a treatment plan can be initiated. Clues are obtained by the patient's history and physical examination and assessment of the location, characteristics, and distribution pattern of the lesion. Once the cause is determined, a multidisciplinary treatment plan can be developed and realistic goals established (Bryant & Nix, 2016).

Skin temperature, texture, and tone need to be assessed by palpation. Skin palpation is especially critical when assessing darkly pigmented skin. Skin with deviation from normal should be compared with the adjacent skin area or contralateral body part. Applying moisture to the area being assessed assists in identifying the color (Edsberg et al., 2016). The shift in racial and ethnic demographics in the United States makes performing a skin assessment of patients an essential skill for healthcare providers. Darker pigmented skin has unique characteristics that require more than a simple visual inspection (Bryant & Nix, 2016).

Table 9.1 provides a comprehensive guide to the morphologic characteristics of skin lesions.

Wound Assessment

The patient with a wound requires a focused assessment that incorporates systemic, psychosocial, and local factors. The differential diagnosis will drive interventions and treatment strategies. The completed assessment will exclude different etiologies as well as treatment options. Let us explore many of these factors more closely.

> ### Key Points
>
> Wound age is a critical component in determining the etiology of the wound as well as its potential for healing.

Anatomic location can provide clues to the etiology. The extent of tissue involvement and damage will guide interventions to promote tissue healing. *Tissue damage* is described as either partial thickness or full thickness:

- A partial-thickness wound has tissue destruction through the epidermis level, extending into but not through the dermis. These wounds heal by re-epithelialization.
- A full-thickness wound indicates tissue destruction through the dermis into the subcutaneous tissue and possibly into the muscle or bone. Healing of full-thickness wounds occur by neovascularization, fibroplasia, contraction, and epithelial migration from the wound edges.

Wound base tissue provides insight into the severity and duration of the wound and whether the wound is healing. A wound with evidence of granulation tissue is healing, unlike a wound with slough, eschar, or necrotic tissue. Nonviable tissue in the wound bed is associated with altered tissue oxygenation, desiccation, or increased bioburden (Bryant & Nix, 2016). Table 9.2 includes wound bed descriptors.

Wound size can be determined by various approaches, each with advantages and disadvantages. Most commonly, a three-dimensional approach (length × width × depth) is performed using a disposable paper or plastic ruler. Additionally, it is important to identify

TABLE 9.1 MORPHOLOGIC CHARACTERISTICS OF SKIN LESIONS

CHARACTERISTIC	DESCRIPTION	EXAMPLES
Distribution		
Localized	Lesion appears in one small area	Impetigo, herpes simplex, tinea corporis
Regional	Lesions involve a specific region of the body	Acne vulgaris, herpes zoster, psoriasis (flexural surfaces and skin folds)
Generalized	Lesions appear widely distributed or in numerous areas simultaneously	Urticaria, disseminated drug eruptions
Shape/Arrangement		
Round/discoid	Coin or fine shaped (no central clearing)	Nummular eczema
Oval	Ovoid shape	Pityriasis rosea
Annular	Round, active margins with central clearing	Tinea corporis, sarcoidosis
Zosteriform (dermatomal)	Following a nerve or segment of the body	Herpes zoster
Polycyclic	Interlocking or coalesced circles (formed by enlargement of annular lesions)	Psoriasis, urticarial
Linear	In a line	Contact dermatitis
Iris/target lesion	Pink macule with purple central papules	Erythema multiforme
Stellate	Star form	Meningococcal septicemia
Serpiginous	Snakelike or wavy line track	Cutaneous larva migrans
Reticulate	Netlike or lacy	Polyarteritis nodosa, lichen planus lesions of erythema infections
Morbilliform	Measles-like, maculopapular lesions that become confluent on the face and body	Measles, roseola
Border/Margin		
Discrete	Well-demarcated or defined, able to draw a line around it with confidence	Psoriasis
Indistinct	Poorly defined, borders merging into normal skin or outlying ill-defined papules	Nummular eczema
Border raised above center	Center of lesion is depressed compared with the edge	Basal cell carcinoma
Irregular	Nonsmooth or notched margin	Malignant melanoma
Advancing	Expanding at margins	Cellulitis

TABLE 9.1 MORPHOLOGIC CHARACTERISTICS OF SKIN LESIONS   (CONTINUED)

CHARACTERISTIC	DESCRIPTION	EXAMPLES
Associated Changes within Lesions		
Central clearing	An erythematous border surrounds lighter skin	Tinea eruptions
Desquamation	Peeling or sloughing of skin	Rash of toxic shock syndrome
Keratotic	Hypertrophic stratum corneum	Calluses, warts
Punctation	Central umbilication or dimpling	Basal cell carcinoma
Telangiectasias	Dilated blood vessels within lesion blanch completely, may be markers of systemic disease	Basal cell carcinoma, actinic keratosis
Pigmentation		
Flesh	Same tone as surrounding skin	Neurofibroma, some nevi
Pink	Light red undertones	Eczema, pityriasis rosea
Erythematous	Dark pink to red	Tinea eruptions, psoriasis
Salmon	Orange-pink	Psoriasis
Tan-brown	Light to dark brown	Most nevi, pityriasis versicolor
Black	Black or blue black	Malignant melanoma
Pearly	Shiny white, almost iridescent	Basal cell carcinoma
Purple	Dark red-blue-violet	Purpura, Kaposi sarcoma
Violaceous	Light violet	Erysipelas
Yellow	Waxy	Lipoma
White	Absence of color	Lichen planus

From Seidel, H. M., Ball, J. W., Dains, J. E., Flynn, J. A., Solomon, B. S., & Stewart, R. W. (2011). *Mosby's guide to physical examination* (ed 7.). Mosby.

tunnels or sinus tracts, as well as undermining, which is tissue destruction under the intact skin of the wound perimeter (Bryant & Nix, 2016).

Wound exudate should be assessed by volume (none, scant, moderate, large, copious) and type (clear, serosanguineous, sanguineous, purulent). Volume and type of exudate varies with the type of wound and can drive the type of dressing that is needed to manage the wound exudate.

Odor can be described as none, faint, or malodorous and is dependent upon wound moisture, amount of nonviable tissue, and how long the dressing has been on. Most wounds have some odor. Some dressings as well as personal body hygiene can impact wound odor (Bryant & Nix, 2016).

Wound edge reveals valuable information regarding chronicity, epithelialization status, and possibly etiology. Wound edges should be attached, moist, and flush with the wound to promote epithelial migration across the wound bed, which promotes healing. Unattached edges, also known as undermining, are present between the dermis and subcutaneous tissue. Closed wound edges are usually dry and rolled. This is premature or "epibole" closure of the wound edge and is common in chronic wounds. Cautery using silver nitrate or surgical debridement is needed to open the edges to promote healing (Bryant & Nix, 2016).

TABLE 9.2 WOUND BED DESCRIPTORS

TERM	DEFINITION
Necrotic, nonviable, or devitalized	Tissue that has died and has lost physical and biological activity
Eschar	Black, brown necrotic, devitalized tissue, can be loose or firmly adherent, hard, soft, or boggy
Slough	Soft, moist, avascular tissue; may be white, yellow, tan, or green; may be loose or firmly adherent
Scab	Crust of hardened blood and serum over the wound
Granulation tissue	Pink/red moist tissue composed of new blood vessels, connective tissue, fibroblasts, and inflammatory cells that fill an open wound when it starts to heal; typically appears deep pink or red; surface is granular, berry-like, or cobblestone
Clean, nongranulating	Absence of granulation, surface appears smooth and red but not granular and berry-like or cobblestone
Epithelial	Regenerated epidermis across the wound surface; pink and dry

From Bryant, R. A., & Nix, D. P. (2016). *Acute and chronic wounds* (ed 5.). Elsevier.

Periwound skin, the skin adjacent to the wound, is described in terms of color, texture, integrity, and temperature. Assessment of the periwound skin will provide clues to the effectiveness of the treatment plan. A macerated periwound suggests that the current dressing choice may not be adequately absorbing the volume of exudate. Dressing application and removal technique can also impact the periwound skin status. Skin stripping in the periwound area, as well as blistering, can indicate inappropriate tape selection or adhesive removal (Bryant & Nix, 2016).

Table 9.3 describes periwound skin.

All wounds have a *bacterial bioburden*, the bacteria living on the surface. The extent and significance of bioburden are dependent on many factors. Local signs of infection should be documented, whether they are present or not. Remember that not all wounds with significant bioburden will display the classic signs and symptoms of infection due to immunosuppression or biofilm presence. Overwhelming bioburden may present as delayed healing despite optimal treatment, discolored or friable granulation tissue, breakdown of the wound base, and foul odor (Bryant & Nix, 2016).

Pain in the wound can indicate infection or deterioration. Pain must be measured at each assessment and dressing change using a validated pain assessment tool.

TABLE 9.3 PERIWOUND CHARACTERISTICS

CRITERIA	DESCRIPTION
Color	Erythema, pale, white, blue, purple
Texture	Moist, dry, indurated, boggy, macerated
Temperature	Warm, cool, cold
Integrity	Denudement, maceration, excoriation, stripping, erosion, papules, pustules

Data from Bryant, R. A., & Nix, D. P. (2016). *Acute and Chronic Wounds*. Elsevier.

Differential Diagnosis

The common differential diagnosis for a coccyx/buttock wound includes the following:

- *Pressure injury*: Localized damage to the skin and underlying tissue usually over a bony prominence or related to a medical or other device are pressure injuries. The injury results from intense or prolonged pressure, or pressure combined with shear. The microclimate, nutrition, comorbidities, and perfusion greatly affect the ability of the soft tissue to tolerate pressure and shear (Edsberg et al., 2016).
- *Incontinence-associated dermatitis* is inflammation of the skin that occurs when urine or stool comes into contact with perineal/perigenital area, inner thighs, buttocks, or adjacent skin folds. Characteristics include inflammation and erythema with or without erosion or denudation (Coloplast, 2011).
- *Herpes simplex* manifests as clusters or isolated shallow lesions or blisters on the genitals, buttocks, or anal area. Herpes simplex is spread by direct contact. Immunosuppression is a risk factor. Initially, the lesions are pink or red. Later, the lesions crust over. The patient reports tingling initially, which can progress to severe pain (MedlinePlus, 2018).

Key Points

You can make a diagnosis based on your physical examination findings, ROS (review of systems), skin, and wound assessment.

Case Study

Your admission information from the ED suggests that the patient has been deteriorating at home for about a week, lying in bed with anorexia and poor hydration, indicating prolonged immobility and compromised nutrition. Her daughter reported that she has not been incontinent. These factors are risks for a pressure injury (Box 9.1). Your physical examination revealed a nonblanchable, purple/maroon area over the coccygeal and right and left inner buttock area. The area is over a bony prominence and is tender to touch. Other than her ammonia level, her labs are normal. There is no anemia or thrombocytosis. You make the diagnosis that she has a pressure injury of the coccyx that extends into the right and left inner buttock area. Using the NPIAP staging guidelines and your physical examination findings, you ascertain that this is a deep tissue injury.

Besides the pressure injury of the coccyx/buttock, the patient presented with vesicular lesions on an erythematous base over the right lower forehead and right inner eye. There is a regional distribution and a dermatomal arrangement. From the history and ROS, you know that Ms. G has had malaise and a low-grade fever in the days leading up to her admission to the hospital. The physical examination is positive for hyperemic conjunctivitis. There is no uveitis or keratitis. You notice that there are vesicular lesions on the side and the tip of the nose. You order an ophthalmology consult. Based on your physical examination finding for the eye lesions, what are your top differential diagnoses?

> ### BOX 9.1 | Deep Tissue Pressure Injury
>
> A deep tissue pressure injury is a localized area of deep red, maroon, or purple discolored skin or a blood-filled blister due to damage of underlying tissue from pressure and/or shear (Edsberg et al., 2016).
>
>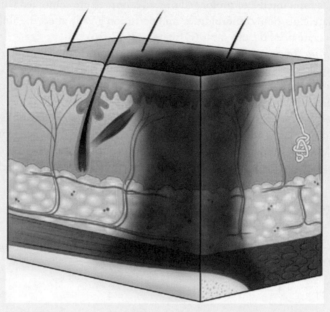
>
> Image from Taylor, C., Lynn, P., Bartlett, J. (2019). *Fundamentals of nursing* (9th ed.). Lippincott Williams & Wilkins.

Differential Diagnosis

Herpes zoster ophthalmicus (HZO) is one possible differential. Herpes zoster (shingles) is caused by varicella zoster virus (VZV) infection. In humans, primary infection with VZV occurs when the virus comes into contact with the mucosa of the respiratory tract or conjunctiva. From these sites, it is distributed throughout the body. After primary infection, the virus migrates along sensory nerve fibers to the satellite cells of dorsal root ganglia where it becomes dormant. Reactivation of VZV that has remained dormant within dorsal root ganglia, often for decades after the patient's initial exposure to the varicella virus (chickenpox), results in herpes zoster. Age is the most important risk factor for the development of herpes zoster, and the likelihood of complication increases with age. Women are more likely to develop herpes zoster than men (Albrecht & Levin, 2019; Roat, 2019).

Possible triggers include the following:

- Re-exposure to the virus
- Acute or chronic disease processes, especially malignancy and infection
- Medications
- Emotional stress

Impetigo is an acute, highly contagious gram-positive bacterial infection of the superficial layers of the epidermis. Skin lesions such as cuts, abrasions, and chickenpox can also become secondarily infected with the same pathogens that produce classic impetigo.

Impetigo occurs most commonly in children, especially those who live in hot, humid climates. Nonbullous impetigo starts with a solitary erythematous macule that quickly evolves into a vesicle or pustule and bursts. The serous contents then dry into a yellow, honey-colored crust over the erosion. This is followed by rapid spread from scratching. The skin of the face and extremities are affected most commonly, but lesions can be found anywhere. Lesions are usually asymptomatic, with occasional pruritus. Little or no surrounding erythema or edema is noted (MedlinePlus, 2018).

Case Study

Based on your physical examination and review of the patient's history and ROS, you are confident in your assessment that your patient has HZO, which is a potentially sight-threatening condition. You have already ordered an ophthalmology consult. HZO involves the ophthalmic division of the fifth cranial nerve. Roughly 50% of patients with HZO will develop direct ocular involvement if antiviral therapy is not initiated promptly. According to Ms. G's daughter, the rash presented yesterday. You noted that there are vesicular lesions along the side of her nose extending to the tip of her nose, which indicate that there is involvement of the nasociliary branch of the trigeminal nerve (V1), innervates the globe. Your early diagnosis and prompt initiation of treatment is essential to prevent progressive corneal involvement and possible vision loss (Albrecht & Hirsch, 2019).

The standard approach to treatment includes oral antiviral therapy to limit virus replication and the possible use of adjunctive topical steroid drops, per the ophthalmologist, to reduce the inflammatory response. Your immediate treatment plan includes the following:

- Famciclovir or valacyclovir for 7–10 days, with intravenous acyclovir given as needed for retinitis
- Pain medicines, for immunocompetent patients·
- Cool-to-tepid wet compresses (if tolerated); can use 5% Burow solution compresses for 30–60 min, 4–6 times a day
- Antibiotic ophthalmic ointment administered twice daily (e.g., bacitracin–polymyxin) to protect the ocular surface
- No topical antivirals (Janniger, 2019)

Topical steroids (e.g., 0.125%–1% prednisolone 2–6 times daily) must be prescribed and managed by an ophthalmologist for corneal immune disease, episcleritis, scleritis, or iritis (Albrecht & Levin, 2019). The ophthalmology consult arrives, confirms your suspicion, and agrees with your plan of care. They also order topical steroids. She remains hospitalized for 4 days. Her mental status improves to her baseline. She is discharged to short-term rehabilitation for intensive rehabilitation services and ongoing wound care. She will follow up with ophthalmology in 2 weeks.

Key Points

Keratitis and uveitis can be severe and need to be managed by an ophthalmologist. The following studies are available but not necessary unless the lesions are atypical:

- Direct fluorescent antibody (DFA) testing of vesicular fluid or a corneal lesion
- Polymerase chain reaction (PCR) testing of vesicular fluid, a corneal lesion, or blood
- Tzanck smear of vesicular fluid (lower sensitivity and specificity than DFA or PCR) (Janniger, 2019)

CLINICAL PEARLS

- Adequate lighting during skin assessment is critical for visualization.
- Always palpate the skin to assess for warmth, coolness, induration, fluctuance, crepitus, bogginess, and tenderness.
- Determine the patient's activity or degree of immobility the days leading up to the admission. This can indicate risk for pressure injury.
- Always describe what you see, especially if you are unsure about correct staging or classification.
- Moisten intact skin to visualize color, especially in darkly pigmented individuals.

REVIEW QUESTIONS

1. Performing a skin assessment on a patient with darkly pigmented skin includes all of the following **except**:
   a. Visual inspection
   b. Skin palpation
   c. Using moisture, such as an alcohol pad to highlight the color of the skin
   d. Lightly brushing a Q-tip over the skin

2. All of the following are good techniques to assess heel redness on a patient with dark skin tones **except**:
   a. Use a flashlight
   b. Use an alcohol wipe to moisten the skin for improved visualization
   c. Ask the patient if his/her heels are red
   d. Have the patient lie prone

3. HZO requires quick diagnosis and initiation of antiviral therapy to limit herpes zoster virus replication and prevent vision loss.
   a. True
   b. False

Answers: 1, d; 2, c; 3, a

REFERENCES

Albrecht, M., & Hirsch, M. (2019). Treatment of herpes zoster in the immunocompetent host. In J. Mitty (Ed.), *UpToDate*. Retrieved August 31, 2019. https://www.uptodate.com/contents/treatment-of-herpes-zoster-in-the-immunocompetent-host

Albrecht, M., & Levin, M. (2019). Epidemiology, clinical manifestations, and diagnosis of herpes zoster. In J. Mitty (Ed.), *UpToDate*. Retrieved August 31, 2019. https://www.uptodate.com/contents/epidemiology-clinical-manifestations-and-diagnosis-of-herpes-zoster

Bryant, R., & Nix, D. (2016). *Acute and chronic wounds*. Elsevier.

Coloplast. (2011). *Skin care, educational pocket guide*. https://www.coloplast.us/Documents/Skin/Skin%20Care%20Pocket%20Guide_M1235N.pdf

Edsberg, L. E., Black, J. M., Goldberg, M., McNichol, L., Moore, L., & Sieggreen, M. (2016). Revised national pressure ulcer advisory panel pressure injury staging system: Revised pressure injury staging system. *Journal of Wound, Ostomy, and Continence Nursing*, 43(6), 585–597.

Janniger, C. (2019). *Herpes zoster guidelines*. Emedicine.medscape.com. https://emedicine.medscape.com/article/1132465-guidelines

MedlinePlus. (2018). *Herpes simplex*. National Library of Medicine (US). [updated November 2, 2018]. https://medlineplus.gov/herpessimplex.html

Roat, M. (2019). *Herpes zoster ophthalmicus. Merck manual professional version*. Retrieved September 1, 2019. https://www.merckmanuals.com/professional/eye-disorders/corneal-disorders/herpes-zoster-ophthalmicus?query=herpes%20zoster%20ophthalmicusrom

Seidel, H. M., Ball, J. W., Dains, J. E., Flynn, J. A., Solomon, B. S., & Stewart, R. W. (2011). *Mosby's guide to physical examination*. Elsevier.

10

Neurological Management

Angela Starkweather   •   Cedric McKoy

INTRODUCTION

This chapter will focus on neurological emergencies and immediate interventions that must be coordinated in order to reduce neuronal injury and maximally restore physiological functioning including cognition, movement, speech, and sensation.

STROKE

Case Study

Mrs. A is a 56-year-old Black female with atrial fibrillation who has been taking warfarin for the past 5 years. She walks about 2 miles/day and denies use of alcohol, tobacco, or other substances. While getting ready to go out to dinner with her husband, she suddenly felt her left arm go numb and was not able to move her fingers or lift her arm. She called her husband to come help her, and upon hearing her symptoms, he immediately called 9-1-1. Her last known well time was 6:05 p.m.

An ambulance arrived within 10 min and the paramedics assessed Mrs. A using the Cincinnati Prehospital Stroke Severity Scale (CPSSS) which was designed to identify patients with large vessel occlusion (Table 10.1). The CPSSS is positive, so they take Mrs. A to the closest major medical center with interventional radiology (IR). In route, her prehospital vital signs were as follows: temperature, 98.7 °F; HR, 80 bpm; blood pressure, 156/88 mm Hg; respiratory rate, 16 per min; and oxygen saturation, 96% on 2 L nasal cannula. On arrival to the emergency room, she is placed on continuous heart rate, blood pressure, and oxygen saturation monitoring. A urinary catheter and rectal temperature probe are placed, and an ECG is obtained. While waiting for the rest of the team to arrive, you complete her physical examination. You find Mrs. A to be confused to time and place. She has a left facial droop, slurred speech, and left motor weakness of the upper limb (0/5) and lower limb (2/5) with decreased tone. Altered sensation to fine touch is detected. Repeat vital signs show the following: temperature, 99.0 °F; pulse, 90 bpm; blood pressure, 164/98 mm Hg; respiratory rate, 18 breaths per minute; and oxygen saturation, 99% on 2 L nasal cannula. Her pupils are equal, round, and responsive to light and accommodation (PERRLA) at 3 to 2 mm without nystagmus but with dysconjugate gaze and right gaze preference.

You use the NIH Stroke Scale (NIHSS) and find left hemiparesis and left visual/spatial neglect, with a score of 22 (Table 10.2). Blood is drawn for CBC, PT, serum electrolyte levels, cardiac biomarkers, and renal function studies, which are all WNL. Her INR is 1.4.

1. What is the likely diagnosis?
2. What are the precipitating factors?
3. What symptoms led you to the diagnosis?
4. What physical findings suggest the diagnosis?
5. What laboratory results support the diagnosis?
6. What additional laboratory tests would you order?
7. How would you treat this patient?
8. What are the possible differential diagnoses?

Based on her symptom presentation, you suspect ischemic stroke; however, other differential diagnoses to consider include a brain tumor, intracerebral hemorrhage, cerebral amyloid angiopathy, encephalopathy (hypertensive or Wernicke), hypoglycemia, complicated migraine, seizure, or conversion and somatoform disorder (Powers et al., 2019). Hypoglycemia was ruled out by the initial glucometer reading, and she has no history of migraine or seizure disorder. Other possible differentials would be adequately evaluated by imaging, followed by other diagnostic testing once the initial differential diagnosis list is more focused.

Mrs. A is immediately taken for a CTA of the head and neck. The stroke team arrives and views the CT scan, noting a hyperdense right middle cerebral artery (MCA), and right M1 cut-off (occlusion). The Alberta Stroke Program Early CT Score (ASPECTS) is 8 (Table 10.3). There is no sign of subarachnoid hemorrhage. The team speaks with Mrs. A and her husband about recombinant tissue plasminogen activator, or r-tPA (Alteplase IV) therapy. You also order a second intravenous site to be secured stat.

TABLE 10.1 CINCINNATI PREHOSPITAL STROKE SEVERITY SCALE

POINTS	DEFICIT
2 points	Conjugate gaze deviation (≥1 on NIHSS item for Gaze)
1 point	Incorrectly answers at least one of two level of consciousness questions on NIHSS (age or current month) **and** does not follow at least one of two commands (close eyes, open and close hand) (≥ on the NIHSS item for Level of Consciousness 1b and 1c))
1 point	Cannot hold arm (either right, left, or both) up for 10 sections before arm(s) fall to bed (≥2 on the NIHSS item for Motor Arm)

NIHSS, National Institutes of Health Stroke Scale.
Reprinted with permission from Katz, B. S., McMullan, J. T., Sucharew, H., Adeoye, O., & Broderick, J. P. (2015). Design and validation of the a Prehospital scale to predict stroke severity: Cincinnati Prehospital stroke severity scale. *Stroke, 46,* 1508–1512.

TABLE 10.2 NIH STROKE SCALE OVER TIME

TEST ELEMENTS	ON ADMISSION	12-HR POST tPA	24-HR POST tPA
Level of consciousness (LOC)	1	0	0
LOC questions	2	1	0
LOC commands	2	1	0
Best gaze	1	1	1
Visual field testing	2	1	1
Facial palsy	2	2	1
Motor function: arm right	0	0	0
Motor function: arm left	4	3	2
Motor function: leg right	0	0	0
Motor function: leg left	3	2	1
Limb ataxia	0	0	0
Sensory	1	1	1
Aphasia	1	1	0
Dysarthria	2	1	1
Extinction and inattention	1	1	1
Total	22	15	9

tPA, tissue plasminogen activator.

TABLE 10.3 ALBERTA STROKE PROGRAM EARLY CT SCORE (ASPECTS)

POINT	REGION(S) INVOLVED
1	Caudate
1	Putamen
1	Internal capsule
1	Insular cortex
1	M1: anterior MCA cortex corresponding to frontal operculum
1	M2: MCA cortex lateral to insular ribbon corresponding to anterior temporal lobe
1	M3: posterior MCA cortex corresponding to posterior temporal lobe
1	M4: anterior MCA territory immediately superior to M1
1	M5: lateral MCA territory immediately superior to M2
1	M6: posterior MCA territory immediately superior to M3

10-point quantitative topographic CT scan score used in patients with middle cerebral artery (MCA) stroke. An ASPECTS score <7 predicts a worse functional outcome at 3 months as well as symptomatic hemorrhage.
Reprinted with permission from Barber, P. A., Demchuk, A. M., Zhang, J., & Buchan, A. (2000). Validity and reliability of a quantitative computed tomography score in predicting outcome of hyperacute stroke before thrombolytic therapy. ASPECTS Study Group. Alberta Stroke Programme Early CT Score. *Lancet*, 355(9216), 1670–1674.

> **Key Point**
>
> The standard window of time to receive r-tPA therapy is within 4.5 hr of stroke onset. If the last known well time is beyond that window, the likelihood of benefit is significantly reduced and risk of hemorrhage increases.

Epidemiology of Stroke

An estimated 7 million Americans older than 20 years have a stroke each year (Virani et al., 2020). On average, someone in the United States has a stroke every 40 s. There are approximately 610,000 first attacks and 185,000 recurrent attacks each year: 87% are ischemic strokes, 10% are intracerebral hemorrhage, and 3% are subarachnoid hemorrhage (American Stroke Association, 2020). The prevalence of stroke in the United States increases with advancing age across sex, race, and ethnic groups. Classic signs and symptoms of stroke include facial droop, arm or extremity weakness, slurred speech, and confusion (Box 10.1). Risk factors are listed in Table 10.4.

Ischemic stroke can be broadly categorized as cardioembolic, small vessel occlusion, larger artery occlusion, or stroke of undetermined etiology. A thrombotic or embolic event causes decreased perfusion to an area of the brain. In thrombosis, the blood flow is obstructed within the blood vessel due to dysfunction of the vessel itself, usually secondary to atherosclerotic disease, and less often from arterial dissection, fibromuscular dysplasia, or an inflammatory condition. An embolic event, usually cardioembolic, blocks blood flow to brain tissue due to debris within circulation that occludes the vessel.

The MCA is the most common artery involved in ischemic stroke and irrigates the lateral cerebral cortex, part of the basal ganglia, and the internal capsule. The length of the MCA is described in segments (M1–M4) based on the distribution of blood flow. Typical signs and symptoms of MCA occlusion include facial paralysis, contralateral hemiparesis, and sensory loss of the face and upper extremity. While the lower extremity may be affected, the upper extremity symptoms usually predominate. Signs of aphasia, dysarthria, neglect, and gaze preference toward the side of the lesion may also be present.

BOX 10.1 Stroke Warning Signs and Symptoms

Sudden onset of any of the following signs and symptoms may indicate stroke:

- Numbness or weakness of face, arm, or leg
- Confusion, trouble speaking or understanding speech
- Trouble seeing in one or both eyes
- Difficulty walking, dizziness, loss of balance or coordination
- Severe headache with no known cause

The pneumonic FAST is also used to help people remember the signs of stroke:

Facial drooping, **A**rm weakness, **S**peech, **T**ime to call 9-1-1

Data from American Stroke Association. (2020). *Stroke warning signs and symptoms*. American Stroke Association.

TABLE 10.4 RISK FACTORS OF STROKE

MODIFIABLE	NONMODIFIABLE
Physical inactivity	Age
Tobacco use	Family history or prior stroke, TIA, or heart attack
Diet (high in saturated fat, salt)	Sex (higher prevalence and death rate among women)
Management of high blood pressure, diabetes mellitus, high blood cholesterol, carotid and peripheral artery disease, atrial fibrillation, sickle cell disease	Race (African Americans with higher risk of stroke)

TIA, transient ischemic attack.

The anterior cerebral artery (ACA) distribution is the medial cerebral cortex as it supplies blood to the frontal, prefrontal, primary motor, and sensory areas and supplemental motor cortices (including Broca area). Due to significant collateral blood flow provided by the anterior circulating artery, ACA infarction is relatively rare. Usual clinical presentation of ACA damage or infarction includes contralateral sensory and motor deficits of the lower extremity; however, depending on the area involved, it can also cause confusion, motor aphasia, and motor hemineglect.

The posterior cerebral artery (PCA) provides blood flow to the occipital lobe and inferior portion of the temporal lobe, as well as the thalamus, internal capsule, and other deep structures of the brain. Superficial PCA infarcts can cause visual (homonymous hemianopsia) and somatosensory (stereognosis, tactile sensation, proprioception) deficits, and rarely amnesia or cortical blindness if the infarction is bilateral. When infarction involves deep segments of the PCA, hemisensory loss and hemiparesis may be present, along with hypersomnolence and ataxia.

The vertebrobasilar arteries supply the cerebellum and brainstem. The vertebrobasilar region involves blood flow from the vertebral and basilar arteries originating in the spinal column and terminating in the Circle of Willis. Infarction of the vertebrobasilar system can cause headache, vomiting, visual-field deficits, nystagmus, ataxia, and vertigo. In addition to infarctions in these regions, cerebellar and lacunar infarctions can result. Cerebellar infarction is characterized by nausea, vomiting, headache, dysarthria, ataxia, and vertigo, while lacunar infarcts usually present as pure motor and sensory loss, hemiparesis, and/or ataxia.

Key Point

Other atypical or nontraditional symptoms of stroke—including loss of consciousness, shortness of breath, pain, and/or headache—are more prevalent among women and often lead to delayed evaluation for stroke.

The main goal of treatment in acute ischemic stroke is to preserve tissue in the ischemic penumbra, the area of tissue where perfusion is decreased but adequate enough to reduce the risk of infarction. By restoring blood flow to the oligemic tissue, the compromised region can be minimized with increased collateral flow to the area.

Contraindications to r-tPA therapy must be evaluated prior to administration and include active internal bleeding, recent head trauma or intracranial surgery, bleeding diathesis, severe uncontrolled HTN, recent stroke, or current ICH or subarachnoid hemorrhage. Serious risks of r-tPA are bleeding (conversion to hemorrhagic stroke) and orolingual angioedema, in which airway management is a priority. If angioedema develops, the IV must be stopped, the airway secured, and administration of methylprednisolone, diphenhydramine, and ranitidine or famotidine immediately provided. As bleeding can be a complication, the AGACNP instructs the team to not place any nasogastric tubes or intra-arterial pressure catheters. In addition, the AGACNP prescribes antihypertensive medications to maintain blood pressure at or below systolic blood pressure (SBP) ≤180 and diastolic blood pressure (DBP) ≤105 mm Hg. If the patient develops severe headache, acute HTN, nausea, or vomiting, or has a worsening neurological examination, the infusion is to be immediately discontinued and an emergency head CT scan will be obtained.

Case Study

You initiate r-tPA at a dose of 0.9 mg/kg (maximum dose 90 mg) over 60 min, with 10% of the dose given as a bolus over 1 min. Within several minutes of starting tPA, Mrs. A begins responding verbally and following commands. The stroke team discusses the possibility of endovascular treatment with Mrs. A and her husband, who is at the bedside. The decision is made to take Mrs. A for endovascular therapy. Angiography confirms a right M1 cut-off. A successful thrombectomy is performed with a combination of a stent-retriever and intra-arterial Alteplase IV r-tPA, with thrombolysis in cerebral infarction (TICI III) recanalization.

She is admitted to the Acute Stroke Unit with 24-hr monitoring, and referral is made for occupational therapy, speech and language therapy, and physical therapy. The nursing staff is instructed to measure blood pressure and perform neurological assessments every 15 min during and after IV r-tPA infusion for 2 hr, then every 30 min for 6 hr, and then hourly until 24 hr after IV r-tPA treatment. In reviewing her case, she received Alteplase IV r-tPA with a door-to-needle time of 45 min, 90 min from symptom onset. You continue to track her progress (Table 10.2).

Key Point

Increase the frequency of blood pressure measurements if SBP >180 mm Hg or DBP >105 mm Hg.

Treatment

Treatment during the acute period is focused on preserving normal perfusion to all body organs and maintaining normothermia and normoglycemia. Sources of hyperthermia (temperature >100.4 °F) should be identified and treated with antipyretic medications administered to lower temperature in hyperthermic patients. Patients with hypo- or hyperglycemia should be treated appropriately to achieve normoglycemia and dysphagia screening instituted prior to feeding. Enteral diet should be started within 7 days of admission after an acute stroke. For patients with dysphagia, it is reasonable to initially use nasogastric tubes for feeding in the early phase of stroke (within first 7 days if safe to place a nasogastric tube) and evaluate for percutaneous gastrostomy tubes for those with longer anticipated nutritional needs. In addition, IPC therapy is started to reduce the risk of deep vein thrombosis (DVT).

Studies have shown that progressive physical therapy for walking training conducted in a clinic or strength and balance exercises conducted at home are superior to delayed recovery initiation of physical therapy, regardless of severity of initial impairment (Duncan et al., 2007; Wonsetler & Bowden, 2017). Participants engaging in early physical therapy are 18% more likely to transition to a higher functional walking level (Nadeau et al., 2013). The Berg Balance Scale and the Stops Walking When Talking test are used to screen the patient's risk of falls, complications with ambulation, and balance.

In addition, the Center for Epidemiologic Studies Depression (CES-D) scale is used to screen for depression. All patients should be assessed regularly for poststroke depression using a standardized scale because of the prevalence and its impact on quality of life (Powers et al., 2019). Patients diagnosed with poststroke depression should be treated with antidepressants in the absence of contraindications and closely monitored to evaluate effectiveness.

For most patients with an acute ischemic stroke with atrial fibrillation, it is reasonable to initiate oral anticoagulation between 4 and 14 days after the onset of neurological symptoms. In patients with noncardioembolic acute ischemic stroke, the selection of an antiplatelet agent should be individualized on the basis of patient risk factor profiles, cost, tolerance, and known efficacy of anticoagulation agents.

Case Study

The next day, Mrs. A undergoes an MRI scan of her brain, which shows minimal infarct burden in her right MCA territory. You assess her again with the NIHSS, and the score is 15.

When Mrs. A's condition is stabilized, you work with her neurologist and PCP to coordinate referral for stroke rehabilitation and a treatment strategy tailored to her specific needs. Her NIHSS score is now 9; besides her left visual/spatial neglect, her cognitive and communication skills are intact. The physical therapist working with Mrs. A recommends rehabilitation for at least 1 week. On evaluation with the Functional Independence Measure (FIM), she does have continued motor and dexterity deficits in her left arm.

You recommend a sleep study to be done after learning that the patient snores and has periods of apnea during sleep, information that was provided by the patient's husband and the nurses caring for her.

You provide recommendations to Mrs. A's PCP regarding medication management. Since she was already taking warfarin for a history of atrial fibrillation, she will be continued on her current dose with INR monitoring. You also recommend a low-fat diet based on her lipid profile, along with regular exercise.

Risk of Recurrence

Obstructive sleep apnea not only increases the risk of initial stroke, it also increases stroke recurrence. Current studies to evaluate whether automatically adjusting continuous positive airway pressure (aCPAP) treatment for obstructive sleep apnea improves clinical outcomes and reduces recurrent vascular events are underway (Brown et al., 2020). In addition to screening for obstructive sleep apnea, it is also recommended that smokers should receive in-hospital initiation of high-intensity behavioral interventions and nicotine replacement therapy to promote smoking cessation.

For patients with hypercholesterolemia, statin therapy can be continued or initiated during the acute phase of stroke. Patients should be managed according to the most recent American College of Cardiology (ACC)/American Heart Association (AHA) Cholesterol Guidelines, which recommend a tiered approach beginning with lifestyle modification, dietary recommendations, and medication recommendations.

Case Study

The comprehensive rehabilitation plan is communicated with Mrs. A and her husband with written documentation to ensure continuity of care. She is discharged to rehabilitation to continue her progress and focus on reducing risk factors of recurrent stroke.

CLINICAL PEARLS

- Head and neck vessels should be thoroughly evaluated to assess for degree of arteriosclerosis via ultrasonography or MRI (high-resolution vessel wall imaging).
- The risk of recurrent stroke is highest during the first 90 days after the initial stroke, and 8% will have recurrence in the first year. Each patient should be assessed for strategies to reduce the risk of recurrence including aggressive HTN management, lipid-lowering therapy, antithrombotic treatment, and carotid interventions, as well as smoking cessation, low-fat diet, daily exercise, and other lifestyle modifications.

SEIZURES

Case Study

Mr. Q is an 18-year-old non-Hispanic White male who presents to the ED via ambulance after being found face down in a pool of vomit by his friend. The two friends were hanging out all night watching movies and fell asleep on the couch. In the morning, his friend tried to wake him up by shaking his shoulder, but Mr. Q started convulsing in all extremities and he remained unconscious. The friend immediately called 9-1-1, and an ambulance arrived to transport him to the nearest hospital. In the ambulance, he received oxygen via face mask. An intravenous line was started with 0.9% normal saline, and he was given 2 mg of lorazepam every 2 min for a total of 6 mg in an attempt to stop the seizure activity.

On presentation to the ED, rapid examination confirms continuing convulsive seizure activity with vital signs as follows: heart rate, 140 bpm; sinus rhythm; blood pressure, 132/80 mm Hg; respiratory rate, 26 breaths per minute on high-flow oxygen; and oxygen saturation, 95%. You quickly decide to order serum electrolytes (a basic metabolic panel) with magnesium and calcium, CBC, ABG, and toxicology to assess for the presence of cocaine, amphetamines, and alcohol. The patient is approximately 60 kg and is given 1.2 g PE (phenytoin equivalent) of IV fosphenytoin over 20 min to treat the ongoing seizure activity. He is placed on continuous monitoring, and a urinary catheter is placed.

Convulsive Status Epilepticus

Seizures are a transient occurrence of signs and symptoms due to abnormal excessive or synchronous neuronal activity in the brain. A seizure may be provoked (known cause) or unprovoked, occurring in the absence of precipitating factors or caused by static or progressive injury. Focal, or partial, seizures start on one side of the body and may not impair consciousness but can progress to involve more areas of the brain. Approximately 70% of first seizures are focal with common causes including head trauma, brain tumor or infection, stroke, or alcohol withdrawal.

In contrast, status epilepticus is a life-threatening prolonged seizure that can be caused by preexisting seizure disorder, acute cerebral injury, or systemic illness (Glauser et al., 2016). In patients with known epilepsy, the most common cause of status epilepticus is a change in medication. Historically, the International League Against Epilepsy (ILAE, 1993) defined status epilepticus as seizure of 30 min duration or longer in which function is not regained between ictal events. However, due to neurological and cardiovascular insults that can occur with prolonged seizure activity, this definition has fallen out of favor and every case of status epilepticus should be managed as a medical emergency (Leitinger et al., 2020). In most cases, immediate treatment with a benzodiazepine will cease seizure activity; however, when continued or recurrent seizure activity is seen, more aggressive management is immediately warranted (Table 10.5).

Nonconvulsive status epilepticus is seizure activity without convulsions and can be sometimes difficult to identify with patients who already have an altered level of consciousness. In fact, this condition is usually associated with unexplained comas or altered level of consciousness and is prevalent in patients with TBI, subarachnoid hemorrhage, and cerebral malignancy. Diagnosis is made by continuous EEG monitoring.

Case Study

You quickly access Mr. Q's electronic medical record to determine whether he has a history of known epilepsy, and you find that he does not. The paramedics are questioned regarding how the seizure started, to identify any signs of a focal seizure, which could indicate a mass lesion.

Mr. Q continues to have tonic-clonic seizure activity and has not regained consciousness. You prepare for intubation out of concern for airway protection, and the need for intubation is confirmed with the ABG analysis. Rapid sequence intubation (RSI) is carried out with assistance from the anesthesia service using alfentanil 1 mg, thiopental 350 mg, and suxamethonium 100 mg. His seizure activity ceases, and he is taken to radiology for a head CT with contrast to assess for a neurological lesion, such as a mass or tumor. You also prepare for a lumbar puncture to assess for meningitis or encephalitis. The scan shows an acute right frontal ICH with vasogenic edema and a prominent tangle of vessels located at the medial aspect of the right frontal hemorrhage. This is suspected to be an arteriovenous malformation (AVM). The patient is transferred to the neuro ICU (NICU) for continued observation. A PT/PTT is ordered for possible surgical correction, and you evaluate his medical history and medication list for coagulation factor deficiency, severe thrombocytopenia, or the need to use reversal agents for anticoagulants (Griffiths et al., 2017).

TABLE 10.5 PHASES OF TREATMENT FOR CONVULSIVE STATUS EPILEPTICUS

Stabilization Phase: 0–5 min

- Airway, breathing, circulation, disability
- Assess oxygenation
  - Provide supplemental oxygen via nasal cannula/mask
  - Consider intubation if respiratory assistance is needed
- Time seizure from onset, monitor vital signs
- Initiate ECG monitoring
- Attempt IV access and collection of laboratory test results
- Obtain finger-stick glucose
  - If glucose <60 mg/dl then
    - Adults: 100 mg thiamine then 50 ml D50 W IV
    - Children >2 years: 2 ml/kg D25 W IV
    - Children <2 years: 4 ml/kg D12 W IV

Initial Therapy Phase: 5–20 min

First-line options (choose one):

- Intravenous lorazepam (0.1 mg/kg/dose, max: 4 mg/dose, may repeat dose once
- Intramuscular midazolam (10 mg for > 40 kg, 5 mg for 13–40 kg, single dose)
- Intravenous diazepam (0.15–0.2 mg/kg/dose, max: 10 mg/dose, may repeat dose once)

If first-line options unavailable, choose one of the following:

- Intravenous phenobarbital (15 mg/kg/dose, single dose)
- Rectal diazepam (0.2–0.5 mg/kg, max: 20 mg/dose, single dose)
- Intranasal midazolam/buccal midazolam

Second Therapy Phase: 20–40 min

Second-line options (choose one and give as a single dose):

- Intravenous fosphenytoin (20 mg PE/kg, max: 1,500 mg PE/dose, single dose)
- Intravenous valproic acid (40 mg/kg, max: 3,000 mg/dose, single dose)
- Intravenous levetiracetam (60 mg/kg, max: 4,500 mg/dose, single dose)

Third Therapy Phase: 40–60 min

Choices include repeat second-line options or intubation with anesthetic doses of either thiopental, midazolam, pentobarbital, or propofol (all with continuous EEG monitoring)

ECG, electrocardiogram; EEG, electroencephalogram; PE, phenytoin equivalent.
Data from Glauser, T., Shinnar, S., Gloss, D., Alldredge, B., Arya, R., Bainbridge, J., Bare, M., Bleck, T., Dodson, W. E., Garrity, L., Jagoda, A., Lowenstein, D., Pellock, J., Riviello, J., Sloan, E., & Treiman, D. M. (2016). Evidence-based guideline: Treatment of convulsive status epilepticus in children and adults. Report of the guideline committee of the American Epilepsy Society. *Epilepsy Currents, 16*(1), 48–61.

Treatment of Intracranial Hemorrhage

Patients with ICH and severe coagulation factor deficiency or severe thrombocytopenia should receive appropriate factor replacement therapy. If INR is elevated due to vitamin K antagonists (most common, warfarin), patients should receive therapy to replace vitamin K–dependent factors and correct the INR and receive intravenous vitamin K.

For patients presenting with ICH and SBP >220 mm Hg, consider aggressive reduction of blood pressure with continuous intravenous infusion and frequent blood pressure monitoring. This is typically managed with labetalol push (initial bolus of 20 mg IV followed by 20–80 mg IV bolus every 10 min; maximum 300 mg), labetalol drip (0.5–2 mg/min as IV loading infusion following an initial 20 mg IV bolus; maximum 300 mg), or nicardipine drip (5–15 mg/hr as IV infusion; some patients may require up to 30 mg/hr).

Case Study

The AGACNP in the NICU assesses Mr. Q on arrival. The head of bed is at 30°, and he remains on mechanical ventilation at a rate of 16 breaths per minute. His vital signs are as follows: temperature, 98.7 °F; BP, 126/76 mm Hg; HR, 88 bpm; and oxygen saturation, 98%. On examination, he opens his eyes to voice but is unable to follow commands and withdraws from noxious stimuli. His GCS score is 8. His pupils are 3 mm, equal in size, and reactive to light bilaterally. Babinski sign is absent. He is diaphoretic, with a regular heart rate and normal S1 and S2, and no appreciable murmurs, rubs, or gallops. His lungs are clear to auscultation bilaterally. He has 2+ dorsalis pedis pulses. He is administered 100 mg IV infusion of phenytoin every 8 hr to control seizure activity, and continuous EEG monitoring is ordered.

An hour later, the nurse caring for Mr. Q reports that he is no longer opening his eyes to verbal stimuli and is not responding to pain. The AGACNP confirms and, given his deteriorating neurological status, prepares for placement of a parenchymal fiberoptic bolt to measure his intracranial pressure (ICP). His initial ICP is 30 mm Hg, and he receives a rapid intravenous bolus of 50 g of mannitol and 500 ml of 3% saline to manage the cerebral edema. A radial arterial catheter is placed, and a norepinephrine intravenous drip is started with instruction to titrate in order to maintain cerebral perfusion pressure (CPP) between 60 and 80 mm Hg.

Key Point

To calculate the cerebral perfusion pressure (CPP), use these equations:

Pulse pressure = Systolic blood pressure − diastolic blood pressure
Mean arterial pressure (MAP) = Diastolic blood pressure + 1/3 (pulse pressure)
Cerebral perfusion pressure (CPP) = MAP − ICP

Case Study

After stabilizing his CPP, Mr. Q is moved to the angiography suite for a four-vessel angiogram, which confirms an AVM in the right frontal lobe, and endovascular embolization is used to reduce blood flow through the AVM. The patient is taken the next day to the OR for microsurgical resection and returns to the NICU for continued observation.

On post-op day 1, Mr. Q's condition is stable. He is awake, alert, and able to nod his head (yes/no) to questions. His ventilator is titrated to continuous positive airway pressure, and he has SCDs for DVT prophylaxis. He is extubated later that day without incident and is titrated to oxygen per nasal cannula, which is subsequently removed. On follow-up evaluation, his GCS score is 15. He is able, oriented to person, place, and time, and follows all commands. He has fluent speech with mild dysarthria. His sensation is intact, and motor strength is noted as weakness of left upper extremity strength of 4/5, with lower extremity strength including hip flexion of 5/5, knee extension of 5/5, and foot dorsiflexion of 5/5. His right upper and lower limb strength are normal. He passes a swallow evaluation and is started on a clear liquid diet with orders placed for physical and occupational therapy. He is transferred to the floor on postoperative day 2, and his medications are all switched to be taken by mouth.

Although Mr. Q presented with a provoked seizure that required immediate intervention with antiepileptic medications, the inciting condition (the AVM) is now removed. However, the AGACNP in the NICU recommends that he continue the medication, phenytoin, until a thorough follow-up can be coordinated with the neurologist, who will decide on continuation or titration. The AGACNP provides Mr. Q with information about AVMs, the surgery that was performed, and follow-up to check on the microsurgical dissection wound in 2 weeks in the neurosurgical follow-up clinic. For prophylaxis of infection, he is prescribed an antibiotic for 1 week. Mr. Q is provided with information about the medical and social consequences of seizures and safety considerations. Activities that lower the seizure threshold, including sleep deprivation, stress, alcohol intake, drug use, and strobe lights, are reviewed. Risks for working at heights and with heavy machinery are discussed with recommendations to avoid tub baths, scuba diving, climbing, or unobserved swimming. Driving restrictions vary by state, and most do not require the healthcare provider to report a history of seizure activity to the motor vehicle administration. The AGACNP discusses the risks of driving with a history of seizures and legal rules and responsibilities for driving and encourages him to self-report and continue to follow-up with the neurologist for continued workup and titration of medications. These discussions are documented in the patient's chart, and he is discharged home with home-based physical and occupational therapy.

CLINICAL PEARLS

With aggressive blood pressure management, close monitoring of end-organ function is indicated (neurological status, electrolytes and other laboratory tests, and urinary output).

HEADACHES

Case Study

Mr. R is a 40-year-old obese Hispanic male with a history of migraine headaches since the age of 18 years, chronic back pain, CHF (last ejection fraction [EF] 55% in 2019), and bipolar disorder who presents with an extremely severe headache. The patient reports being diagnosed with migraine at the age of 18 years. He is depressed and has insomnia but denies suicidal intention. He has continued to have chronic headaches for the past 20 years with worsening severity and frequency in the last few months. The pain varies from 4 to 10/10 with some improvement by OTC NSAIDs, but his other medication used to treat the migraines (tramadol) no longer works. The pain is mostly throbbing in the bilateral frontal area and behind the eyes, and he notes + photosensitivity and reports nausea/vomiting with the migraine attacks. Over the past month, he has had projectile vomiting with the headaches. He also complains of word-finding difficulty, memory problems, and chronic neck and back pain that is controlled with gabapentin.

His past medical history includes HTN, headache, and bipolar affective disorder. He takes the following medications:

- Bupropion (Wellbutrin) 200 mg tables
- Gabapentin (Neurontin) 300 mg capsule
- Ziprasidone (Geodon) 80 mg capsule
- Nicotine (NicoDerm CQ) 14 mg/24 hr patch
- Zolpidem (Ambien) 10 mg tablet
- Lisinopril (Zestril) 10 mg tablet
- Aripiprazole (Abilify) 15 mg tablet
- Cyclobenzaprine (Flexeril) 10 mg tablet
- Divalproex (Depakote) 500 mg tablet
- Furosemide (Lasix) 10 mg tablet
- Ibuprofen (Motrin) 400 mg tablet
- Trazodone (Desyrel) 50 mg tablet
- Tramadol (Ultram) 50 mg tablet

He has no known allergies.

Mr. R's social history reveals that he is unemployed and lives with his mother. He has smoked 1 pack per day for the past 20 years but is currently trying to quit and is on a nicotine patch. His family history is as follows: mother, DM type 2; and father, CHF (died at the age of 55 years).

His review of systems is documented as the following:

- Constitutional: The patient denies fever chills or weight loss. Headaches have been more severe and frequent, + photosensitivity, + nausea, and vomiting.
- HEENT: Episodes of blurry vision but denies congestion, sore throat, or otalgia.
- Respiratory: Denies shortness of breath, wheezing, or sputum production.

- Cardiovascular: Denies chest pain, palpitations, DOE, edema, or syncope.
- Gastrointestinal: The patient has been throwing up with projectile vomiting for the past month when migraine headaches worsen. He denies abdominal pain, hematemesis, or diarrhea.
- Genitourinary: He denies dysuria or urgency.
- Musculoskeletal: He reports intermittent weakness.
- Psychiatric/behavioral: He reports depressed mood.

His current vital signs are as follows: temperature, 100.0 °F; BP, 154/88 mm Hg; HR, 72 bpm; and oxygen saturation, 94% on room air. On physical examination, Mr. R is alert and oriented x 3, but has difficulty naming two of four familiar objects and gets three correct on a six-item recall. His pupils are 4 to 3 mm and sluggish, and his extraocular movement (EOM) is intact. His jaw moves without crepitus or pain. His CN II-VII is intact with full sensation throughout all dermatomes. Motor strength shows 4/5 on right biceps/triceps and hip flexion/knee extension/foot dorsiflexion. Left upper and lower extremities are 5/5 throughout. He has full range of cervical motion without crepitus or pain. His cardiovascular system shows normal S1 and S2 without appreciable murmurs, rubs, or gallops. His lungs are clear to auscultation bilaterally. He has 1+ dorsalis pedis pulses.

Headaches

Headaches are one of the most common reasons that patients seek medical assistance, with lifetime prevalence of 66% in the United States, including up to 16% for migraines, 78% for tension headaches, and 1% for cluster headaches. While most headaches are benign and resolve with common analgesics, such as acetaminophen or NSAIDs, there are red flag symptoms to consider, including thunderclap onset, fever and meningismus, papilledema with focal signs or reduced level of consciousness, or acute glaucoma. Other signs that are urgent include temporal arteritis, papilledema without focal signs or reduced level of consciousness, systemic illness, or new headache with cognitive changes in an elderly patient.

When presented with headache, diagnosis is focused on whether the pattern, frequency, and duration are consistent with a primary headache or secondary headache. Possible indicators of a secondary headache include onset after the age of 50 years, unexplained focal signs, unusual aura symptoms or headache precipitants, and atypical headaches. In addition, secondary headaches may arise from neck movement as well as jaw symptoms, which should both be assessed during the physical examination. Medication overuse is a common problem, especially for patients with a history of headaches, and can be managed in the outpatient setting to monitor use and systematically titrate medications. In most cases, acute management of noncomplex migraine is managed with a triptan and NSAID or antiemetic. Tension-type headaches are typically treated with analgesics, and patients may benefit from preventative therapies, such as amitriptyline or topiramate, as well as nonpharmacological interventions such as acupuncture. Cluster headache is the most common of the trigeminal autonomic cephalalgias, and patients usually report excruciating unilateral pain in an orbital, supraorbital, or temporal distribution lasting up to 3 hr for each attack, with a frequency of up to eight per day at predictable times (Burish & Rozen, 2019). The attacks occur in bouts of weeks to months and may repeat multiple times in a year. Usually abortive therapy is used with subcutaneous or intranasal sumatriptan. In addition, high-flow oxygen via a nonrebreather mask at 12–15 L/min for up to 20 min may provide relief. Transitional therapy is used to get patients through a crisis period while starting prevention management, usually with prednisolone tapered over 2 weeks. Preventative therapy may include verapamil. Patients should be evaluated with ECG before starting verapamil, as well as with dosage increase, to assess for prolonged P to R wave interval. With any patient presenting with a new headache, it is important to provide a thorough examination to assess for any possible mass lesion, which often presents with headache, nausea, projectile vomiting, and/or altered level of consciousness.

Key Point

For any change in headache pattern or new pattern of headache in people older than 50 years, imaging should be considered.

Case Study

Due to the change in Mr. R's headache severity and frequency, an MRI of the head is ordered to rule out a brain lesion, such as tumor, arterial aneurysm, AVM, or abscess. Laboratory tests are ordered, including a comprehensive metabolic panel, CBC, and PT/PTT, and an ECG is obtained. The MRI shows a large heterogeneously enhancing tumor in the corpus callosum with severe mass effect. To monitor his condition overnight, he is transferred to the neuro stepdown unit with continuous monitoring of vital signs and cardiology consultation for surgical clearance. He is scheduled for craniotomy and microsurgical removal of the tumor. He is provided with a clear liquid diet for the evening with orders for nothing after midnight, SCD for DVT prophylaxis, and a second-generation antibiotic to be administered prior to surgery. His histopathology revealed a grade 3 anaplastic oligodendroglioma.

His recovery from surgery is uneventful, and physical and occupational therapy is ordered to assess his level of independence. He remains with mild right-sided weakness, word-finding difficulty, and memory problems that will require home-based physical and occupational therapy. The consultation from the on-service oncologist recommends radiation therapy and adjuvant temozolomide chemotherapy, and he is scheduled for follow-up as an outpatient the following week. He is provided with instructions on resuming his home medications and follow-up in the neurosurgical clinic in 2 weeks for removal of staples from his craniotomy incision. Documentation of the hospital stay and surgery are sent to his primary healthcare provider for continuity of care and management of his CHF, mental health, and headaches.

REVIEW QUESTIONS

1. A stroke involving the ACA would characteristically cause which of the following?
   a. Facial droop
   b. Upper extremity weakness
   c. Sensory loss of the face and upper extremity
   d. Motor deficits of the lower extremity

2. In a patient with increased ICP (over 20 mm Hg), which of the following would be prescribed to reduce cerebral edema?
   a. Labetalol push
   b. Mannitol push
   c. Norepinephrine drip
   d. A benzodiazepine

3. A red flag condition associated with headache includes which of the following?
   a. Fever and meningismus
   b. Temporal arteritis
   c. Papilledema without focal signs
   d. Systemic illness

Answers: 1, d; 2, b; 3, a

REFERENCES

American Stroke Association. (2020). *Stroke warning signs and symptoms*. American Stroke Association.

Brown, D. L., Durkalski, V., Durmer, J. S., Broderick, J, P., Zahuranec, D. B., Levine, D. A., Anderson, C. S., Bravata, D. M., Yaggi, H. K., Morgenstern, L. B., Moy, C. S., & Chervin, R. D. (2020). Sleep for Stroke Managemenet and Recovery Trial (Sleep SMART): Rationale and methods. *International Journal of Stroke*, 1747493020903979. https://doi.org/10.1177/1747493020903979

Burish, M. J., & Rozen, T. D. (2019). Trigeminal autonomic cephalalgias. *Neurology Clinics*, 37(4), 847–869.

Duncan, P. W., Sullivan, K. J., Behrman, A. L., Azen, S. P., Wu, S. S., Nadeau, S. E., Dobkin, B. H., Rose, D. K., Tilson, J. K., & LEAPS Investigative Team. (2007). Protocol for the Locomotor Experience Applied Post-Stroke (LEAPS) trial: A randomized controlled trial. *BMC Neurology*, 7, 39.

Glauser, T., Shinnar, S., Gloss, D., Alldredge, B., Arya, R., Bainbridge, J., Bare, M., Bleck, T., Dodson, W. E., Garrity, L., Jagoda, A., Lowenstein, D., Pellock, J., Riviello, J., Sloan, E., & Treiman, D. M. (2016). Evidence-based guideline: Treatment of convulsive status epilepticus in children and adults. Report of the guideline committee of the American Epilepsy Society. *Epilepsy Currents*, 16(1), 48–61.

Griffiths, C. L., Vestal, M. L., Livengood, S. J., & Hicks, S. (2017). Reversal agents for oral anticoagulants. *Nurse Practitioner*, 42(11), 8–14.

International League Against Epilepsy. (1993). Guidelines for epidemiologic studies on epilepsy: Commission on Epidemiology and Prognosis, International League Against Epilepsy. *Epilepsia*, 34, 592–596.

Leitinger, M., Trinka, E., Zimmermann, G., Granbichler, C. A., Kobulashvili, T., & Siebert, U. (2020). Epidemiology of status epilepticus in adults: Apples, pears and oranges – a critical review. *Epilepsy & Behavior*, 103, 106720.

Nadeau, S. E., Wu, S. S., Dobkin, B. H., Azen, S. P., Rose, D. K., Tilson, J. K., Cen, S. Y., Duncan, P. W., & LEAPS Investigative Team. (2013). Effects of task-specific and impairment-based training compared with usual care on functional walking ability after inpatient stroke rehabilitation: LEAPS trial. *Neurorehabilitation & Neural Repair*, 27(4), 370–380.

Powers, W. J., Rabinstein, A. A., Ackerson, T., Adeoye, O. M., Bambakidis, N. C., Becker, K., Biller, J., Brown, M., Demaerschalk, B. M., Hoh, B., Jauch, E. C., Kidwell, C. S., Leslie-Mazwi, T. M., Ovbiagele, B., Scott, P. A., Sheth, K. N., Southerland, A. M., Summers, D. V., & Tirschwell, D. L. (2019). Guidelines for the early management of patients with acute ischemic stroke: 2019 update to the 2018 guidelines for the early management of acute ischemic stroke. A guideline for healthcare professionals from the America Heart Association/American Stroke Association. *Stroke*, 50, e344–e418.

Virani, S. S., Alonso, A., Benjamin, E. J., Bittencourt, M. S., Callaway, C. W, Carson, A. P., Chamberlain, A. M., Chang, A. R., Cheng, S., Delling, F. N., Djousse, L., Elkind, M. S. V., Ferguson, J. F., Fornage, M., Khan, S. S., Kissela, B. M., Knutson, K. L., Kwan, T. W., Lackland, D. T., …Tsao, C. W., & American Heart Association Council on Epidemiology and Prevention Statistics Committee and Stroke Statistics Subcommittee. (2020). Heart disease and stroke statistics – 2020 update: A report from the American Heart Association. *Circulation*, 141, e139–e596.

Wonsetler, E. C., & Bowden, M. G. (2017). A systematic review of mechanisms of gait speed change post-stroke. Part 2: Exercise capacity, muscle activation, kinetics, and kinematics. *Topics in Stroke Rehabilitation*, 24(5), 394–403.

11

Musculoskeletal Management

Sandra Barnosky   •   Arthur Kasimer-Colon

HIP FRACTURES

Case Study

You are an APRN working in the ED. Mr. P is an 81-year-old male who presents to the ER via ambulance after a mechanical fall at home. The patient tripped over a throw rug and fell onto his left side. He was unable to get up, so he used Medic alert for assistance. He denies hitting his head or losing consciousness. He is complaining of left-sided pain especially in his hip region.

His past medical history is significant for type 2 diabetes, currently on insulin therapy; HTN; myocardial infarction; COPD; OSA-CPAP–compliant obstructive sleep apnea; benign prostatic hypertrophy; osteoarthritis; and osteoporosis with an atraumatic clavicle fracture 1 year ago. Past surgical history includes multiple right wrist surgeries with fusion of wrist, left wrist open reduction and internal fixation (ORIF), and intestinal resection. Current medication include Toprol 50 mg daily, aspirin 81 mg daily, NPH insulin 50 units every morning, Janumet XR 100/1,000 daily, Tamsulosin 0.4 mg at bedtime, Lasix 40 mg daily, potassium 20 mg daily, Dulera inhaler 2 inhalations daily, and Proair inhaler 2 puffs Q6 hours as needed. He has no known drug allergies. He does not currently use tobacco but has a 30 pack-year smoking history having quit at age 50. He has some social alcohol use with three drinks weekly. He denies any substance use. He has not had anything to eat or drink since 8 p.m. last evening besides a small sip of water with his morning pills, which he has taken, and the time is now 10 a.m.

His review of symptoms reveals the following: He denies any fever or chills. He has no difficulty swallowing. He wears glasses. He denies chest pain or palpitations. He endorses DOE. He is unable to ambulate stairs at baseline due to arthritis. He has no cough or sputum. He endorses swelling in his right lower leg greater than the left. He denies any abdominal pain, weight loss, or heart burn. He has normal bowel movements. He does have urinary frequency related to diuretic usage but denies burning or pain with urination. He has chronic low back pain (LBP) and right knee pain worse than left knee pain, especially with walking and standing. The patient typically ambulates with a four-wheeled walker.

His physical examination is as follows: temperature, 98.2 °F; pulse, 88 bpm; respiratory rate, 20 per min; blood pressure, 158/86 mm Hg. His stated weight and height are 273 pounds and 5′ 1″, respectively. His lung sounds are clear throughout all lung fields. The cardiovascular examination reveals a regular rate and rhythm, normal S1, S2, and no murmur, gallop, or rub. His abdomen is soft, rounded, and nontender with normal bowel sounds. The examination of his neck reveals that he has no pain with flexion or extension of his cervical spine or side to side turning, and it is nontender to midline palpation. The examination of his extremities reveals a scar to his right dorsal hand and wrist with limited flexion mobility, and he has full ROM of his fingers, elbow, and shoulder. He has a palpable radial pulse with normal sensation. Left upper extremity reveals a scar at dorsal wrist with full ROM of fingers, hand, wrist, elbow, and shoulder. His left lower extremity appears shortened compared with the right. His foot and leg are externally rotated. There is 1+ edema to the foot. He complains of pain in his hip when performing a log roll maneuver (repetitive internal and external rotation of the femur). He refuses to range his hip or knee due to severe pain. He has full ROM of the ankle. Sensation is intact to the dorsal and plantar foot with a palpable dorsal pedis pulse. He has an intact flexor and extensor hallucis longus and tibialis anterior. His right lower extremity has no visible deformity or shortening and he has no pain with hip log roll. He has full ROM of his hip, knee, ankle, and foot and an intact flexor and extensor hallucis longus and tibialis anterior.

Based on the information, list your top differential diagnosis. What tests do you need to order to rule out your diagnosis?

Joint Pain

The causes of joint pain range from common to rare and from minor to life threatening. Missed fractures resulting in incorrect weight bearing recommendations or missed joint infections can lead to worsening joint damage or untreatable infections that can overwhelm the body. Careful review of traumatic vs. nontraumatic history as well as physical examination helps to narrow the diagnosis.

Differentials may include hip fracture; a tear to a ligament, tendon, or muscle; tumor or metastasis; or infection/septic arthritis. Findings for common differentials are included in Table 11.1.

Diagnostic Imaging

Diagnosis requires plain radiographs of the involved hip and pelvis. If a patient has pain but imaging shows no fracture, further imaging may be needed. Other scans you may consider for possible occult fracture include

1. Bone scan
2. MRI
3. CT scan

TABLE 11.1 COMMON DIFFERENTIALS FOR JOINT PAIN	
DIFFERENTIAL	FINDINGS
Hip fracture	Hip or groin pain Leg rotated and/or shortened
Ligament, tendon, or muscle injury	Hip, leg, or groin pain No fracture on x-ray Possible swelling or bruising
Tumor or metastasis	Hip, leg, or groin pain History of cancer Possible fall *after* feeling pain or "hearing crack" Mass, lesion, or tumor on x-ray
Infection/septic arthritis	Hip or groin pain Fever Abnormal laboratory test results/inflammatory markers Possible recent infection (urinary tract, dental abscess, pneumonia, etc.)

Data from Stern, S. D., Cifu, A. S., & Altkorn, D. (2015). *Symtom to diagnosis: An Evidence-based guide* (3rd ed.). McGraw-Hill Education.

CT scans are usually the quickest and least costly examination; however, magnetic resonance images are shown to be 100% sensitive in confirming a hip fracture when plain radiographs are negative. MRI is the scan of choice for detecting occult fractures. Bone scan of the hip is 98% sensitive in confirming the presence of a hip fracture (Ramponi et al., 2018).

Case Study

You order a supine low AP pelvis, dedicated left hip, and left shoot through cross-table lateral x-ray series. In addition, you order a CBC with differential, a basic metabolic panel, PT/INR, type and screen, and ECG. Images obtained in the ED are as seen in Figures 11.1–11.3.
   What is your next step?

Etiology and Risk Factors

Hip fractures are becoming increasingly common due to the aging population. They are more common in women (80%) than in men and more common in white patients than in black patients. They are associated with significant morbidity and mortality. They occur most often in elderly patients after ground-level falls or low-energy trauma. Decreased bone mineral density is also a major factor. It is important to know that the United States has the highest incidence of fractures worldwide. In terms of healing potential, intracapsular femoral neck fractures have a lower healing potential, as the fracture is bathed in synovial fluid, which limits callus formation. A systematic approach is recommended to assess, diagnose, and treat a patient with a hip fracture (Egol et al., 2015).

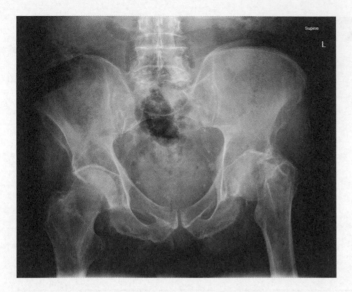

Figure 11.1 AP pelvic x-ray of left displaced femoral neck fracture.

CLINICAL PEARLS

- Early physical assessment and evaluation of radiological findings are essential.
- Pre-injury mobility and overall health are essential for guiding operative vs. non-operative treatment.
- Early medical stabilization for operative treatment is important in decreasing mortality and improving patient outcomes.

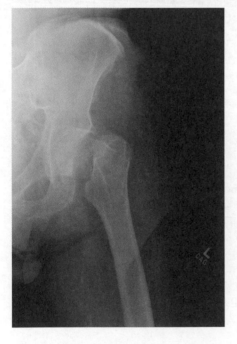

Figure 11.2 AP hip x-ray of the left hip again demonstrating a displaced femoral neck fracture.

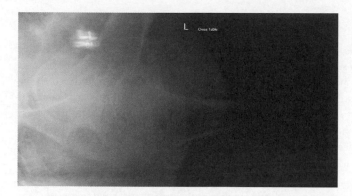

Figure 11.3 Cross-table lateral x-ray of the displaced left femoral neck fracture.

Prognosis

.   Outcomes differ depending on whether the fracture needs surgical vs. nonsurgical treatment and additionally by the various types of surgical treatment. Surgical treatment can be used as a palliative procedure as well as to increase the potential for mobility. Mortality from hip fracture is 25%–30% at 1 year (Keene et al., 1993).

Hip Fracture Types

Femoral neck fractures occur at junction between the head and the neck within the capsule of the hip joint. There is an interruption in the blood supply of the femoral head when the fracture is displaced, which can lead to osteonecrosis in 20% of these injuries. For this reason, femoral neck fractures typically require a hemiarthroplasty. Nondisplaced fractures have lower risk of disruption of blood flow (Ramponi et al., 2018).

Intertrochanteric hip fractures occur between the greater and lesser trochanters of the proximal femur. There is a good blood supply to this area, so they usually heal well. These can be fixed with either a sliding hip screw or a cephalomedullary nail depending on fracture displacement.

Subtrochanteric hip fractures occur in the proximal femoral shaft just distal to the lesser trochanter. These fractures can be seen not only in the elderly but also in high-energy trauma patients. Due to the muscular attachments, these fractures tend to displace significantly. These are often treated with long cephalomedullary nails. There can be complications of malunion or nonunion of these fractures.

Presentation

Patients typically present with groin pain and inability to bear weight on the affected leg after a fall, or they complain of groin or hip pain that radiates to the knee. When lying supine, the affected leg will typically appear shortened and externally rotated on physical examination if the fracture is displaced. Pain will worsen with both external and internal rotation of the hip joint (log roll). The patient may refuse to perform or have pain with distal motion, especially of the knee. Patients rarely initially present with ecchymosis or swelling in the hip area, although, depending on body habitus, a deformity to the proximal femur may be notable (Ramponi et al., 2018). A full body survey should be done to assess the unaffected extremities and body for any associated trauma that may not be apparent to the patient given the substantive known injury.

Preoperative Management

Evaluation of mental status, significant chronic and acute medical problems, and suitability for the patient to undergo surgical repair is needed. Advanced directives, patient goals, and prior activity level should be considered and factored into the decision to undergo surgical fixation. Immediate surgical repair (within 48 hr) is associated with reduced pain and decreased LOS (Orosz et al., 2004). It also allows for earlier ambulation and mobility, which may prevent further deconditioning or other medical issues associated with immobility. However, immediate surgical repair does not reduce mortality or long-term functionality.

Case Study

Mr. P is an elderly man, who is ambulatory at baseline, presented to the emergency setting with a closed, displaced fracture of his left femoral neck. For most patients, this type of injury leads to operative treatment for different reasons. In Mr. P's case, he is ambulatory at baseline. Choosing not to have surgical repair would lead to extended weeks of non–weight bearing. Given his comorbidities, including his BMI, this would likely result in the patient being on strict bed rest as he likely cannot support his full weight on one leg or tolerate the pain of sitting in a chair with an unfixed fracture. Even if Mr. P was nonambulatory at baseline, fixation of his fracture could still be warranted as a palliative procedure for pain control, which can increase quality of life. For many patients, the risks associated with surgical intervention are less than the risks associated with prolonged immobility.

You determine that Mr. P needs surgical intervention. Do you need to call any consultants in for additional evaluation? What tools can you use to help assess risk in the preoperative patient? You can use the American College of Surgeons National Surgical Quality Improvement Program (ACS NSQIP) Surgical Risk Calculator and the American Society of Anesthesiologists (ASA) classification. What are typical surgical options for hip fractures? Are any more or less invasive procedures available? What will you recommend for Mr. P?

Risk Assessment

The ACS NSQIP® Surgical Risk Calculator (Figure 11.4) is a revolutionary tool that quickly and easily estimates patient-specific postoperative complication risks for almost all operations (MDedge:Surgery, 2013). The Surgical Risk Calculator allows clinicians to enter a total of 22 preoperative patient risk factors about their patients. The calculator then estimates the potential risks of mortality and eight important postoperative complications and displays these risks in comparison to an average patient's risks. The ACS NSQIP Surgical Risk Calculator yields excellent prediction results for death, overall complications, and serious complication rates, as well as six additional postoperative complications: pneumonia, heart problems, surgical site infection, UTI, blood clots, and kidney failure. In addition, the Surgical Risk Calculator estimates a customized length of hospital stay for the patient. However, other hard-to-measure factors may increase a patient's risk of postoperative

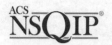
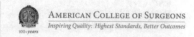

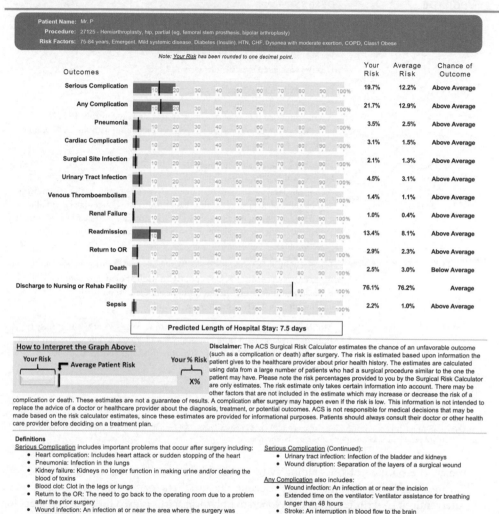

Figure 11.4 American College of Surgeons NSQIP Surgical Risk Calculator results.

complications, so the web-based risk calculator includes an important novel feature: a Surgeon Adjustment Score that allows surgeons to increase the risk of an operation based on their subjective assessment of a patient. This feature enables surgeons to better counsel patients using the modeled estimate along with the surgeon's experience and evaluation of the patient.

The ASA Physical Status classification system (Table 11.2) was initially created in 1941 by the American Society of Anesthetists, an organization that later became the ASA known

TABLE 11.2	AMERICAN SOCIETY OF ANESTHESIOLOGISTS PHYSICAL STATUS CLASSIFICATION SYSTEM
GRADE	**DESCRIPTION**
ASA PS 1	Normal, healthy patient No organic, physiologic, or psychiatric disturbance Excludes the very young and very old Healthy with good exercise tolerance
ASA PS 2	Patients with mild, systemic disease No functional limitations A well-controlled disease of one body system such as controlled HTN or diabetes without systemic effects, cigarette smoking without COPD, mild obesity, or pregnancy
ASA PS 3	Patients with severe systemic disease Some functional limitation A controlled disease of more than one body system or one major system with no immediate danger of death, such as controlled congestive heart failure (CHF), stable angina, an old heart attack, poorly controlled HTN, morbid obesity, chronic renal failure, or bronchospastic disease with intermittent symptoms
ASA PS 4	Patients with severe systemic disease that is a constant threat to life At least one severe disease that is poorly controlled or at end stage with a possible risk of death, such as unstable angina, symptomatic COPD, symptomatic CHF, or hepatorenal failure
ASA PS 5	Moribund patients who are not expected to survive >24 hr without surgery Imminent risk of death from diseases like multiorgan failure, sepsis syndrome with hemodynamic instability, hypothermia, and poorly controlled coagulopathy
ASA PS 6	A patient declared brain dead whose organs are being removed for donor purposes

Data from American Society of Anesthesiologists. (2014). *ASA phyical status classification system.* https://www.asahq.org/standards-and-guidelines/asa-physical-status-classification-system.

today. The purpose of the grading system is simply to evaluate the degree of a patient's "sickness" or "physical state" before selecting the anesthetic or before performing surgical intervention. Describing patients' preoperative physical status is used for recordkeeping, for communicating between colleagues, and to create a uniform system for statistical analysis for the entire healthcare team. The grading system is not intended for use as a measure to predict operative risk (American Society of Anesthesiologists, 2014).

Nonsurgical Management

What difference in complications would you expect in the surgical vs. nonsurgical patient?

The majority of hip fractures in the elderly are managed surgically; however, patients or families may refuse surgery or be deemed medically unfit to undergo surgical fixation. Patients and/or their families who opt for nonsurgical management may require skeletal traction until early fracture consolidation or clinical resolution of pain is noted. The clinician can try early mobilization with the patient remaining non–weight bearing on the affected extremity to help decrease complications. Complications for nonsurgical patients are pneumonia, ACS, and cerebrovascular accident, in addition to UTI, pressure sores, and wound infection. Nonsurgical patients have twice the odds of developing complications compared with surgically treated patients. Nonsurgical patients also had longer lengths of stay when compared with their surgical counterparts. In advanced dementia patients, those who were surgically repaired had a significantly lower risk of death and a median increased survival at 1 year compared with nonsurgical patients. Hospice should be considered in nonsurgical patients who are profoundly impaired (Berry et al., 2018).

Surgical Options

For true non-displaced intracapsular hip fractures, the surgeon may decide either to fix the fracture with individual screws (percutaneous pinning) or place a single larger screw that slides within the barrel of a plate. This compression hip screw will allow the fracture to become more stable by having the broken area impact on itself. For displaced fractures, patients will do better if some of the components of the hip are replaced. In some cases, this can mean a replacement of the ball or head of the femur (hemiarthroplasty). In other cases, this can mean the replacement of both the ball and socket or head of the femur and acetabulum (total hip replacement).

Most intertrochanteric fractures are managed with either a compression hip screw or an intramedullary nail. The compression hip screw is fixed to the outer side of the bone with bone screws and has a large secondary screw (lag screw) that is placed through the plate into the neck and head of the hip. The design of the device allows for impaction and compression at the fracture site. This may increase the stability of the area and promote healing. The intramedullary nail is placed directly into the canal of the bone through an opening made at the top of the greater trochanter. A lag screw is then placed through the nail and up into the neck and head of the hip.

At the subtrochanteric level, most fractures are managed with a long intramedullary nail together with a large lag screw, or they are managed with screws that capture the neck and head of the femur or the area immediately underneath it, if it has remained intact. Plates and screws can also be utilized either as stand alone treatments or in addition to other methods of fixation.

Pain

Throughout the patient's hospital course, pain is a consistently pivotal symptom to monitor and address. Depending on fracture morphology and patient condition, pain may be a determining reason for surgery or nonoperative treatment. Pain should be treated in a multimodal approach and, given the specific population prone to hip fracture, must be consistently monitored and tailored to each patient. Narcotics and nonnarcotic medications are often used concurrently with the goal of getting the patient off narcotic pain medications as quickly as possible. It is important to remember that narcotics can increase delirium in the elderly; however, so can uncontrolled pain. Monitoring pain through an appropriate, validated pain scale throughout the patient's stay is imperative to successful treatment.

Pain after an injury or surgery is a natural part of the healing process. Older adults are at risk for underassessment of pain. Risk factors for inadequate pain control are age, gender, dementia, multiple comorbidities, ED crowding/busyness, hospital unit census, and staffing. Postoperative pain control remains difficult in the aging population, and opioid analgesia dominates current pain management strategies. Elderly persons can experience higher peak effect and longer duration of action of opioids due largely to decreased renal and hepatic clearance as well as a change in body composition. This puts them at increased risk of respiratory depression, constipation, delirium, pulmonary complications, and oversedation. Medications are often prescribed for short-term pain relief after surgery or an injury. Many types of medicines are available to help manage pain, including opioids, NSAIDs, and local anesthetics. You may use a combination of these medications to improve pain relief, as well as to minimize the need for opioids. Although opioids help relieve pain after surgery or an injury, they can be addictive. Opioid dependency and overdose have become critical public health issues in the United States. Despite pain-induced complications such as delirium, many healthcare providers are reluctant to prescribe opioid analgesics to elderly patients for fear of potential opioid-induced adverse effects. Postoperative pain has been associated not only with delirium but also with prolonged bed rest following surgery. This affects participation with physical therapy (PT) and postoperative ambulation. This can lead to an increase in risk of thromboembolism and functional impairment, which in turn may result in significantly longer hospital lengths of stay, long-term functional impairment, and other costs. Use of IV acetaminophen was consistently a statistically significant predictor of decreased LOS, decreased pain scores, lower narcotic usage, and fewer missed PT sessions when controlling for all other variables. Multimodal pain management has also proven effective (Bollinger et al., 2015).

Case Study

Mr. P undergoes operative fixation, followed by ongoing assessment of his heart, pulmonary and neurovascular status, especially of the postoperative limb. Post procedure, he is admitted to the surgical floor with frequent checks of his vital signs, telemetry monitoring, strict monitoring of intake and output, daily CBC and electrolytes, and renal function. Immediately postoperative, you focus on pain relief and rehabilitation, including physical therapy. You order low-dose opioids for the first 24–48 hr but attempt to quickly transition to Tylenol when pain is minimal to help reduce development of delirium. You avoid NSAIDs due to his DM and CKD. He undergoes early mobilization and is out of bed on day 1. He remains on the surgical floor for 3 days post procedure with stable vital signs, blood loss anemia that is stable and does not require transfusion, and stable renal function. Due to the high risk, medication for thromboembolism prophylaxis is started on postoperative day 1 according to the hospital's fragility fracture pathway, in addition to restarting the patient's home medications. Patients may require drugs such as Lovenox for 4-6 weeks as their mobility is decreased secondary to trauma, surgical intervention, and decompensation/rehabilitation. You place Mr. P on Lovenox. He is discharged to a rehabilitation facility for 2 weeks for additional physical and occupational therapy.

LOW BACK PAIN

Case Study

You are an APRN working the evening shift in the ED. Mr. C is a 37-year-old male who presents to the ED via personal automobile with a chief complaint of LBP. The patient states he was helping a friend move a couch over the weekend and felt acute right-sided back pain when lifting. The patient denies falling or direct trauma to the lower back or previous issues with his lower back. The patient states the pain was sharp and radiated down his right buttock. The patient said he tried to lie down and use a heat pack with minimal relief. The patient said he has tried to take "a few doses" of Tylenol without significant relief. He states he has been able to complete his ADLs but has issues with long periods of sitting and improves with standing.

His past medical history is significant only for borderline cholesterol, for which he takes no medications, and he is a current one-half pack per day smoker × 5 years. The patient had a left ankle ORIF in high school after a sports injury. The patient takes no current medications. He states he drinks alcohol socially with four drinks weekly and denies any substance use. The injury occurred Saturday, and it is now Monday morning.

His review of symptoms reveals the following:

- He denies any recent fever, chills, or night sweats.
- Cardiac: He denies chest pain, palpitations, DOE, cough, or productive sputum. There is no edema appreciated.
- Gastrointestinal/urinary: He denies abdominal pain, weight loss, heart burn, and bowel or bladder dysfunction/incontinence/dysuria.
- Musculoskeletal: He endorses pain in his right lower back that radiates to the buttock and to the back of his knee. It worsens with sitting and improves with standing. The patient typically walks without assistive device.

His physical examination is as follows: temperature, 98.6 °F; pulse, 72 bpm; respiratory rate, 16 breaths/min; blood pressure, 135/84 mm Hg. His lung sounds are clear throughout all fields. The cardiovascular examination reveals a regular rate and rhythm, normal S1/S2, and no murmur, gallop, or rub. His abdomen is soft, flat, and nontender with normal bowel sounds. In his neck, he has no pain with flexion or extension of the cervical spine or side-to-side turning. There is no pain to posterior cervical midline palpation. In his thoracic spine, he has no pain with flexion or extension or side-to-side turning and no tenderness to midline palpation. In his lumbar spine, he has pain with flexion/extension and side-to side turning but no pain to midline palpation of the lumbar spine. No saddle anesthesia is noted. He has appropriate rectal tone. A bilateral upper extremity examination reveals no pain with active or passive ROM of the shoulder, elbow, or wrist. Deltoid, biceps, triceps, wrist flexion/extension, grip strength, and intrinsics are all 5/5 strength. Hoffman's test is negative bilaterally. He has a palpable radial artery pulses. Sensation is intact to radial/medial/ulnar distributions. The examination of his lower extremities reveals 4/5 right hip flexion with the examination being limited secondary to pain. Right hip flexion elicits pain that passes through the right gluteus and down the back of the right leg terminating just about the posterior knee. Right lower extremity sensation is diminished but intact to deep and superficial perineal as well as tibial nerve distributions. Strength, sensation, and pulses are otherwise normal to bilateral lower extremities except above. No clonus is appreciated bilaterally. You elicit normal reflexes to bilateral lower extremities.

Based on the initial information given, list your top differential diagnoses. What tests should you order to rule your differentials in or out?

Etiology and Differentials for LBP

LBP is one of the leading complaints in U.S. emergency departments and urgent care centers, yet LBP diagnosis and treatment remains challenging. The cause of LBP can range from muscle strain to fracture. About 50%–80% of the U.S. population will be affected by LBP in their lifetime. A provider's primary goal is to detect serious pathology that requires urgent intervention while triaging LBP that can be worked up and treated in the outpatient setting. In primary care settings, the prevalence of serious pathologies was found to be less than 1%; however, the prevalence in the ED is not well documented (Galliker et al., 2019). LBP is ranked as the fifth reason patients seek care from healthcare providers. LBP is prevalent among all age groups, from adolescents to older adults. LBP is also the leading reason for disability among patients under the age of 45, and 60%–80% of those with LBP have ongoing complaints after 1 year (Metzger, 2016).

Major differentials for LBP include muscular strain, acute fracture, spinal stenosis, disk herniation, discogenic back pain, and infection. Due to the multiple causes of LBP, treatment can also vary widely. It is important to carefully elicit a detailed history and perform a thorough physical examination. Since the treatment spectrum can vary from outpatient follow-up to urgent surgery, it is important to efficiently rule differential diagnoses in or out to ensure appropriate disposition. You may implement CDR such as Waddell signs (Box 11.1) to help with your differential.

There are several forms of LBP: nonspecific low back pain (NSLBP), LBP without radiculopathy, LBP with radiculopathy caused by herniated disk or extrusion, LBP with radiculopathy due to spinal stenosis, critical conditions of the lumbar spine such as tumor/cancer/fracture or trauma, and chronic LBP:

- Nonspecific LBP is a mechanical type of pain that varies with the patient's physical activity and posture. It is not caused by any recognizable pathology, structural deformity, osteoporosis, or radicular syndrome. It can be related to degenerative changes in disks or joints, or presence of osteophytes, especially in the working age group (Metzger, 2016).
- LBP without radiculopathy is back pain that does not radiate down the lower extremities. There is no associated numbness, tingling, or weakness. It may be a result of muscle strain or arthritis.
- LBP with radiculopathy caused by herniated disk or extrusion involves compression of the nerve roots and can result in numbness, tingling, pain, and/or weakness. Patients

---

BOX 11.1 Waddell Signs

- A system designed to evaluate for potential nonorganic or psychogenic back pain symptoms
- To be clinically significant, three or more of the following positive signs must be present:
  - Nonanatomic/superficial tenderness
  - Pain with simulated rotation of the spine or axial compression
  - Patient unable to straight leg raise even with concurrent distraction
  - Hypersensitivity or overreaction to physical examination
  - Nondermatomal regional disturbances

may also have only radicular symptoms without actual LBP. The symptoms usually follow a nerve root dermatomal distribution. The most common lumbar disk areas that herniate are L3-4, L4-5, and L5-S1.

- LBP with radiculopathy due to spinal stenosis results from an arthritic enlargement of the facet joints and posterior elements of the spine. This can cause a mass effect and compress the lumbar nerve roots. Spinal stenosis can be considered central canal stenosis, neural foramina stenosis, or both. It is more common in older patients. Symptoms of pain radiating from the buttocks into legs, caused by neurogenic claudication, is usually worsened with standing or walking. The pain starts proximally and radiates distally, which is the opposite of vascular claudication (Metzger, 2016).

- Critical conditions of spine include tumor/neoplasm, infection, hematoma, and trauma/fracture fall. Missing a critical condition can result in irreversible neurologic damage, paralysis, permanent bowel and bladder dysfunction, and other irreversible conditions (Edward (Ted) Parks, 2018).

- Chronic LBP is defined as pain extending beyond 12 weeks and occurring on at least half the days extending beyond 6 months (Kuebler & Oskouei, 2020). Chronic LBP is more prevalent in men than in women as well as in older age groups (Dupuis & Duff, 2019).

Presentation

The type of LBP the patient is experiencing will influence the clinical symptoms. Obtaining a detailed history is an important part in determining what type LBP the patient is experiencing and possible cause. History should include the patient's description of symptoms, length of symptomology, location of pain, degree of pain, any trauma precipitating symptoms, previous back problems, and presence or absence of lower extremity symptoms (unilateral/bilateral/area of symptoms). Determine what activities improve or worsen symptoms, for example, walking, sitting, standing, flexion, extension, or lying down. Review modalities the patient has tried for treatment, such as medication, heat, ice, massage, or physical therapy.

Physical Examination

A basic physical examination should always be performed and should include cardiovascular, respiratory, abdominal, genitourinary, musculoskeletal, neurologic, and skin assessments. The cardiovascular examination should include assessing the heart rate and rhythm and the listening for murmurs. Consider whether the patient has peripheral edema or any signs of aortic aneurysm, peripheral vascular disease, CAD, or decreased perfusion. The respiratory examination should include lung sounds. The abdominal assessment should include auscultation for bruits, light and deep palpation, and rectal tone if the patient has decreased sensation or bowel/bladder incontinence. Skin assessment includes looking for rashes such as varicella zoster or signs of infection such as erythema/abscess (Pfieffer, 2019). The physical examination should include inspection and palpation of the spine for alignment, tenderness, and reproducible pain. Motor assessment should include gait assessment, which may include heel walking, toe walking, and tandem gait assessments; flexion and extension of the full spine, including cervical, thoracic, and lumbar/sacral; and ROM of upper and lower extremities, including wrist flexion/extension, thumb flexion/extension (extensor and flexor pollicis longus), hand intrinsics, hip flexion/extension, knee flexion/extension, foot plantar/dorsiflexion, great toe range (extensor and flexor hallucis longus); and strength testing of biceps, triceps, and deltoid. Muscle strength testing is graded on a scale from 0 to 5 and is reviewed in Box 11.2 (Metzger, 2016).

BOX 11.2 | Muscle Strength Grading Scale

5: Normal strength
4: Movement possible against some resistance by examiner
3: Movement possible against gravity but not against resistance by examiner
2: Movement possible when removed from gravity
1: Muscle flicker but no movement
0: No muscle contraction

Reflex testing and a tactile sensory examination can determine any dermatomal deficits. Other neurological tests, such as straight leg raise, are important to perform when looking for nerve root impingement. Babinski reflex and clonus are signs of upper motor neuron dysfunction.

A weak straight leg raise without other positive findings lacks diagnostic utility. It is performed by having the patient lie down supine and the provider gently lifting the leg by flexing the hip with the knee in extension. The test is considered positive when the leg is lifted greater than 40° and the patient experiences pain along the leg. A positive result indicates compression of lower lumbar nerve roots (L4-S1). It is important to distinguish nerve root compression from hamstring tightness.

A crossed straight leg test is performed by flexing the uninvolved limb and keeping the knee on the side being examined in extension while performing hip flexion. A crossed straight leg test is positive in the involved limb if pain is present at 40° of flexion (Metzger, 2016).

Diagnostic Tests

Laboratory and diagnostic tests are usually not routinely performed with acute back pain unless the patient has red flag symptoms. Red flags include local or systemic infection, tumor or history of malignancy, acute or periacute trauma, and signs and symptoms of cauda equina. Radiographs are the standard for initial workup of most orthopedic injuries. Pain exceeding 1 month that does not respond to nonoperative management and red flags on physical examination are both indications for radiographs in a nonacute setting. In the acute care setting, such as the ER, plain radiographs are a standard diagnostic in the workup of LBP. If the patient has pain but imaging is negative for acute fracture or abnormality that explains the presenting symptomology, then advanced imaging may be needed.

Key Points

Physical examination red flags require laboratory and diagnostic tests:

- infection (fever and chills)
- tumor (history of malignancy)
- trauma (history of higher energy injury)
- cauda equina syndrome (new bowel/bladder changes)

Scans you can order to diagnose the potential causes of LBP include CT scans and MRI. CT scans are best suited to confirm or rule out acute fracture and are less clinically useful than an MRI with the workup of LBP in the absence of acute fracture (Dupuis & Duff, 2019). MRIs are highly sensitive and specific examinations but should only be used in coordination with red flag physical examinations and patient history due to the high rate of abnormal findings present in the asymptomatic population (Moore, 2020). Consideration should be taken for patients with implants of any kind prior to obtaining an MRI, as they may or may not be MRI compatible. If needed, a CT myelogram may be of diagnostic use.

CT scans or MRI can be done for patients that present with suspicious neurologic changes. CT is preferred for bony concerns or to investigate potential metastases in the setting of known/suspected malignancy (Metzger, 2016). Also, if a patient cannot undergo MRI, a CT or CT myelogram may be performed. MRI is preferred, given its sensitivity and specificity, when infection is suspected or if certain neurologic findings are present (Dupuis & Duff, 2019). WBC count, estimated sedimentation rate (ESR), and CRP can be ordered if infectious process is suspected.

Diagnosis

Nonspecific LBP accounts for 80% of LBP cases. The diagnosis can be used after differentials and red flags are ruled out (Pfieffer, 2019).

Radicular LBP involves impingement of the nerve roots. Physical examination as well as diagnostic studies such as electromyography (EMG) can be useful in the diagnosis. Lumbar disk herniation is frequently seen in acute back pain especially after lifting or straining. MRI and CT scan can be helpful in the diagnosis.

Spinal infection patients can present with fever, vertebral tenderness, back pain that worsens with activity, and neurological symptoms. Laboratory studies as well as MRI are useful in confirming this diagnosis. The abdomen should also be assessed to determine if the infection has spread.

Ankylosing spondylitis is usually found in a patient younger than 40 years of age. Pain is usually gradual with improvement with exercise, no improvement with rest and pain at night. Elevated levels of ESR and CRP are also usually found. Imaging may reveal bamboo spine, a radiographic feature that occurs as a result of vertebral body fusion (Pfieffer, 2019).

Compression fracture describes a type of fracture in which a spinal vertebrae caves in on itself due to compression—or pressure—on the bone. There are several types of compression fractures, each with different risks and treatment options. The most common cause of a spinal compression fracture is osteoporosis. In vertebrae weakened by osteoporosis, a slight increase in stress, or even the normal amount of axial loading placed on them, can cause them to break. Compression fractures occur most often in the lower portion of the thoracic spine or in the upper portion of the lumbar spine (thoracolumbar junction), where stresses tend to be highest on the vertebrae.

There are three types of compression fractures: wedge, crush, and burst (Figure 11.5). A wedge fracture is the most common type of compression fracture. It usually occurs in the front of the cylinder-shaped vertebra, causing the front of the vertebra to collapse but leaving the back of the bone intact, resulting in a wedge shape. A wedge compression fracture is usually a mechanically stable fracture but can lead to spinal deformity, such as a hunchback posture. A crush fracture is characterized by a fracture throughout the entire vertebra, not just the front. In this type of compression fracture, the bone tends to collapse in on itself, and these fractures are usually mechanically stable. A burst fracture is named, because as the vertebra collapses, it breaks out in multiple directions, often sending pieces of shattered

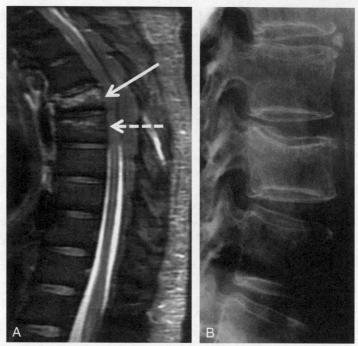

Figure 11.5 Common vertebral fracture morphologies. A, Burst fracture (solid arrow) and wedge fracture (dashed arrow). B, Crush fractures. (A, From Sanelli, P., Schaefer, P., & Loevner, L. (2016). *Neuroimaging: The Essentials.* Lippincott Williams & Wilkins and B, From Vigorita, V. J. (2016). *Orthopedic Pathology.* Lippincott Williams & Wilkins.)

bone into the surrounding tissues of the spine or the spinal canal. This type of fracture is usually more serious and more likely to be unstable. A burst fracture may require immediate medical attention because, of the three types, it has the highest potential for cord impingement. Symptoms of compression fracture typically include pain and a forward curving of the spine that results in a hunched appearance (kyphosis) and the loss of height. Symptoms may also include a loss of ROM and reduction of sensation in the extremities depending on the vertebral level(s) affected (Spivak, 2015).

Compression fractures can be caused by traumatic injury, such as a hard fall. But many cases of compression fracture develop as a result of osteoporosis. A person with osteoporosis may develop compression fractures during routine daily activities and may not realize the extent of their injuries until they experience severe deformity of the spine (Spivak, 2015).

Case Study

You order plain AP and lateral radiographs of Mr. P's lumbar spine. Figure 11.6 shows the images obtained in the ED.

Based on Mr. P's examination and history, you then order an MRI. Figure 11.7 shows the sagittal view and a corresponding axial image of the L4-5 disk space, which reveals, most significantly, a right-sided, paracentral disk herniation at the L4-5 level. Given the MRI findings and in correlation with Mr. P's physical examination, you determine that you should try conservative treatment with nonnarcotic pain control trial. You give him 975 mg oral Tylenol and 30 mg Toradol IV. After medication, Mr. P feels his pain is under much better control.

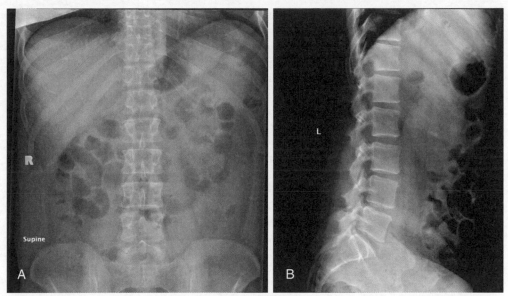

Figure 11.6 Lumbar spine radiographs obtained in the ED. A, Anteroposterior view. B, Lateral view.

> **Key Points**
>
> Treatment of LBP usually requires a multimodal approach.

Treatment

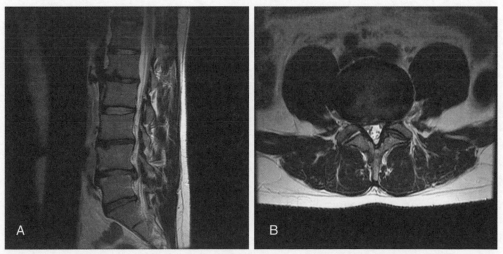

Figure 11.7 Magnetic resonance imaging of Mr. P's lower back. A, Sagittal and (B) axial views show a right paracentral disk herniation at the L4-5 level.

Pharmacologic treatment can include nonopioid analgesics, opioids, skeletal muscle relaxants, and adjuvant medications. NSAIDs and acetaminophen are used frequently. Caution should be used with NSAIDs if the patient has a history of GI, cardiovascular, or renal problems. Hepatic disorder and alcohol use should be reviewed prior to acetaminophen recommendations. NSAIDs are used short term for 2–4 weeks (Metzger, 2016).

When you prescribe NSAIDs, you should also provide patient education. Risks of GI bleeding, dyspepsia, HTN, kidney toxicity, heart failure, cardiovascular events, and asthma exacerbation should be discussed. Opioid analgesics carry the risk of misuse and dependence. They should not be used longer than 3 days for acute pain. They are not recommended for patients with chronic back pain. They are not recommended as a first line for nonmalignant pain, and they lack long-term documented efficacy. Skeletal muscle relaxants are used with some patients to help with pain associated with muscle spasm. Potential adverse reactions include dizziness and sedation, and use in patients over age 65 can be risky. Other adjuvant medications include antidepressants and anticonvulsants for subacute and chronic back pain. Duloxetine is approved for chronic musculoskeletal pain. Neurontin, topiramate, and pregabalin can be used for subacute and chronic back pain with radicular symptoms; however, use is usually considered off label. Common side effects include dizziness, somnolence, dry mouth, changes in vision, and GI disturbance including diarrhea and constipation (Pfieffer, 2019).

Nonpharmacologic treatment includes physical therapy, exercise, acupuncture, massage, spinal manipulation, and transdermal electrical stimulation. Referral to these areas usually occurs after several weeks of initial pharmacologic therapy, approximately at the 3-week mark (Metzger, 2016).

Referrals to Specialty

Primary care or urgent care/emergency providers can manage common LBP diagnosis. Findings consistent with cauda equina syndrome require immediate referral and hospitalization. Disk herniation, spinal stenosis, spinal fracture, and suspected infection require referral to surgical specialty. Ankylosing spondylitis is usually managed by rheumatology (Pfieffer, 2019).

Case Study

Since Mr. P did well with pain control in the ED and was able to ambulate around the unit, per nursing protocol with minimal pain. You make the decision to send him home with instructions for rest, icing, and stretching. In addition, you prescribe him Tylenol ATC and a long-acting, twice-daily NSAID, Celebrex. You give him a referral to the Comprehensive Spine Center (CSC) for outpatient follow-up in 2–3 weeks. If he fails conservative treatment, oral steroids, or fluoroscopy-guided corticosteroid injection, surgical intervention may be warranted. You educate Mr. P regarding red flag symptomology that warrants emergent assessment for surgical decompression at the nearest ED/Urgent Care.

At his follow-up appointment with the CSC, his pain is greatly improved and he has returned to his normal functional status and is back to work. You offer him a physical therapy referral to provide healthy back program that may help prevent future exacerbation of the injury. He will seek outpatient follow-up as needed in the future.

CLINICAL PEARLS

- LBP affects 50%–80% of population in lifetime, $100 billion in annual cost. Therefore, it is essential to efficiently work up each patient to avoid unnecessary, expensive imaging and workup.
- Muscle strain is most common cause of LBP.
- Risk factors for LBP include
  - Obesity
  - Smoking
  - Gender
  - Lifting
  - Vibration
  - Prolonged sitting
  - Job dissatisfaction
- Red flags must be assessed for every patient with LBP. Positive findings require radiographs and a specialty referral.
- Ninety percent of LBP resolves within 1 year.
- Treatment should always be dictated by cause of pain.
- A multimodal approach should be taken.

REVIEW QUESTIONS

1. A patient is able to perform at left lower extremity SLR with 5/5 strength and without significant pain. However, the patient has a diminished left-sided Achilles reflex and a 4/5 strength on planar flexion. During his examination, there is also decreased sensation to light touch to the left lateral foot. The rest of the examination is benign.

   Which of the following nerve roots is most likely compromised?
   a. S1
   b. S2
   c. L3
   d. L4

2. Appropriate initial pharmacological treatment for a patient's acute LBP should include which of the following?
   a. Oxycodone and Valium
   b. Acetaminophen
   c. Oxycontin
   d. B and C

3. In the early morning hours, a 74-year-old male presents to the emergency department complaining of right buttock and hip pain. Several hours before his arrival, he states he fell in the bathroom. He recalls standing without his walker and fell when attempting to turn and leave the bathroom. He denies loss of consciousness or head trauma. He lives with his son who was at the scene quickly and found the patient awake, alert, and moving all extremities. The patient did not attempt to ambulate after the fall and EMS was called. Other than right hip tenderness, his examination is unremarkable. The patient is vitally stable.

Which of the following is most likely to assist you in initial workup?
   a. CT scan of the pelvis
   b. Thorough physical examination
   c. Pelvic x-ray
   d. MRI of the pelvis with IV contrast

4. A 37-year-old male presents for evaluation of new onset lower back pain. All of the following are nonorganic signs of LBP (Waddell signs) EXCEPT:
   a. Positive straight leg raise even with patient distraction
   b. Pain with simulated rotation or axial loading of the spine
   c. Diffuse tenderness with palpation throughout the paraspinal musculature of the low back
   d. Nondermatomal pattern of lower extremity numbness

5. A 57-year-old man with a history of intermittent LBP for 3 years reports a day and a half of increased, severe lower back pain. He does not recall any precipitating trauma and states the pain started after a coughing fit. The patient states that over the last day he has had difficulty urinating and is only able to produce small amounts at a time with a lot of effort. His examination reveals saddle anesthesia, generalized bilateral lower extremity weakness, diminished lower extremity reflexes, and a loss of rectal tone. Which is the most appropriate initial management?
   a. Tapered oral steroid course and outpatient follow-up in 1 week for re-examination
   b. Outpatient referral for L1 epidural steroid injection
   c. 2 weeks of NSAIDs and referral to physical therapy
   d. Urgent MRI of the lumbar spine

6. All of the following are ways to prevent hip fractures due to falls in the elderly EXCEPT:
   a. Regular, low impact, physical exercise and muscle strengthening
   b. Regular hearing and eye examinations
   c. Wear smooth-soled shoes so you can shuffle along the floor easily
   d. Use an appropriate fitting assistive device and receive training and therapy from skilled therapists

Answers: 1, a; 2, a; 3, b; 4, a; 5, d; 6, c

REFERENCES

American Society of Anesthesiologists. (2014). *ASA physical status classification system*. Accessed February 8, 2020. https://www.asahq.org/standards-and-guidelines/asa-physical-status-classification-system

Berry, S., Rothbaum, R., Kiel, D., Lee, Y., & Mitchell, S. (2018). Association of clinical outcomes with surgical repair of hip fracture vs nonsurgical management in nursing home residents with advanced dementia. *JAMA Internal Medicine*, 178(6), 774–780.

Bollinger, A., Butler, P., Nies, M., Sietsema, D., Jones, C., & Endres, T. (2015). Is scheduled intravenous acetaminophen effective in the pain management protocol of geriatric hip fracture? *Geriatric Orthopedic Surgery & Rehabilitation*, 6(3), 202–208.

Dupuis, M., & Duff, E. (2019). Chronic low back pain: Evidence-informed management considerations for nurse practitioners. *The Journal for Nurse Practitioners*, 15(8), 583–587.

Edward (Ted) Parks, M. (2018). *Practical office orthopedics*. McGraw-Hill Education.

Egol, K. A., Koval, K. J., & Zuckerman, J. D. (2015). Femoral neck fractures. In *Handbook of fractures* (5th ed., pp. 371–380). Wolters Kluwer.

Galliker, G., Scherer, D., Trippolini, M., Rasmussen-Barr, E., LoMartire, R., & Wertli, M. (2019). Low back pain in the emergency department: Prevalence of serious spinal pathologies and diagnostic accuracy of red flags. *The American Journal of Medicine*, 133(1), 60–86. Accessed January 20, 2020.

Keene, G. S., Parker, M. J., & Pryor, G. A. (1993). Mortality and morbidity after hip fractures. *British Medical Journal*, 307(6914), 1248–1250.

Kuebler, K. K., & Oskouei, A. (2020). Collaborating with a spinal interventionalist in the management of low back pain. *The Journal for Nurse Practitioners*, 16(1), 23–27.

MDedge:Surgery. (2013). New ACS NSQIP surgical risk calculator offers personalized estimates of surgical complications. Accessed December 10, 2019. https://www.mdedge.com/surgery/article/77540/new-acs-nsqip-surgical-risk-calculator-offers-personalized-estimates-surgical

Metzger, R. L. (2016). Evidence-based practice guidelines for the diagnosis and treatment of lumbar spine conditions. *The Nurse Practitioner Journal*, 41(12), 30–37.

Moore, D. (2020). *Low back pain - introduction*. Orthobullets. Accessed March 2, 2020. https://www.orthobullets.com/spine/2034/low-back-pain--introduction

Orosz, G. M., Magaziner, J., Hannan, E. L., Morrison, R. S., Koval, K., Gilbert, M., McLaughlin, M., Halm, E. A., Wang, J. J., Litke, A., Silberzweig, S. B., & Siu, A. L. (2004). Association of timing of surgery for hip fracture and patient outcomes. *The Journal of the American Medical Association*, 291(14), 1738–1743.

Pfieffer, M. L. (2019). Evaluating and managing low back pain in primary care. *The Nurse Practitioner Journal*, 44(8), 40–47.

Ramponi, D., Kaufmann, J., & Drahnak, G. (2018). Hip fractures. *Advanced Emergency Nursing Journal*, 40(1), 8–15.

Spivak, J. M. (2015). *Types of spinal compression fractures*. Spine-Health. Accessed February 22, 2020. https://www.spaine-health.com/conditions/osteoporosis/types-spinal-compression-fractures

Stern, S. D., Cifu, A. S., & Altkorn, D. (2015). *Symtom to diagnosis: An Evidence-based guide* (3rd ed.). McGraw-Hill Education.

12

Cardiology

Paula McCauley • Anantha Sriharsha Madgula

INTRODUCTION

Cardiology is a significant system with a broad depth and breadth of topics that ANCPs will encounter. Using a case-based approach and current guidelines, we have addressed a few of the most common topics in this chapter including ACS, arrhythmias, heart failure, and diseases of the aorta and valves.

ACUTE CORONARY SYNDROME

Case Study

Mr. C is a 55-year-old male with past medical history of type 2 diabetes mellitus and HTN who was brought to the emergency department with chest pain.

The chest pain started about 30 min earlier when he was watching television. He does endorse that his symptoms initially started 6 months ago when he noticed chest pain with moderate exertion. Now, he can only walk half a block or one flight of stairs before his chest pain occurs. It had been relieved with rest in the past, but over the last week he had episodes of chest pain even at rest. Prior to today, the pain had never lasted more than 5–10 min and improved spontaneously. As this episode was unrelenting, he decided to call 911. His chest pain is of crushing type that is predominantly substernal in location and 8/10 in intensity and radiates down his left arm.

Upon emergency medical system (EMS) arrival, an ECG was done that revealed 2 mm ST elevation in leads II, III, and aVF.

What is your diagnosis? How would you initially manage this patient? What would you want to avoid in this patient? What is your differential diagnosis for Mr. C?

Given Mr. C's typical chest pain character and risk factors (elderly male, HTN, diabetes) along with ST segment elevations, he might be having an STEMI. Initial management of all STEMIs may begin in the field before the patient is brought to the hospital if the EMS is activated. The initial management for this patient would include administering a full dose of aspirin, 325 mg once. If the patient has chest pain, 0.4 mg of sublingual nitroglycerin can be given every 5 min for up to three doses, except in those patients in whom an inferior myocardial infarction (MI) is suspected (as in Mr. C).

Your differential diagnosis for acute chest pain includes the following:

* Pulmonary embolism
* Aortic dissection
* Acute pericarditis

Key Points

ST elevations in leads II, III, and aVF are concerning for STEMI of the inferior myocardium which incorporates the right ventricle. In this situation, nitroglycerin should be used very carefully as it can cause significant hypotension due to preload dependence of the RV. If the patient becomes hypotensive, he must be given intravenous fluids such as normal saline to improve blood pressure immediately.

Definition

ACS can be categorized as STEMI and non–ST elevation myocardial infarction (NSTEMI). The distinction is based on findings of an ECG. ACS is caused by erosion or rupture of a plaque in the coronary arteries that causes complete or near complete occlusion of coronary arteries (Anderson & Morrow, 2017; O'Gara et al., 2013).

STEMI is characterized by elevation of ST segments of at least 1 mm in two or more contiguous leads except in V2 and V3. In V2 and V3, there must be an elevation of at least 2 mm or greater in men and 1.5 mm or greater in women (O'Gara et al., 2013). Box 12.1 lists ECG leads that reflect the changes associated with the region they reflect.

Diagnosis of STEMI

The pathogenesis behind STEMI is plaque rupture with complete occlusion of the coronary artery. This results in a transmural infarction of the affected region of the heart causing ST segment elevations. Time is of the essence to open this closed blood vessel in order to minimize permanent damage of the myocardium. There are other conditions that can present with ST segment elevations including myocarditis and pericarditis (Anderson & Morrow, 2017).

Pericarditis is the inflammation of the pericardium, which is the heart lining. The pericardium can be divided into two layers: the parietal pericardium on the outside and visceral pericardium on the inside. Inflammation of this tissue can present with chest pain that is acute and sharp. The pain is positionally variant with exacerbation when lying down and improvement when sitting. ECG would demonstrate ST segment elevation in all the leads, as opposed to regional elevations in STEMI.

BOX 12.1 Regions of ST segment changes

1. Inferior region: ST changes in leads II, III, and aVF.
2. Anterior region: ST changes in leads I and aVL, V1, V2, V3.
3. Lateral region: ST changes in V4, V5, V6.
4. Posterior region: ST depressions in V1, V2, V3 and ST elevations in II, III, aVF.
5. STEMI equivalents: new left bundle branch block (LBBB).

Data from O'Gara, P. T., Kushner, F. G., Ascheim, D. D., Casey, D. E., Chung, M. K., de Lemos, J. A., Ettinger, S. M., Fang, J. C., Fesmire, F. M., Franklin, B. A., Granger, C. B., Krumholz, H. M., Linderbaum, J. A., Morrow, D. A., Newby, K., Ornato, J. P., Ou, N., Radford, M. J., Tamis-Holland, J. E., ...Zhao, D. X. (2013). 2013 ACCF/AHA guideline for the management of ST-elevation myocardial infarction: Executive summary. A report of the American College of Cardiology Foundation/American Heart Association Task Force on practice guidelines. *Journal of the American College of Cardiology, 61*(4), 485–510. https://doi.org/10.1016/j.jacc.2012.11.018 and Thygesen, K., Alpert, J. S., Jaffe, A. S., Chaitman, B. R., Bax, J. J., Morrow, D. A., White, H. D., & Executive Group on behalf of the Joint European Society of Cardiology (ESC)/American College of Cardiology (ACC)/American Heart Association (AHA)/World Heart Federation (WHF) Task Force for the Universal Definition of Myocardial Infarction. (2018). Fourth universal definition of myocardial infarction (2018). *Journal of the American College of Cardiology, 72*(18), 2231–2264. https://doi.org/10.1016/j.jacc.2018.08.1038

Case Study

When Mr. C arrives to the emergency department, the following vitals are obtained: temperature, 99 °F; HR, 95 beats/minute; RR, 22 breaths/minute; blood pressure, 100/68 mm Hg. His medications include metformin 500 mg twice daily and amlodipine 5 mg daily. In his review of systems, he denies headaches, dizziness, nausea, vomiting, visual disturbances, anxiety, palpitations, abdominal discomfort, change in bowel habits, lower extremity pain, or swelling.

- His physical examination reveals the following: a middle-aged male lying down on the ED bed holding his fists to his chest in acute distress
- HEENT: pupils are equal, reactive to light
- Cardiac: normal rate, normal rhythm, normal S1, S2 heard, no murmurs appreciated
- Lungs: normal breath sounds heard, crackles are heard at bilateral bases
- Abdomen: unremarkable
- Extremities: warm, well perfused, pulses are equal peripherally, no edema

He smokes about 1 pack of cigarettes a day, drinks wine occasionally, and denies any illicit substance abuse.

The cath lab was already alerted on his way to the hospital. The patient is immediately taken to the cath lab for an emergency percutaneous coronary intervention (PCI).

When should Mr. C be taken to the cath lab and why? What if your hospital does not have a cath lab? Should he be given any medications before going to the cath lab?

Acute Management of STEMI

Once diagnosed, opening the occluded blood vessel as soon as possible is very important to minimize permanent damage to the myocardium. This can be done with thrombolytics or by PCI. PCI is preferred over thrombolytics if time permits (Anderson & Morrow, 2017; O'Gara, 2013).

Key Points

The ideal time from first medical contact until PCI is less than 90 min, and outcomes are best when done within 12 hr of onset of chest pain.

The ideal door to balloon time is less than 90 min and directly correlates to the volume of salvageable myocardium. This directly correlates to the volume of salvageable myocardium. If a patient presents to a hospital that does not perform PCI, the patient should be transferred to a PCI capable facility and the time from first medical contact to PCI should be less than 120 min. Patients with PCI should receive a full dose of aspirin and heparin before thrombolytic therapy. Patients also receive P2Y12 inhibitors such as clopidogrel, prasugrel, or ticagrelor before thrombolytic therapy (Anderson & Morrow, 2017; O'Gara et al., 2013).

Key Points

Checking serum troponin levels before taking to initial angiography delays care unnecessarily. If the clinical picture is not clear, then they may be of value.

When PCI is not available, thrombolytic therapy is recommended within 12 hr from onset of symptoms.

Nitroglycerin is given sublingually for pain relief in ACS patients. It acts by reducing the preload and also dilating the coronary vessels, temporarily increasing the blood flow. Nitrates should be avoided in patients with inferior STEMI as these patients are preload dependent.

Case Study

Mr. C undergoes a left heart catheterization via right femoral access; the angiogram showed 100% occlusion of the right coronary artery and a drug eluting stent is placed. He has nonobstructive disease in his left anterior descending (LAD). Mr. C is admitted to the coronary ICU for 24 hr. When you see him, he reports that his chest pain is now completely gone.

Why did you admit him to the coronary care unit (CCU)? What medications do you want to start on Mr. C and for how long? What laboratory tests would you obtain on Mr. C? What imaging tests would you want to obtain? Why were serum troponin levels not checked before he was taken to the cath lab? In addition to medications, what counseling is important to reduce his risk for more CAD?

You admit him to the ICU for the first 24 hr post-STEMI for high acuity monitoring for reperfusion arrhythmias. You start Mr. C on aspirin 81 mg daily and the P2Y12 inhibitor ticagrelor and high-intensity statin therapy. Because underlying renal insufficiency may put patients at risk for contrast-induced nephropathy, you follow his BUN and creatinine post. He is on metformin, which you will hold for 3 days after the procedure to minimize renal impact. You obtain an echocardiogram to establish a new baseline heart function before discharge.

Medical Management of ACS

Beta-blockers are a class of medications that block the beta receptors in the heart and decrease the heart rate and as a result the myocardial oxygen demand. They should be started within 24 hr of an ACS if not contraindicated as they have demonstrated mortality benefit. They should be avoided in patients with evidence of decreased cardiac function such as low blood pressure, pulmonary congestion, or cardiogenic shock (Anderson & Morrow, 2017).

High-intensity statin therapy should be initiated in all patients with STEMI. Cholesterol, being a negative acute phase reactant, can be transiently low after a STEMI. Even if the cholesterol is normal, the patient should be started on a high-intensity statin. If they cannot tolerate statins due to severe myopathy, PCK9 inhibitors are good alternatives (Anderson & Morrow, 2017).

Angiotensin-converting enzyme inhibitors (ACE-Is) should also be initiated in STEMI patients. They block the renin angiotensin aldosterone system, which should help with remodeling of the heart. They have been studied extensively and have a proven mortality benefit, especially in patients with reduced left ventricular (LV) function [2]. They should be administered within 24 hr of STEMI. The main contraindications to ACE-Is are poor renal function and hyperkalemia. If patients experience cough as a side effect from ACE-Is, they can be switched to angiotensin receptor blockers (ARBs) (Anderson & Morrow, 2017).

Diabetes Management

In patients with type 2 diabetes and Cardiovascular Disease, there was a reduction in CVD outcomes with glucagon-like peptide-1 (GLP-1) receptor agonists. In patients deemed to be at high risk for contrast-induced AKI (CI-AKI) who are taking metformin and who are to undergo CT with administration of iodinated contrast material, the 2018 ACR guidelines recommend that the drug should be temporarily discontinued at the time of, or prior to, the study and should be withheld for at least 48 hr.

Case Study

Mr. C remains in the hospital for another 48 hr. His transthoracic echocardiography reveals a reduced EF of 40% with inferior wall hypokinesis. Lifestyle modifications after STEMI are very important. Because smoking confers a very high risk for progression of his CAD, you recommend smoking cessation counseling. Level 1 cardiac rehabilitation is initiated, including education for dietary modifications, exercise, smoking cessation, and medications. Ticagrelor 90 mg bid, enteric-coated aspirin 81 mg daily, metoprolol succinate 25 mg daily, atorvastatin 80 mg daily, and lisinopril 5 mg daily are introduced during his stay and his vital signs remain stable. He is discharged home on day 3 on these medications with a referral for outpatient cardiac rehabilitation to continue. He will follow up with you in 2 weeks as an outpatient.

ATRIAL FIBRILLATION

Case Study

You are the nurse practitioner in cardiology at the local medical center. Mr. E is a 69-year-old male with HTN, COPD, and type 2 diabetes mellitus who was referred to your clinic for evaluation and to discuss options for elective cardioversion for new-onset atrial fibrillation (AF). He has a past medical history of CAD with one prior infarct, which was treated with a PCI and placement of a drug-eluting stent (DES) to his LAD coronary artery. He has preserved ventricular function (ejection fraction, or EF) of 50% on a Transthoracic echocardiogram last year. His recent echocardiogram has also demonstrated mild to moderate aortic stenosis (AS). He also has a long-standing history of COPD with a 40 pack-year smoking history.

During his review of systems, he relates several recent episodes of not "feeling right" for the past week, excessive fatigue, and more dyspnea than usual on exertion. He notices when he has palpitations he gets exhausted more quickly.

His medications include furosemide 20 mg daily, atenolol 50 mg daily, and aspirin 81 mg daily. He is allergic to calcium channel blocking drugs.

His physical examination reveals the following: temperature, 98.6 °F; heart rate, 108 and irregular; respiratory rate, 16; and blood pressure, 130/85. His jugular venous pressure (JVP) is 9 cm with the head of the bed at 45°. On pulmonary examination, he has a prolonged expiratory phase and no crackles. His cardiac examination reveals a lateral PMI, variable S1 and single S2, and a II/VI holosystolic murmur heard best at the upper sternal border which radiates to his neck. He has 1+ peripheral edema and no clubbing or cyanosis. His ECG reveals AF with ventricular response of 124 and ST depression in I, AVL, and V2-V6.

Can you provide reasons based on cardiac pathophysiology for the worsening exercise intolerance and increased dyspnea when not in Normal Sinus Rhythm?

Definition

AF is a common heart rhythm disorder caused by degeneration of the electrical impulses in the atria resulting in a rapid, chaotic rhythm. AF may have hemodynamic consequences with a decrease in cardiac output due to ineffective atrial systole and increased pulmonary venous pressure, which may result in heart failure. Hemodynamic effects also include nonphysiologic tachycardia, increased valvular regurgitation, and irregularity in ventricular systole with either a slow or rapid ventricular response (January et al., 2014).

According to the 2014 AHA/ACC/Heart Rhythm Society (HRS) clinical practice guidelines, AF can be classified based on the duration of episodes:

- Paroxysmal AF begins suddenly and ends spontaneously within 7 days of onset.
- Persistent AF occurs for longer than 7 days and ends spontaneously.
- Long-standing persistent AF is uninterrupted for more than a year.
- Permanent AF persists despite treatment to restore normal sinus rhythm or has not been treated.

AF is associated with morbidity and mortality. It can produce symptoms that affect quality of life, creates a substantial risk of thromboembolic stroke, and is associated with an increased risk of heart failure as well as risk of dementia and mortality (January et al., 2014).

Key Points

Most patients presenting with AF are not critically ill, although it may cause life-threatening hemodynamic compromise. For any unstable patient presenting with AF, the recommended therapy is rapid electrical cardioversion according to the Advance Cardiovascular Life Support guidelines (Neumar et al., 2015).

Management

There are three goals in the management of AF:

- control of the ventricular rate,
- minimization of thromboembolism risk, and
- restoration and maintenance of sinus rhythm.

In addition to improving symptoms, the potential benefits of restoring and maintaining sinus rhythm include avoidance of the development of atrial cardiomyopathy, improvement in heart failure, and improvement in overall quality of life. A rhythm control strategy may require the use of antiarrhythmic drugs that may produce significant side effects and procedures that carry potentially life-threatening or disabling complications.

Large, multicenter randomized studies have compared rate control with rhythm control in patients with AF (Coleman et al., 2015; de Denus et al., 2005). Both treatment strategies use appropriate anticoagulation according to established guidelines. The evidence from trials comparing rhythm control with ventricular rate control strategies has shown no significant difference in quality of life, incidence of stroke, or mortality at a follow-up of approximately 5 years (Coleman et al., 2015; de Denus et al., 2005).

Case Study

Upon further discussion and consultation with your favorite EP cardiologist, you decide to send Mr. E for elective cardioversion. He has not been anticoagulated and so potential thrombus must be ruled out. You order a transesophageal echocardiogram (TEE). Your management decisions will include consideration for anticoagulation and antiarrhythmic control.

Assessment of Stroke and Bleeding Risks

There are CDRs associated with stroke risk and bleeding risk that have been developed and revised over the past several years (Table 12.1). You will utilize these to help guide decisions for anticoagulation, along with informed discussion with the patient. Recommendations for anticoagulant therapy should be individualized on the basis of shared decision-making, discussion of the absolute risks and relative risks of stroke and bleeding, and the patient's values and preferences. Reevaluation of the need for and choice of anticoagulant therapy at periodic intervals is recommended to reassess stroke and bleeding risks.

When discussing the benefits and risks of anticoagulation, discussion would include that for most people, the benefit of anticoagulation outweighs the bleeding risk. For people with an increased risk of bleeding, the benefit of anticoagulation may not always outweigh the bleeding risk, and careful monitoring of bleeding risk is important (January et al., 2014).

Key Points

Do not withhold anticoagulation solely because the person is at risk of having a fall (January et al., 2014).

Using these CDRs, you consider anticoagulation for men with a CHA2DS2-VASc score of 1 and offer anticoagulation to all people with a CHA2DS2-VASc score of 2 or above. For patients with AF and an elevated CHA2DS2-VASc score of 2 or greater in men or 3 or greater in women, oral anticoagulants are recommended. For patients with AF and a CHA2DS2-VASc score of 0 in men or 1 in women, it is reasonable to omit anticoagulant therapy patients with AF unless they also have moderate to severe mitral stenosis or a mechanical heart valve (Go et al., 2001). Aspirin has no role.

TABLE 12.1 CLINICAL DECISION RULES FOR ANTICOAGULATION

TYPE OF RISK	CLINICAL DECISION RULES
Stroke	For patients with atrial fibrillation, use the CHA(2)DS(2)-VASc stroke risk score to assess stroke risk in people with any of the following: • Symptomatic or asymptomatic paroxysmal, persistent, or permanent AF • Atrial flutter • A continuing risk of arrhythmia recurrence after cardioversion back to sinus rhythm (January et al., 2014)
Bleeding	Providers may use the HAS-BLED score to assess the risk of bleeding in people who are starting or have started anticoagulation. Other considerations are the need for modification and monitoring of the following risk factors: • Uncontrolled HTN • Poor control of INR • Concurrent medication, such as concomitant use of aspirin or an NSAID • Harmful alcohol consumption (January et al., 2014)

Choices for AC include warfarin and NOACs which include dabigatran and rivaroxaban, apixaban, and edoxaban. The latter three are also referred to as DOACs as they are factor Xa inhibitors. NOACs are recommended over warfarin in NOAC-eligible patients with AF except for those with moderate to severe mitral stenosis or a mechanical heart valve. Warfarin is recommended for these patients (Coleman et al., 2015).

Key Points

Rate control is the first-line strategy for people with AF, except in people

- whose AF has a reversible cause
- who have heart failure thought to be primarily caused by AF
- with new-onset AF
- with atrial flutter whose condition is considered suitable for an ablation strategy to restore sinus rhythm
- for whom a rhythm control strategy would be more suitable based on clinical judgment (January et al., 2014)

Rate Control

A standard beta-blocker or a rate-limiting calcium channel blocker is initial monotherapy to people with AF. The choice of drug should be based on the person's symptoms, heart rate, comorbidities, and preferences. Consider digoxin monotherapy for people with nonparoxysmal AF only if they are sedentary. This is important as digoxin works by increasing the vagal tone, which diminishes in a mobile patient. If monotherapy does not control symptoms, and if continuing symptoms are thought to be due to poor ventricular rate control, consider combination therapy with any two of the following: a beta-blocker, diltiazem, or digoxin (January et al., 2014).

Rhythm Control

Rhythm control may be achieved using pharmacologic or electrical cardioversion.

Decisions for cardioversion will be based on the duration of AF. For patients who have been in AF for more than 48 hr and are not adequately anticoagulated, electrical or pharmacologic cardioversion should be delayed until appropriate measures are taken to reduce the thromboembolic risk. Most of the time, it is not possible to conclude with certainty the exact duration of AF as patients may remain asymptomatic.

There are two approaches to reduce thromboembolic risk in these patients:

1. Administer oral anticoagulation for at least 3 weeks before electrical or pharmacologic cardioversion, or
2. Use a TEE-guided electrical cardioversion method when cardioversion cannot be postponed or an expedited approach is preferred. In these cases, once a therapeutic level of anticoagulation has been achieved with an oral agent, intravenous heparin, or subcutaneous enoxaparin, cardioversion may be performed. The TEE may be performed to exclude the presence of an intracardiac thrombus (Coleman et al., 2015).

Hemodynamic Instability

For patients with AF or atrial flutter of more than 48 hr' duration or unknown duration that requires immediate cardioversion for hemodynamic instability, anticoagulation should be initiated as soon as possible and continued for at least 4 weeks after cardioversion unless contraindicated. Amiodarone therapy may be considered with these patients, starting 4 weeks before and continuing for up to 12 months after electrical cardioversion to maintain sinus rhythm. It is important to discuss the benefits and risks of amiodarone with the patient (January et al., 2014).

Catheter Ablation

AF catheter ablation may be reasonable in patients with symptomatic AF and HF with reduced LV ejection fraction to potentially lower mortality rate and reduce hospitalization for HF. Surgical procedures such as the Cox-Maze, left atrial appendectomy, and the Watchman device are other options for invasive treatment. These may require more invasive approaches with longer recovery time. Developments in these procedures continue to evolve, becoming less invasive using robotic or catheter-based approaches.

Drug Treatment for Long-Term Rhythm Control

Assess the need for drug treatment for long-term rhythm control, taking into account the patient's preferences, associated comorbidities, and risks of treatment and likelihood of recurrence of AF. If drug treatment for long-term rhythm control is needed, consider a standard beta-blocker as first-line treatment unless there are contraindications. If beta-blockers are contraindicated or unsuccessful, consider alternative drugs for rhythm control, taking comorbidities into account (January et al., 2014).

Class Ia antiarrhythmic drugs including quinidine, procainamide, and disopyramide have become less commonly prescribed than in the past because of their side effect profiles. The class Ic agents, flecainide and propafenone, are usually well tolerated and are appropriate first-line options for the treatment of AF in patients without structural heart disease, LV hypertrophy, or marked pre-existing conduction disease. QT prolongation is an expected effect of these medications and requires frequent monitoring when the drug is initially begun.

Amiodarone is generally reserved for patients with AF for whom other antiarrhythmic drugs have been contraindicated, ineffective, or poorly tolerated. This is primarily because amiodarone has potential time-dependent and dose-dependent organ toxicities that can affect the liver, thyroid, lungs, and eyes (January et al., 2014).

Special Considerations

Patients treated for ACS normally require DAPT with aspirin plus a platelet P2Y12 receptor inhibitor. For patients with AF at increased risk of stroke, the addition of warfarin or an NOAC may be required, resulting in triple therapy for primary prevention. One option is to consider the use of an oral anticoagulant plus a P2Y12 inhibitor without aspirin. If triple therapy is used, a period of 4–6 weeks' duration is considered, as this is the period of greatest risk of stent thrombosis.

Case Study

Mr. E has a significant risk for stroke when using the CHA2DS2-VASc score and no risk for bleeding when assessed with HAS-BLED. His symptoms have been present for several days; thus his risk for thrombus is high. You choose to start a heparin infusion and perform a TEE before cardioversion. His TEE does not reveal any atrial thrombus and you successfully cardiovert him to sinus rhythm, resume his beta-blocker, and start apixaban.

CLINICAL PEARLS

1. The treatment of AF is complex with frequently updated guidelines.
2. Therapy for AF focuses on three goals: minimize thromboembolic stroke risk, control ventricular rate, and control the atrial rhythm in selected patients.
3. Any unstable patient presenting with AF should undergo immediate electrical cardioversion as documented in the Advance Cardiovascular Life Support guidelines.
4. Elective cardioversions are safe and effective with attention to appropriate anticoagulation strategies, including a TEE when needed.
5. Guidelines for specific topics include
    Stroke prevention of people with nonvalvular AF
    Rate control strategies
    Rhythm control strategies
    Left atrial ablation strategies
6. A pathway called the "Atrial Fibrillation Overview" is available from the National Institute for Health and Care Excellence (NICE).

HEART FAILURE

Case Study

Mr. E is admitted to the intermediate unit after his cardioversion for post-procedure recovery. His EF on the TTE is down from his previous findings and is now found to be 20%–25%. There is no significant wall motion abnormality. He also is found to have moderate AS. Did his physical examination demonstrate any concern for heart failure? How do you explain his drop in EF?

Definition

HF is a complex clinical syndrome that results from any structural or functional impairment of ventricular filling or ejection of blood. The cardinal manifestations of HF are dyspnea and fatigue, limited exercise tolerance, fluid retention, pulmonary and/or splanchnic congestion, and/or peripheral edema. HF affects nearly 6.2 million Americans. It is the primary diagnosis for hospital discharge in about 1 million and a secondary diagnosis in about 2 million hospitalizations annually. Patients admitted with HF have a 20%–30% risk of death within a year. Although survival has improved, the absolute mortality rates for HF remain approximately 50% within 5 years of diagnosis (Yancy et al., 2017).

Key Points

Because some patients present without signs or symptoms of volume overload, the term "heart failure" is now preferred over "congestive heart failure."

Etiology

HF may result from disorders of the pericardium, myocardium, endocardium, heart valves, or great vessels or from certain metabolic abnormalities, but most patients with HF have symptoms due to impaired LV myocardial function. The etiology of HF has been categorized into ischemic cardiomyopathy (ICM) or nonischemic cardiomyopathy (NICM). NICM may include cardiomyopathies due to volume or pressure overload, such as HTN or valvular heart disease (Yancy et al., 2017).

Classification

The ACC, the AHA, and the New York Heart Association (NYHA) have developed functional classifications and stages of heart failure. Table 12.2 lists classifications of heart failure. Therapeutic interventions are aimed at modifying risk factors, treating structural heart disease, and reducing morbidity and mortality. Most patients with acute decompensated heart failure (ADHF) are admitted for symptomatic treatment of congestion with intravenous diuretics, respiratory failure, cardiogenic shock, incessant ventricular tachycardia, or the need for urgent diagnostic or therapeutic procedures (Yancy et al., 2017).

Case Study

Mr. E has HTN and ischemic heart disease. His review of symptoms includes DOE, fatigue, and edema. His EF has decreased significantly since the last echo. He also has AS. Are there other review of symptoms that you need to explore?

TABLE 12.2 CLASSIFICATION OF HEART FAILURE

CLASS	DESCRIPTION
HFrEF	Heart failure with reduced left ventricular ejection fraction (EF ≤ 0.40)
HFpEF	Heart failure with preserved left ventricular ejection fraction (EF ≥ 0.50)
HFmrEF	Heart failure with midrange ejection fraction (EF <0.50 but >0.40)

Physical Findings

HF is largely a clinical diagnosis based on a comprehensive history and physical examination. Risk factors known at the time of hospitalization include age, duration of HF, and frequency of hospitalization. HTN, diabetes mellitus, metabolic syndrome, and atherosclerotic disease are important risk factors for HF (Yancy et al., 2017). Chronic renal dysfunction and right ventricular dysfunction predict higher risk. Of the biomarkers measured clinically, natriuretic peptide levels are the most robust predictors of readmission and death (Hollenburg et al., 2019).

Symptoms that need to be explored that are more specific to HF include fatigue, DOE, orthopnea, PND, and weight gain. Determining and quantifying changes in the patient's normal activity and changes that have occurred with the progression of symptoms is important. Symptoms of chest pain or any anginal equivalent may point toward an ischemic etiology.

Physical findings of HF have been categorized as warm or cold and wet or dry and reflect the patient's pulmonary and peripheral examination. A warm and wet clinical profile characterizes more than 80% of patients admitted with reduced EF and almost all with preserved EF except those with restrictive or hypertrophic cardiomyopathies. These patients have edematous, warm extremities, and pulmonary congestion and are often hypertensive. The cold and wet profile describes congestion accompanied by the clinical evidence of hypoperfusion, narrow pulse pressure, hypotension, cool extremities, oliguria, and reduced alertness. Altered mental status, impaired concentration, and very low urine output may also be present (Hollenberg et al., 2019).

The JVP reflects elevated right-sided filling pressures and is a sensitive indicator of elevated left-sided filling pressures. Rales, when present, usually indicate higher filling pressures than baseline. Extensive pitting edema, ascites, or large pleural effusions reflect large extravascular reservoirs that may take many days to develop (Yancy et al., 2013).

Diagnostic Tests

There is no specific/sensitive test for HF. Initial labs should include serum electrolytes, BUN, creatinine, lipid profile, liver function, and TSH. Natriuretic peptide biomarkers have been used increasingly to establish the presence and severity of HF. In general, both natriuretic peptide biomarker values, brain natriuretic peptide (BNP) and N-terminal prohormone of BNP (NT-proBNP), can be used in patient care settings. In patients treated with angiotensin receptor–neprilysin inhibitor (ARNI), NT-proBNP levels should be utilized as use will cause elevation in BNP levels.

A chest radiograph, though not specific for HF, is an important diagnostic used to assess heart size and pulmonary congestion. An echocardiogram will assess ventricular function, size, wall thickness, wall motion abnormalities, and valvular disease.

Invasive hemodynamic monitoring with a pulmonary artery catheter could be performed to guide therapy in patients who have respiratory distress or clinical evidence of impaired perfusion in whom the adequacy of intracardiac filling pressures cannot be determined from clinical assessment. Right heart and left heart catheter may be considered in patients who are congested to determine if filling pressures are elevated. Right atrial pressure (RAP) >10 mm Hg and pulmonary capillary wedge pressure >22 mm Hg are consistent in 75%–80% of patients with chronic HFrEF (Yancy et al., 2013).

Case Study

You are concerned that Mr. E's reduction in EF may be related to prolonged tachycardia-mediated stress and hope that restoring a regular rhythm will improve his EF. While he is hospitalized, you choose to be more aggressive with his diuresis due to his DOE and edema. Mr. E takes 20 mg of furosemide at home, and you increase this to 40 mg for the time being and chose to deliver it intravenously. You order daily weights and strict intake and output. His renal function is normal and electrolytes also WNL. What other measures for HF will you institute? What is the conversion of oral to intravenous furosemide, torsemide, and bumetanide?

Guideline-Directed Medical Therapy

Guideline-directed medical therapy (GDMT) has been developed and revised over the past several years, and optimal therapy should be achieved, which is reaching either the target or the highest tolerated dose for a given patient. Early stages of HF treatment include ACE-I or ARB, beta-blockade, and diuretics, if needed. Addition of an aldosterone antagonist should be considered with a reduced EF and advancing functional class. If the HF progresses to NYHA functional class II–IV with reduced EF, changing from ACE-I or ARB to ARNI should be considered. Use hydrazine and nitrates if the patient is African American and is unable to tolerate ACE-I or ARB (Yancy et al., 2013). SGLT-2 inhibitors represent a rapidly emerging group of drugs that have been shown to reduce hospitalization rates in patients with HFrEF. Although they are not a part of GDMT, they are very promising.

Implantable Cardioverter-Defibrillator

Implantable cardioverter-defibrillator (ICD) therapy is recommended for primary prevention of sudden cardiac death to reduce total mortality in selected patients with NICM. It is also considered for ischemic heart disease at least 40 days post-MI with LVEF of 35% or less and NYHA class II or III symptoms on chronic GDMT or for those with a LBBB.

Cardiac Resynchronization Therapy

Cardiac resynchronization therapy (CRT) may be considered for patients who have LVEF of 35% or less, sinus rhythm, a non-LBBB pattern with a QRS duration of 150 ms or greater, and NYHA class III/ambulatory class IV symptoms on maximally tolerated GDMT. CRT includes placement of an ICD along with biventricular pacemaker to synchronize contraction of both ventricles and potentially improve EF. Evaluation for advanced therapies should be considered in patients refractory to GDMT and includes heart transplant or ventricular assist devices as well as palliative care or hospice (Yancy et al., 2013).

> ### Key Points
>
> Hospitalization is a pivotal opportunity to decrease risk and improve clinical trajectory in patients who respond well to diuresis and who have not previously received adequate trials of GDMT.

The introduction of GDMT in patients hospitalized for HF with reduced EF is a key target and has been well documented to reduce risk. It should include introduction of ACE-I and beta-blockers, and it has recently added the recommendation for introduction of ARNI while in the hospital (Hollenberg et al., 2019). Neurohormonal antagonists have improved outcomes for HFrEF. When possible, continuation of GDMT through hospitalization or initiation before discharge is associated with substantially better outcomes (Yancy et al., 2017). Many institutions now have GDMT clinics where these patients are followed very closely in an ambulatory setting to reduce readmission.

Diuretic Use

National Heart, Lung, and Blood Institute–sponsored trials of ADHF have specified goals of resolution of edema, orthopnea, and jugular venous distention. The ultimate goals should aim to reduce JVP to <8 cm, relieve dyspnea at rest, and resolve residual orthopnea, PND, or edema. Establishing an effective diuretic regimen is crucial for addressing congestion. Patients usually require the first dose of intravenous (IV) diuretics at presentation or in the ED, and IV diuretics are continued throughout the hospitalization until effective decongestion warrants transition to oral diuretics before discharge (Hollenberg et al., 2019).

Recommendations for diuretics include administering an equivalent oral dose as IV at 1–2.5 times the total daily dose for patients who have been on loop diuretic therapy as an outpatient. If not on diuretics as an outpatient, initial furosemide dose will vary according to patients' fluid overload, kidney function, and age. Generally, the starting dose is 40–80 mg IV daily dose with additional IV bolus every 8–12 hr or by continuous IV infusion.

Acetazolamide 250–500 mg/day may also be considered in refractory patients. The escalation or modification of the diuretic dose depends on the diuretic response, target weight, kidney function, and other patient-related factors such as hemodynamic factors, comorbidities, and serum electrolytes (Hollenberg et al., 2019).

The treatment plan for care especially if on diuretics should include daily electrolytes with appropriate corrections. Daily weights, intake and urine output, kidney function by measurement of serum creatinine, and BUN should be monitored.

Comorbidities

Addressing comorbidities is an important aspect of treatment in patients with HF. Iron infusions should be used if anemia is present Additionally, optimal treatment of HTN and diabetes and a formal sleep assessment and treatment of obstructive sleep apnea with continuous positive airway pressure are addressed in the guidelines for treatment of HF (Hollenberg et al., 2019).

Valvular Disease

Valvular heart disease should also be evaluated in patients with HF. Mitral regurgitation or stenosis and AS are most commonly associated with HF.

Mitral Disorders

Mitral regurgitation (MR) may be surgically addressed if the cause is from primary MR or if it is secondary to connective tissue disorders, rheumatic heart disease, cleft mitral valve, and radiation heart disease. In patients in whom MR is secondary to severe LV dysfunction or CAD, treating the underlying cause is most important. Surgical intervention should be considered if the EF is <30%. Mitral valve surgery for MS patients is recommended if NYHA class III/IV with severe MS (Nishimura et al., 2014).

Aortic Disorders

Aortic valve replacement is recommended in symptomatic patients with severe AS and the following:

- Decreased systolic opening of a calcified or congenitally stenotic aortic valve;
- An aortic velocity 4.0 m/s or greater or mean pressure gradient 40 mm Hg or higher;
- Symptoms of HF, syncope, exertional dyspnea, angina, or presyncope by history or on exercise testing (Nishimura et al., 2014).

Discharge Planning and Palliative Care

Goals of hospitalization include not only clinical response but also the assessment and optimization of therapy to address the long-term trajectory after discharge.

GDMT for HF follows an interdisciplinary approach. For the inpatient care of the patient, the team should include the attending physician and the inpatient nurse, a pharmacist, and a discharge coordinator. Consultation for physical therapy or nutrition should be included in the formal plan and initiated early during hospitalization. Planning for discharge should be initiated at admission with consideration regarding long-term goals of care, identification of gaps in patient understanding and adherence, medical and prescription coverage, and optimization of the chronic regimen. ACNP can play a pivotal role in the care of the hospitalized HF patient by developing comprehensive quality programs and care plans. Successful transition from the hospital back into the residential setting is critical and general checklists have been provided to assist when discharging Medicare patients. These are useful when developing these programs and transitioning any HF patient care.

Advanced Care Planning

Approximately 20%–30% of patients have no improvement in their signs and symptoms during hospitalization. In addition, 15%–20% of clinical trial patients have worsening HF that needs rescue therapy with additional diuretics, IV vasoactive agents, or mechanical circulatory or respiratory support. Goals of care and review of the long-term trajectory of the patient who continues to worsen may require accelerated discussion regarding prognosis, selection, and arrangement of post-discharge care options including home healthcare, SNF, long-term care facilities, palliative care at home, or hospice. Integration of palliative care principles was outlined by an expert consensus document (Hollenberg et. Al. 2019) with emphasis on the importance of palliative care coexisting with active and invasive treatments up to the point of transition to hospice care. Data show that referral to palliative care for these patients remains underutilized and needs to occur early in the diagnosis.

Case Study

You initiate ACE-I on Mr. E along with resumption of his BB and diuretics. Since his EF is <35%, you discuss possible ICD/CRT but agree to defer with outpatient follow-up. The differential for his HF includes potential worsening from prolonged tachycardia, which is currently controlled after cardioversion. For the AF, he will continue on the beta-blockage and apixaban. For his CAD, you will continue a high-intensity statin and aspirin. He receives dietary teaching for a low-sodium, heart-healthy diet. He will monitor his weight daily and notify you if he gains more than 2 lbs in 1 day or 5 lbs in a week. You provide him with the Medicare discharge planning checklist (https://www.medicare.gov/pubs/pdf/11376-discharge-planning-checklist.pdf). He will follow up in 1 week with you in the GDMT clinic with plans for close monitoring of symptoms and up-titration of his mediations as tolerated over the next several weeks. Considerations of care will include initiation of ARNI as well as an outpatient echocardiogram to evaluate for any improvement in EF, progression of AS, and further discussion of consideration for ICD/CRT.

CLINICAL PEARLS

- The pathway to improve outcomes after HF hospitalization begins with admission, continues through the process of decongestion and transition to oral therapies before the day of discharge, and connects through the first post-discharge follow-up.
- The clinical trajectory of HF should be assessed continuously during admission. Three main in-hospital trajectories have been defined: improving toward target, stalled after initial response, or not improved/worsening. These translate into different management strategies throughout hospitalization and post-discharge.
- Evaluation of the long-term course of HF should be part of the initial comprehensive assessment, reviewed on the day of transition to oral therapy, and reassessed at the first follow-up visit for persistent or new indications of high risk leading to consideration of advanced therapies or revision of goals of care.
- Key risk factors modifiable during hospitalization include the degree of congestion as assessed by clinical signs and natriuretic peptides and the lack of appropriate GDMTs. Improvement in these factors is associated with improved prognosis, but failure to improve, including failure to tolerate GDMT for HF, is associated with a much worse prognosis.

- Common comorbidities, including diabetes, anemia, and kidney, lung, and liver disease, should be assessed during initial evaluation and addressed throughout hospitalization and discharge planning.
- The day of transition from intravenous to oral diuretic therapy should trigger multiple considerations related to the overall regimen for discharge, verification of completion of patient education components, caregiver education, and plans for discharge.
- The discharge day should be a time to review and communicate with identified providers rather than to initiate new therapies.
- The elements of the hospitalization events and plans that are most crucial for continuity of care after discharge should be documented in a format that is available to all members of the outpatient team and easily accessible when a patient calls or returns with worsening symptoms.
- Principles of palliative care applied by the in-hospital care team or by palliative care specialists may be particularly relevant when an unfavorable trajectory warrants communication about prognosis, options, and decision-making with patients and families.
- The first follow-up visit should address specific aspects, including volume status, hemodynamic stability, kidney function and electrolytes, the regimen of recommended therapies, patient understanding, adherence challenges (including insurance/coverage issues), and goals of care (Hollenberg et al., 2019).

AORTIC DISSECTION

Case Study

Mrs. S is an 89-year-old white female who resides at home with her daughter, who presents to the ED reporting 7/10 intermittent, aching, generalized chest pain, radiating to mid back which started about 3 hr ago. She notes that she has never felt this pain before and it is different from her arthritis pain. About 2 hr later she started to feel weak, faint, and nauseous. She laid down and attempted to take a nap, but was unable to get to sleep due to the aching pain. She decided to tell her daughter, who felt that it was appropriate to seek medical attention.

Her past medical history includes type 2 diabetes with peripheral neuropathy, HTN, hyperlipidemia, CAD, arthritis, sleep apnea, breast cancer treated with chemotherapy and radiation, hypothyroidism, and depression. She is allergic to penicillins, which cause anaphylaxis. Her immunizations include pneumococcal pneumonia >10 years ago and the influenza vaccine in October 2019. Her current medications are metoprolol 50 mg PO BID, lisinopril 40 mg PO daily, gabapentin 300 mg TID, Lantus 12 units SC every morning, Humalog per sliding scale TID before meals, Lipitor 40 mg every evening, levothyroxine 150 µg at 0630 daily, St. John's wort 150 mg daily, and Tylenol 650 mg every 6 hr PRN.

Her father and paternal grandfather were both deceased by age 65 years secondary to myocardial infarction. Both also had diabetes and CAD. Her mother died at age 92 and had COPD, HTN, diabetes, breast cancer, arthritis, and GERD.

Her sister, who is 87, has diabetes, GERD, IBS, and depression. Her brother, who is 80, has HTN, BPH, GERD, depression, and hypothyroidism.

Mrs. S is a retired social worker who has two daughters and one son and enjoys gardening, playing cards, and playing bingo. She walks to the senior center, which is approximately a quarter of a mile from home, four times per week and helps serve lunch.

She endorses a 25 pack-year smoking history (cigarettes); she did quit 14 years ago. She drinks two glasses of red wine about two times per week, usually with dinner.

She has had the following surgeries and procedures: right hip replaced in 2012, bilateral cataract surgery in 2009, a cholecystectomy in 1961, and bilateral mastectomy with reconstructive surgery in 2005.

You elicit the following information with your review of systems:

- General: denies fever, fatigue, or unexpected weight changes
- Neuro: denies dizziness or lightheadedness, but feels faint and has a mild headache
- HEENT: endorses intermittent blurry vision; denies discharge from eyes, ears, or nose; denies eye or ear pain; denies tinnitus; denies congestion; denies trouble chewing/swallowing
- Cardiac: endorses 7/10 intermittent, aching, generalized chest pain, sudden onset, radiating to neck and upper back which started about 3 hr ago; it is aggravated by movement and not relieved when resting; nothing has helped improve it
- Respiratory: denies SOB, DOE, orthopnea, cough, or hemoptysis; denies flu-like symptoms
- GI: denies vomiting or changes in bowel habits; endorses persistent nausea
- GU: denies dysuria, frequency, hesitancy, urgency, or foul-smelling urine
- Musculoskeletal: endorses intermittent joint pain; denies tenderness
- Integumentary: fungal rash under abdominal folds, otherwise no skin changes; denies appearance of lesions

Her physical examination revealed the following:

- Height, 167.64 cm (66 in); weight, 96 kg (211.2 lbs)
- Vital signs: temperature, 99 °F; HR, 120 bpm; RR, 26 breaths/min; BP, 189/105 mm Hg; Spo2, 93% on RA
- General: She is tachypneic but able to converse in full sentences and appears well-developed and well-nourished for her stated age.
- Neurological: Her eyes open spontaneously. She tracks and focuses. Her visual acuity is intact and speech is clear and appropriate. She reports generalized weakness and is alert and oriented to person and time with disorganized thinking. Pupils, equal, round and reactive to light results are 3 mm brisk. She has a right facial droop. Her tongue is midline. She is moving all extremities with equal strength, and sensation is intact.

- Cardiac: She has sinus arrhythmia with frequent PVCs. You appreciate a III/IV diastolic murmur. Pulses are 1+ to both upper and lower extremities, and she has generalized nonpitting trace edema. She has a right carotid bruit and abdominal aorta bruit.
- Respiratory: She is tachypneic; her lungs are clear bilaterally with diminished sounds to both bases. Chest wall excursion is symmetric, and respirations are nonlabored.
- GI: She has normal bowel sounds. Her abdomen is soft and mildly tender diffusely on palpation. There are no visible pulsations and no masses felt.
- GU: She has clear amber urine with light sediment.
- Musculoskeletal: She has no inflammation, tenderness, or edema to joints. She is hypermobile with loose joints and a ROM appropriate for her age.
- Integumentary: Her skin is hyperelastic, dry, and fragile, with scattered bruising.

Based on her presentation and physical examination, what are your top differentials, including must-not-miss? What are your next steps? What will you order?

Based on the information you have received, your must-not-miss diagnoses include STEMI, aortic dissection, and PE. Other top differentials would include acute infectious/inflammatory pulmonary process.

Your diagnostics should include an ECG to rule out STEMI/NSTEMI; a CXR, which may assist in your differential for aortic dissection and other pulmonary or thoracic concerns; and computed tomography with arterial contrast enhancement (CTA) of chest and abdomen for evaluation for aortic disease, PE, and abdominal aortic aneurysm (AAA). Laboratory tests would include CBC to evaluate for infections/inflammation, anemia, a metabolic panel for electrolyte abnormalities, renal dysfunction, cardiac enzymes, lactic acid, and pro-BNP.

Pertinent results you obtain from Mrs. S's tests include the following:

- CBC: WBC, 9.7 10*3/ul; Hbg, 7.6 g/dl; Hct, 25.6%; MCV, 85 fl; PLT, 133 10*3/ul
- Chemistry: Na, 139 mmol/L; K, 5.1 mmol/L; chlor 92 mmol/L, HCO_3, 27 mmol/L; BUN, 10 mg/dl; creatine, 0.8 mg/dl; glucose, 189 mg/dl; Ca, 9.1 mg/dl; Mg, 2.4 mg/dl; Phos, 4.2 mg/dl; lactic, 3.1
- Cardiac enzymes: troponin, 1.7 ng/ml; CK, 1319 U/L; CKMB, 4.7; pro-BNP, 350 pg/ml; d-dimer, 20 ng/ml
- UA: glucose, negative; ketones, negative; blood, negative; pH, 5.7; specific gravity, 1.010; protein, negative; leukocytes, negative; nitrite, negative
- ECG: HR, 90 bmp; normal PR, QRS, sinus rhythm, normal axis; no ST or T wave abnormalities

You order a CXR.

Your interpretation is as follows:

- Widened mediastinum
- Diffuse enlargement of the aorta, with poor definition of the aortic contour
- Enlarged cardiac silhouette

You are concerned that there is aortic dissection.

Do you have enough data for diagnosis? What test is most sensitive and specific for a more definitive diagnosis? Your patient has an emergent chest CT with arterial contrast enhancement (CTA) and the radiologist calls you with his impression. There is thickening of the aortic wall and displacement of intimal calcifications with dissection of the descending thoracic aorta suggesting type B aortic dissection.

CLINICAL PERALS

CT scanning has a reported sensitivity of 83%–95% and specificity of 87%–100% for the diagnosis of acute aortic dissection (Erbel et al., 1989).

Transthoracic echocardiogram has a very high sensitivity and specificity. It is non-invasive and can be performed at the bedside if the patient is stable (Agabegi & Agabegi, 2016).

Aortic angiography is the best test for determining the extent of the dissection if surgery is indicated (Agabegi & Agabegi, 2016).

Etiology and Types

An aortic dissection occurs in a weakened area of the aortic wall resulting in a tear of the innermost layer of the aorta (intima) that allows blood to flow between the layers of the aortic wall and force them apart (Ziganshin et al., 2014). There are two types of aortic dissections per the Stanford Classification: type A and type B. Type A involves dissection of the ascending aorta and requires immediate surgical intervention, and type B involves dissection of the descending aorta and is usually managed medically initially unless complications arise (Ziganshin et al., 2014). Types A and B can be categorized by DeBakey classification as type I through type III. Types I and II are dissections of the ascending and descending aorta and dissection of the ascending aorta, respectively. These types are also type A. Type III involves only the descending aorta and is the same as type B.

Congenital causes include familial aortic dissections, adult polycystic kidney disease, Turner syndrome, osteogenesis imperfecta, bicuspid aortic valve, and coarctation of the aorta. Other causes include cocaine use, chronic high blood pressure, pregnancy, deceleration injuries in chest trauma, and cardiologic procedures such as valve replacements, CABG, cardiac catheterization, and/or angiogram. Connective tissue disorders such as Marfan syndrome, Ehlers-Danlos syndrome, and metabolic disorders can also cause aortic dissections (Ziganshin et al., 2014). Ehlers-Danlos syndrome is a group of inherited heterogeneous disorders that decrease the tensile strength and integrity of other connective tissue (Castori & Voermans, 2014). This group of connective tissue disorders is characterized by easy bruising, delayed wound healing, and atrophic scarring caused by abnormal collagen synthesis, which lead to hyperextensibility of the skin, hypermobility of the joints, and tissue fragility (Castori & Voermans, 2014).

Treatment

Acute type A dissection is surgical emergency. Initial treatment for type B dissection would also include a cardiothoracic/vascular surgery consultation to determine if surgery is warranted. Surgery would be considered for complications such as refractory pain, rapidly expanding false lumen, or impending or frank rupture. If indicated, the approach may be an endovascular vs. open surgical approach. You would obtain a cardiology consult for medical management and arrange a detailed management plan post-acute medical and/or surgical interventions.

The majority of type B dissections are managed medically and your goals are to prevent further extension of the dissection and decrease the risk of rupture. Medical management will include beta-blockers. In this case, the first-line medication is esmolol (Brevibloc), which is a short-acting intravenous antiarrhythmic/beta-blocker; the starting dose is 50 µg/kg IV bolus followed by an infusion at 50 µg/kg/min to lower the patient's heart rate and diminish the force of LV ejection (Hagan et al., 2000). Pain control with morphine sulfate can be initiated, and the patient should be on Nothing by mouth status. A bedside echocardiogram should be obtained to assess valve patency and determine cause of murmur, assess thickness of the heart wall, determine ventricular ejection, and assess cardiac involvement. An antiemetic such as ondansetron can be used to control nausea and prevent retching, which may exacerbate the dissection. Hemodynamic parameters include blood pressure control and maintaining a MAP above >65 mm Hg. Arterial line insertion is indicated for closer hemodynamic monitoring. Troponin should be trended to monitor enzyme activity and the Critical Care Team should be consulted.

Case Study

Due to early recognition of the patient's presenting symptoms and rapid evaluation, you prevent rupture and further complications related to aortic dissection. Your patient is admitted to the ICU and placed on esmolol. Adequate BP control is attained and she is transitioned to oral metoprolol. She has an initial AKI, but this resolves with hemodynamic support. She is discharged home in good condition. She will need follow-up in 1 week and then close follow-up for the next year.

REVIEW QUESTIONS

1. Mr. M is a 58-year-old man who presents to the ED with chest pain. Which of the following would be your initial diagnostic test?
    a. CXR
    b. ECG
    c. Serum cardiac markers
    d. Cholesterol levels

2. Mr. S is a 68-year-old man who presents to your office complaining of 3 hr of substernal chest pain. He endorses 2 weeks of progressive dyspnea with exertion. Which is the most important next step in management?
   a. Aspirin 325 mg
   b. Sublingual nitroglycerin
   c. Administration of a beta-blocker
   d. Chest radiograph

3. A 66-year-old woman comes into your cardiology clinic for follow-up for newly diagnosed asymptomatic atrial fibrillation. Which of the following is the most common complication of her atrial fibrillation?
   a. Sudden death
   b. Stroke
   c. Shock
   d. Dyspnea

4. A 55-year-old man is seen in the ED with 3 hr of substernal chest pain radiating to his left arm. He has no other associated symptoms and the pain is relieved with sublingual nitroglycerin. His ECG has no acute changes. You share this information with him and he requests to be discharged. Which of the following statements is most accurate?
   a. The patient may be safely discharged home.
   b. If a repeat ECG in 60 min is normal, ACS is essentially ruled out and the patient may be safely discharged.
   c. He should be advised that half of heart attack patients have a nondiagnostic ECG and serial cardiac biomarker levels should be assessed.
   d. You should have him undergo an exercise stress test as an outpatient to further assess for CAD.

5. Mrs. B is a 75-year-old woman who presents to the ED with dyspnea, fatigue, and palpitations. Her blood pressure is 85/50 mm Hg and her ECG reveals a narrow complex tachycardia with a heart rate of 140 beats per minute. She is cool and diaphoretic. Which of the following would you choose for treatment of this patient?
   a. Diltiazem
   b. Metoprolol
   c. Amiodarone
   d. Cardioversion

6. Mr. R is a 75-year-old man who sees you regularly in clinic for CHF with impaired systolic function. His EF is 40%. You have initiated GDMT. Which of the following drugs may lower his mortality risk?
   a. Metoprolol
   b. Digoxin
   c. Aspirin
   d. ACE-I

7. Which of the following is most likely to have caused the CHF in a 55-year-old man who has CHF with impaired systolic function?
   a. Diabetes
   b. Atherosclerosis
   c. Alcohol
   d. Valvular heart disease

8. A 55-year-old man is noted to have CHF and states that he is comfortable at rest but becomes dyspneic with any exertion. On echocardiography, he is noted to have an ejection fraction of 45%. Which of the following is the more accurate description of this patient's condition?

    a. Diastolic dysfunction

    b. Systolic dysfunction

    c. Dilated cardiomyopathy

    d. Angina

Answers: 1, b; 2, a; 3, b; 4, c; 5, d; 6, d; 7, b; 8, b

REFERENCES

Agabegi, E. D., & Agabegi, S. S. (2016). *Step-up to medicine*. Wolters Kluwer.

Anderson, J. L., & Morrow, D. A. (2017). Acute myocardial infarction. *N Engl J Med*, 376(21), 2053–2064. https://doi.org/10.1056/NEJMra1606915.

Castori, M., & Voermans, C.N. (2014). Neurological manifestations of Ehlers-Danlos syndrome(s): A review. *Iranian Journal of Neurology*, 13(4), 190–208.

Coleman, C. M., Khalaf, S., Mould, S., Wazni, O., Kanj, M., Saliba, W., & Cantillon, D. (2015). Novel oral anticoagulants for DC cardioversion procedures: Utilization and clinical outcomes compared with warfarin. *Pacing and clinical electrophysiology*, 38, 731–737.

de Denus, S., Sanoski, C. A., Carlsson, J., Opolski, G., & Spinler, S. A. (2005). Rate vs rhythm control in patients with atrial fibrillation: A meta-analysis. *Arch Intern Med*, 165, 258–262.

Erbel, R., Engberding, R., Daniel, W., Roelandt, J., Visser, C., & Rennollet, H. (1989) Echocardiography in diagnosis of aortic dissection. *Lancet*, 1(8636), 457.

Go, A. S., Hylek, E. M., Phillips, K. A., Chang, Y., Henault, L. E., Selby, J. V., & Singer, D. E. (2001). Prevalence of diagnosed atrial fibrillation in adults: National implications for rhythm management and stroke prevention. The Anticoagulation and Risk Factors in Atrial Fibrillation (ATRIA) study. *Journal of the American Medical Association*, 285, 2370–2375.

Hagan, P.G., Nienaber, C.A., Isselbacher, E.M., Bruckman, D., Karavite, D.J., Russman, P.L., Evangelista, A., Fattori, R., Suzuki, T., Oh, J. K., Moore, A. G., Malouf, J. F., Pape, L. A., Gaca, C., Sechtem, U., Lenferink, S., Deutsch, H. J., Diedrichs, H., Marcos y Robles, J., …Eagle, K. A. (2000). The International Registry of Acute Aortic Dissection (IRAD): New insights into an old disease. *Journal of the American Medical Association*, 283(7), 897.

Hollenberg, S. M., Warner Stevenson, L., Ahmad, T., Amin, V. J., Bozkurt, B., Butler, J., Davis, L. L., Drazner, M. H., Kirkpatrick, J. N., Peterson, P. N., Reed, B. N., Roy, C. L., & Storrow, A. B. (2019). 2019 ACC expert consensus decision pathway on risk assessment, management, and clinical trajectory of patients hospitalized with heart failure: A report of the American College of Cardiology solution set oversight committee. *Journal of the American College of Cardiology*, 74, 1966–2011.

January, C. T., Wann, L. S., Alpert, J. S., Calkins, H., Cigarroa, J. E., Cleveland, J. C., Jr, Conti, J. B., Ellinor, P. T., Ezekowitz, M. D., Field, M. E., Murray, K. T., Sacco, R. L., Stevenson, W. G., Tchou, P. J., Tracy, C. M., Yancy, C. W., & American College of Cardiology/American Heart Association Task Force on Practice Guidelines. (2014). 2014 AHA/ACC/HRS guideline for the management of patients with atrial fibrillation: A report of the American College of Cardiology/American Heart Association Task Force on practice guidelines and the Heart Rhythm Society. *Journal of the American College of Cardiology*, 64, 2246–2280.

Neumar, R. W., Shuster, M., Callaway, C. W., Gent, L. M., Atkins, D. L., Bhanji, F., Brooks, S. C., de Caen, A. R., Donnino, M. W., Ferrer, J. M., Kleinman, M. E., Kronick, S. L., Lavonas, E. J., Link, M. S., Mancini, M. E., Morrison, L. J., O'Connor, R. E., Samson, R. A., Schexnayder, S. M., …Hazinski, M. F. (2015). Part 1: Executive summary 2015 American Heart Association guidelines update for cardiopulmonary resuscitation and emergency cardio vascular care. *Circulation*, 132(Suppl. 2), S315–S367.

Nishimura, R. A., Otto, C. M., Bonow, R. O., Carabello, B. A., Erwin, J. P., III, Guyton, R. A., O'Gara, P. T., Ruiz, C. E., Skubas, N. J., Sorajja, P., Sundt, T. M., III, & Thomas, J. D. (2014). 2014 AHA/ACC guideline for the management of patients with valvular heart disease: Executive summary. A report of the American College of Cardiology/American Heart Association Task Force on practice guidelines. *Journal of the American College of Cardiology*, 63, 2438–2488.

O'Gara, P. T., Kushner, F. G., Ascheim, D. D., Casey, D. E., Chung, M. K., de Lemos, J. A., Ettinger, S. M., Fang, J. C., Fesmire, F. M., Franklin, B. A., Granger, C. B., Krumholz, H. M., Linderbaum, J. A., Morrow, D. A., Newby, L. K., Ornato, J. P., Ou, N., Radford, M. J., Tamis-Holland, J. E., ...Zhao, D. X. (2013). 2013 ACCF/AHA guideline for the management of ST-elevation myocardial infarction: a report of the American College of Cardiology Foundation/American Heart Association Task Force on practice guidelines. *Journal of the American College of Cardiology, 61*(4), e78–e140. https://doi.org/10.1016/j.jacc.2012.11.019

Thygesen, K., Alpert, J. S., Jaffe, A. S., Chaitman, B. R., Bax, J. J., Morrow, D. A., White, H. D., & Executive Group on behalf of the Joint European Society of Cardiology (ESC)/American College of Cardiology (ACC)/American Heart Association (AHA)/World Heart Federation (WHF) Task Force for the Universal Definition of Myocardial Infarction. (2018). Fourth universal definition of myocardial infarction (2018). *Journal of the American College of Cardiology, 72*(18), 2231-2264. https://doi.org/10.1016/j.jacc.2018.08.1038

Yancy, C. W., Jessup, M., Bozkurt, B., Butler, J., Casey, D. E., Jr, Colvin, M. M., Drazner, M. H., Filippatos, G. S., Fonarow, G. C., Givertz, M. M., Hollenberg, S. M., Lindenfeld, J., Masoudi, F. A., McBride, P. E., Peterson, P. N., Stevenson, L. W., Westlake, C. (2017). 2017 ACC/AHA/HFSA focused update of the 2013 ACCF/AHA guideline for the management of heart failure: A report of the American College of Cardiology/American Heart Association Task Force on clinical practice guidelines and the Heart Failure Society of America. *J Am Coll Cardiol, 70*, 776–803.

Ziganshin, B. A., Dumfarth, J., & Elefteriades, J. A. (2014). Natural history of Type B aortic dissection: Ten tips. *Annals of Cardiothoracic Surgery, 3*(3), 247–254. http://doi.org/10.3978/j.issn.2225-319X.2014.05.15

13

Pulmonary Management

Jamie Gooch • Heather Wilson

ASTHMA

Case Study

You are the APRN covering the hospitalist service when your pager goes off requesting immediate help in room 204. On arrival you find Ms. T, a 26-year-old woman admitted 2 days ago with nephrolithiasis. She is sitting up in bed, propping herself up with extended arms, and appearing to be in distress. You note that she is tachypneic, using accessory muscles, and appears focused on her breathing. Her nurse informs you that approximately 5 min after receiving a small dose of IV morphine for pain, the patient rang the call bell complaining that she could not breathe. Although she appeared distressed, her O_2 sat at the time was 98%, her HR was 104 bpm, and her BP was 122/65 mm Hg. Her nurse noted wheezing throughout all lung fields and four- to five-word dyspnea. He administered Ms. T's rescue albuterol inhaler for which there was a standing order. After 5 min, Ms. T's symptoms had not improved, so the inhaler was administered again, and her nurse called you.

Upon review of Ms. T's chart, you note a PMH pertinent for eczema, current tobacco abuse (4 pack-years), and asthma controlled with a PRN short-acting beta-agonist (SABA) rescue inhaler. This is her first hospital admission.

Your initial differential diagnoses and evidence are as follows:

1. Acute asthma exacerbation is the most likely diagnosis. Ms. T. has a history of asthma for which she is prescribed an SABA. Additionally, her use of tobacco, a known trigger for asthma exacerbation, puts her at increased risk for hospitalization (Thomson et al., 2004). We know from her nurse that she received a dose of IV pain medication immediately before her symptoms began. Strong emotions such as fear, anger, and frustration are also triggers for an asthma attack (National Asthma Education and Prevention Program, 2007). Her initial presentation is pertinent for wheezing and a complaint of dyspnea, which further support the diagnosis.

2. Anaphylaxis: The RN reports that shortly before Ms. T developed sudden onset dyspnea, she had received a dose of IV morphine. This is a new medication for her, and as such it is possible that she has an undiagnosed allergy making

anaphylactic reaction a possibility. The incidence of anaphylaxis in people diagnosed with asthma is twice that of people who do not carry the diagnosis (González-Pérez et al., 2010). Additionally, tachycardia and feelings of panic and impending doom often precipitate anaphylaxis (Simons, 2010).

3. Other: COPD or pneumonia is the least likely diagnosis. Acute COPD exacerbation can mimic an acute asthma exacerbation. Ms. T does have a history of tobacco abuse, which is a known risk factor for COPD; however, her age and low pack-year history as well as the absence of previous COPD history make this differential less likely. Although PNA can present with hypoxia and dyspnea, Ms. T has no signs of infection. In the absence of history of cough, presence of leukocytosis, or fever, pneumonia is less likely.

It has been 10 min since her last metered-dose inhaler (MDI) administration, and the patient does not appear to be improving. You suspect a severe asthma exacerbation and order repeat vital signs, continuous pulse oximetry, and continuous O_2 with nebulized albuterol and ipratropium (Table 13.1). You then continue to perform a focused physical exam and review common asthma triggers to consider in her assessment and treatment (Table 13.2). Ipratropium bromide is recommended in severe asthma exacerbations, as is magnesium sulfate if patients are not responding to initial treatment (Global Initiative for Asthma, 2019).

TABLE 13.1 TREATMENT OF ACUTE ASTHMA EXACERBATION

DEGREE OF SEVERITY	TREATMENT
Mild	SABA via MDI or continuous nebulizer Usually may be cared for at home
Moderate	Repeated SABA + oral systemic corticosteroids Office, urgent care, or ED visit
Severe	Repeated or continuous SABA + IV systemic corticosteroid ± adjunctive therapies ED visit and possible hospitalization
Severe, not responding to initial treatment	SABA + anticholinergic, IV systemic corticosteroids Consider magnesium sulfate or heliox if unresponsive to other medications, intubation for impending respiratory failure (PaO_2 < 60, or normal or rising CO_2) ICU admission likely

ED, emergency department; ICU, intensive care unit; IV, intravenous; MDI, metered-dose inhaler; SABA, short-acting beta-agonist.

TABLE 13.2 ASTHMA TRIGGERS

TYPE	EXAMPLES
Environmental	Pollen, dust, pollutants, tobacco and smoke, animal dander
Emotional	Stress, anxiety, strong emotions, fear, anger
Other	Exercise, infection, cold air

Assessment and Treatment

Initial assessment of the patient presenting with asthma includes determining the severity of the attack by evaluating pertinent signs and symptoms, conducting a thorough physical examination and performing tests of pulmonary function (PFTs or spirometry) if the patient is able (National Asthma Education and Prevention Program, 2007). Symptomatic assessment occurs simultaneously with initiation of treatment and includes evaluation of dyspnea, respiratory rate, heart rate, oxygen saturation, and lung function (GINA, 2019). Treatment goals center around correcting hypoxemia and relieving the airway obstruction and inflammation. This is accomplished through the use of supplemental O_2 if hypoxemia is present, administration of intermittent or continuous SABA with or without an anticholinergic, and systemic IV corticosteroids. Routine screening with CXR is not indicated unless pneumothorax is suspected, nor are empiric antibiotics in the absence of suspected infection (GINA, 2019).

Case Study

Your physical exam reveals the following:

- HR, 132 bpm; RR, 26 breaths per min; BP, 102/65 mm Hg with inspiration; O_2 sat, 89%
- Gen: Distressed appearing young adult sitting upright in bed
- Skin: Warm, + perspiration, nail bed cyanosis present
- CV: RRR, tachycardic HR 132, + pulsus paradoxus
- Lungs: Minimal wheezing with quiet breath sounds, no rales or rhonchi; + use of accessory muscles; one- to two-word dyspnea; + tachypnea
- Neuro: Drowsy and confused; follows commands after repeated instructions

What findings from her examination are concerning to you? What is the significance of the drop in her BP? Her lung examination appears to have quieted. Is this a hopeful sign? Is she improving? Why or why not?

Assessment of Impending Respiratory Collapse

A quieting lung examination or the absence of wheezing in the presence of acute asthma exacerbation is an ominous sign, especially when coupled with the onset of drowsiness or confusion. These findings are highly suspicious for severe airflow obstruction with hypercarbia and impending respiratory collapse and require immediate transfer to the ICU (GINA, 2019).

Additionally, Ms. T's examination is notable for a drop of 20 points in her systolic blood pressure. This is pulsus paradoxus—a drop in systolic blood pressure of >10 mm Hg during inspiration—and is caused by increased negative intrathoracic pressure as the patient strains to breathe against obstructed airways resulting in decreased left ventricular preload and consequently reduced left ventricular output (Hamzaoui et al., 2013).

Case Study

On your reevaluation, you note that despite repeated administration of albuterol with ipratropium, she has not responded. You recognize this is an emergent situation that necessitates immediate intubation and transfer to the ICU for management. Prior to her transfer, you order magnesium sulfate, which has been shown to reduce hospital admissions and improve lung function in adults experiencing acute asthma exacerbations not responding to first-line therapies (Kew et al., 2014). You ask the RN to page the CRNA on call STAT to intubate Ms. T at bedside.

What orders will you enter while awaiting intubation? Is a CXR necessary?

Status Asthmaticus

Severe refractory asthma, better known as status asthmaticus, is an emergent situation requiring immediate life-saving interventions. Mainstays of treatment include continuous nebulized SABA plus an anticholinergic, IV corticosteroids, and magnesium sulfate or heliox, in addition to emergent intubation. Serial VS, pulse oximetry, and ABGs should also be obtained.

A CXR is not indicated unless you suspect lung injury or complication like pneumothorax.

CLINICAL PEARLS

- Early recognition and intervention are the mainstays of treatment for acute asthma exacerbation. This includes close monitoring and frequent VS, including SpO_2, and PFTs if the patient is able to cooperate.
- Initial treatment with SABA (either via MDI or nebulizer) is indicated for all those presenting with acute asthma exacerbation. An anticholinergic (e.g., ipratropium) may be added if the initial SABA is ineffective in emergent situations.
- Diminished wheezing and presence of drowsiness are ominous factors indicative of hypercarbia and impending respiratory collapse requiring immediate intubation.
- Initial treatments for acute asthma exacerbation refractory to rescue inhaler include continuous SABA and IV glucocorticoids.
- CXR is not indicated in workup of acute asthma exacerbation unless there is other evidence for infectious process (e.g., leukocytosis, fever, purulent sputum) or pneumothorax (e.g., chest pain) exists.

PNEUMONIA

Case Study

Mr. R, a 46-year-old man, presents to the Fast Track in the ED with his spouse. He complains of an intermittent, nonproductive cough for 1 week, shortness of breath with stair climbing, and a high fever of 102.3 °F, which has persisted despite around-the-clock acetaminophen. During his interview, you note that he is fuzzy on the details of his recent illness and that his husband must frequently help him with the answers. He reports that Mr. R has been mostly confined to the couch and has not been eating or drinking much. His PMH includes hyperlipidemia, STEMI s/p drug-eluting stent (DES) 4 years ago, and recent discharge from University Hospital 2 weeks ago, where he underwent single-vessel CABG and was intubated for 3 days post-op.

His current mediations include daily aspirin 81 mg, Lipitor 20 mg QHS, metoprolol 25 mg bid, and lisinopril 10 mg QD. He has also begun taking Tylenol 650 mg Q 6H for fever and NyQuil QHS for his cough.

On examination, you note the following:

- VS: HR, 114 bpm; BP, 90/58 mm Hg; RR, 28 breaths per min; and SpO_2, 89% on RA
- CV: RRR; no m/r/g; midline incision well healed and without signs of infection
- Lungs: CTA except for inspiratory crackles noted posteriorly in the area of the RML; no wheeze or rhonchi; + nonproductive cough; + egophony; equal expansion bilaterally
- Skin: Warm to touch, dry, poor turgor; nail beds pink, and without clubbing
- Neuro: Pleasant mood, awake and alert, but appears mildly confused; provider must repeat some questions to elicit answers

What are your top differentials based on his presentation?
What diagnostics/laboratory tests will you order to help you narrow down your diagnosis?
You order a CXR and laboratory tests, which result as the following:

- CXR report: Upright portable AP image. Adequate inspiration and penetration. Mediastinal wires noted and are closed and well aligned. No pneumothorax, pulmonary edema, or pleural effusion noted. Image positive for a right middle lobe consolidation with air bronchograms
- Laboratory tests: WBC, 15 K/µl; Hgb, 14 g/dl; platelets, 250 K/µl; sodium, 132 mmol/L; BUN, 30 mg/dl; creatinine, 2.4 mg/dl

Based on Mr. R's HPI, history, and physical exam, your most likely differentials and evidence are as follows:

1. Pneumonia: CAP vs. ventilator-associated pneumonia (VAP). Mr. R's presentation is pertinent for shortness of breath, persistent fever, and cough, which are highly suspicious for a respiratory infection. Infiltrate on CXR or via ultrasound is required to confirm the diagnosis of pneumonia (Kaysin & Viera, 2016). Infiltrates may be observed in the form of opacification of lung tissue, presence of air bronchograms, or lobar consolidation. The patient's history in conjunction with his right middle lobe consolidation and air bronchograms make pneumonia the most likely diagnosis. Mr. R was recently hospitalized and intubated for 3 days. This further expands our differential to include risk for a VAP, so this must also be considered in conjunction with CAP.
2. Pulmonary embolism (PE): Mr. R is short of breath, tachycardic, and hypoxic, all of which are concerning for possible PE. He also has had a recent hospital stay and an increased period of immobility, which also increase his risk for

DVT and subsequent PE. Evaluation for PE can include VQ scan or CTA of the chest. In Mr. R's case, a VQ scan is most appropriate because of his AKI (creatinine of 2.4 mg/dl) and the contrast dye, which can be nephrotoxic, needed for obtaining the CTA.

3. CHF: His presentation of shortness of breath, borderline hypotension, and history of CAD and recent CABG put heart failure in our list of differentials. Mr. R's CXR, however, without evidence of pulmonary edema (a typical "bat wing" pattern in CHF) or pleural effusion, makes this differential less likely.

After ordering a BNP, cardiac enzymes, and a VQ scan, you are able to rule out cardiac dysfunction and PE from your list of potential differential diagnoses. As such, you determine that Mr. R is most likely suffering from CAP or VAP.

What are your next steps? Based on his presentation and current diagnostics, is hospital admission indicated? You can use the CURB-65 risk assessment tool (Table 13.3) to identify the likelihood that the diagnosis is pneumonia (Lim et al., 2003). CURB-65 and the Pneumonia Severity Index (PSI) are both clinical decision-making tools that can be useful in determining whether or not a patient presenting with PNA should be admitted to the hospital.

Based on Mr. R's CURB-65 score of 3 (confusion +1, uremia +1, low BP +1) and his clinical presentation, you decide to admit him to the progressive care unit and to treat him for bacterial pneumonia. Because of his recent intubation, you recognize that it is prudent for you to adjust his antibiotic regimen to not only cover organisms associated with CAP but also for organisms that are known to be prevalent in VAP.

What antimicrobial regimen will you order?

TABLE 13.3 CURB-65 CRITERIA

CRITERIA	YES	NO
Confusion	1+ point	0 points
Uremia (BUN >19 mg/dl or 7 mmol/L)	1+ point	0 points
Respiratory rate ≥30 breaths/min	1+ point	0 points
Systolic blood pressure <90 mm Hg or diastolic blood pressure ≤60 mm Hg	1+ point	0 points
Age ≥65 years	1+ point	0 points
Score	**Disposition**	
0–1: Mortality risk, 1.5%	Outpatient care	
2: Mortality risk, 9.2%	Inpatient vs. observational admission	
≥3: Mortality risk, 22%	Admission for score of 4 or 5; inpatient admission with consideration for ICU	

BUN, blood, urea, nitrogen; ICU, intensive care unit.
Data from Lim, W. S., Van der Eerden, M. M., Laing, R., Boersma, W. G., Karalus, N., Town, G. I., Lewis, S. A., & Macfarlane, J. T. (2003). Defining community acquired pneumonia severity on presentation to hospital: An international derivation and validation study. *Thorax, 58,* 377–382.

Treatment for Pneumonia

Typical bacterial pathogens that cause CAP include *Streptococcus pneumoniae, Haemophilus influenzae, Moraxella catarrhalis,* and human rhinovirus. VAP develops at least 48 hr after endotracheal intubation, and the most common pathogens are gram-negative bacilli, *Staphylococcus aureus,* and *Pseudomonas aeruginosa.* Methicillin-resistant *S. aureus* (MRSA) and other forms of drug resistance are a great concern. Consideration of antibiotic coverage is provided in Table 13.4.

Case Study

Due to Mr. R's risk for VAP and recent stay in the ICU, you decide to start broad-spectrum antimicrobial therapy with coverage for *Pseudomonas*, MRSA, and gram-negative bacilli (IDSA, 2016).

After settling on a plan of care, you return to Mr. R's bedside and review the diagnosis of CAP vs. VAP with him and his spouse. You explain that he will be admitted based on his current vital signs and laboratory test results. Additionally, you order O_2 via nasal cannula at 2 L/min to titrate to an O_2 sat >92% and a 500-cc bolus of NS to be given over 15 min due to his hypotension, followed by a continuous infusion at 150 ml/hr, and first doses of his antimicrobials to be administered prior to his leaving the ED.

TABLE 13.4 INFECTIOUS DISEASE SOCIETY OF AMERICA COMMUNITY-ACQUIRED PNEUMONIA TREATMENT

CHARACTERISTICS	TREATMENT
Non-ICU	Respiratory fluoroquinolone or beta-lactam + macrolide
ICU	Beta-lactam + azithromycin or fluoroquinolone
Pseudomonas	Antipseudomonal, antipneumococcal beta-lactam + ciprofloxacin or levofloxacin or beta-lactam + aminoglycoside + azithromycin or beta-lactam + aminoglycoside + antipneumococcal fluoroquinolone
With MRSA	Add vancomycin or linezolid

ICU, intensive care unit; MRSA, methicillin-resistant *Staphylococcus aureus.*

CLINICAL PEARLS

- Infiltrate on CXR or other imaging is required for diagnosis of pneumonia (Mandell et al, 2007).
- Treatment for patients presenting with severe CAP should include sputum and blood culture, urinary *Legionella* and *Streptococcus pneumoniae* antigen testing (Mandell et al, 2007).
- First dose of antibiotic should be given while patient is still in the ED (Mandell et al, 2007).
- Treatment for VAP is strongly predicated on each institution's local antibiogram (IDSA, 2016).

ACUTE RESPIRATORY DISTRESS SYNDROME

Case Study

You are the APRN in the ICU and are called for a consult in the ED. The patient is a 72-year-old female with a PMH of HTN, DM, CAD s/p coronary artery bypass grafts 6 years ago, and history of heart failure with preserved ejection fraction who presented to the hospital 3 days ago with a complaint of cough and fevers. The ED attending states the patient is becoming restless, and the oxygen saturations are decreasing to 85%.

Her past medical history includes HTN, hyperlipidemia, diabetes mellitus, and heart failure with preserved ejection fraction. Her surgical history includes a laparoscopic cholecystectomy 5 years ago. She has no known drug allergies. Her current medications include metoprolol 25 mg BID, aspirin 81 mg daily, Lipitor 80 mg daily, and metformin 1000 mg BID.

Her review of systems is positive for increasing fatigue and fevers up to 102 °F at home. She also complains of a dry, nonproductive cough. She does report shortness of breath that is worse with exertion; however, she denies chest pain, palpitations, orthopnea, or nocturnal dyspnea. She denies lower extremity edema, abdominal pain, nausea, vomiting, or urinary symptoms.

Her physical examination reveals that she is neurologically intact. Her mucus membranes are dry, and she has tenting of the skin. Her heart sounds include S1S2 regular with no murmurs, rubs, or gallops and no jugular vein distention (JVD). Her lungs reveal rhonchi to the left base with dullness to percussion. Her abdomen is soft, nontender with normal bowel sounds, and no hepatosplenomegaly. Her lower extremities have no edema, and she has palpable pulses throughout. Her bilateral patellas appear slightly mottled. Her vital signs are as follows: temperature, 102 °F; HR, 123 bpm; RR, 30 breaths per minute; BP, 88/50 mm Hg; and SpO_2, 95% on 2 L nasal cannula.

Based on the above information, your initial differential diagnoses and data supporting those diagnoses are as follows. Are there any must-not-miss diagnoses based on the patient's history and examination?

1. Bacterial pneumonia: Evidence supporting this diagnosis include her presenting symptoms of cough, fever, and shortness of breath. Her physical examination lends to this diagnosis with adventitious lung sounds to the left base, and patient has documented hypoxia.
2. Severe sepsis: Evidence supporting this diagnosis includes the presence of hyperthermia, tachypnea, tachycardia, and hypotension. She also has signs of hypoperfusion on physical examination with mottling of her lower extremities.
3. CHF exacerbation: Evidence that may support this is her preexisting cardiac history or CABG as well as her documented history of diastolic heart failure. However, her physical examination does not support volume overload. She has dry mucous membranes, no JVD, and no lower extremity edema. This diagnosis is less likely.

You are reviewing her diagnostic tests, which reveal the following: Na, 135 mmol/L; K, 3.7 mmol/L; CL, 100 mmol/L; CO_2, 18; BUN, 30 mg/dl; creatinine, 1.6 mg/dl; and lactic acid, 2.4. Her ABG is as follows: pH, 7.4; PCO_2, 28 mm Hg; PO_2, 80 mm Hg; HCO_3, 22 mEq/l on 2 L nasal cannula. Blood cultures and urinalysis with reflex to culture were sent.

What is your interpretation of the ABG? Based on your interpretation of her ABG, you determine that she has compensated respiratory alkalosis.

Her chest radiograph reveals left lower lobe consolidation with air bronchograms.

What is your admitting diagnosis now with these additional diagnostic criteria? Where should she be admitted?

Sepsis

CAP can lead to severe sepsis, diagnosed by hyperthermia, tachypnea, tachycardia, hypotension, and hypoperfusion on physical examination, as well as the signs of hypoperfusion evident in laboratory tests, including AKI and lactic acidosis. A documented infiltrate on chest radiograph supports a diagnosis of sepsis. Review the CURB-65 scoring to aid in admission placement.

Case Study

The patient is admitted to the ICU on broad-spectrum antibiotics, a beta-lactam and azithromycin, as well as a bolus infusion of a 30 ml/kg of crystalloid for indication of severe sepsis followed by a crystalloid infusion of 100 ml/hr. You are called 2 hr later by the registered nurse because the patient is having increasing shortness of breath and hypoxia with oxygen saturation dropping to the 70s. When you go to evaluate the patient, she is sitting upright in bed. Her respiratory rate is in the 40s with the use of accessory muscles. She has already been placed on a 100% NRB. You order an ABG and the results are as follows: pH, 7.25; PCO_2, 55 mm Hg; PO_2, 58 mm Hg; and HCO_3, 20 mEq/l.

This ABG shows an uncompensated respiratory acidosis. With this patient's respiratory distress and marked tachypnea, you would expect the ABG to reveal a respiratory alkalosis. The respiratory acidosis is a sign of impending respiratory failure, especially with the patient's profound hypoxemia. Your next steps would be to prepare for intubation. After intubation, you obtain a stat chest radiograph. Interpret the image in Figure 13.1 using the techniques you learned in Chapter 5.

You use the patient's ABG results to calculate her PaO_2/FiO_2 ratio. Her PaO_2 is 58 mm Hg, and her FiO_2 is 100% (expressed as a decimal, it is 1), so her PaO_2/FiO_2 ratio is 58.

From this new diagnostic information, you diagnose her with acute respiratory distress syndrome (ARDS) because of septic shock from pneumonia.

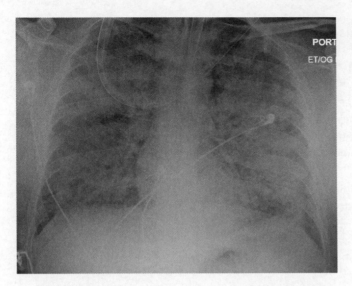

Figure 13.1 This chest radiograph reveals diffuse bilateral infiltrates.

Diagnostic Criteria of ARDS

ARDS is an acute form of lung injury that is characterized by widespread inflammation and is associated with mortality rates as high as 30%–40% (Harman, 2020). ARDS is usually a diagnosis of exclusion, with the key being that cardiogenic pulmonary edema must be excluded as the cause of respiratory failure. ARDS is a form of noncardiogenic pulmonary edema, and this is an important distinction. Clinical diagnosis can be made using the Berlin criteria. For diagnosis, all the following must be present:

- Worsening symptoms within 1 week of initial presentation
- Bilateral opacities on chest radiograph or CT scan
- Exclusion of cardiogenic pulmonary edema as a cause
- A moderate to severe impairment in oxygenation as evidenced by the PaO_2/FiO_2 (P/F) ratio

In addition, the P/F ratio is used to categorize the severity of ARDS using the criteria included in Table 13.5.

The treatment for ARDS is mostly supportive care, as there has been no identified medication to treat or lessen the clinical course in patients with ARDS. Patients require supplemental oxygen and possibly mechanical ventilation. The National Heart, Lung and Blood Institute, National Institutes of Health was formed to study the treatment

TABLE 13.5 SEVERITY OF ACUTE RESPIRATORY DISTRESS SYNDROME	
SEVERITY	**CRITERIA**
Mild	PaO_2/FiO_2 >200 mm Hg but less than 300 mm Hg
Moderate	PaO_2/FiO_2 >100 mm Hg but less than 200 mm Hg
Severe	PaO_2/FiO_2 <100 mm Hg

for ARDS and is the clinical guideline with a mechanical ventilator protocol for patients with ARDS. The end targets for mechanical ventilation in ARDS include maintaining an arterial pH between 7.30 and 7.45 and an oxygenation goal of PaO_2 of 55–80 or SpO_2 of 88%–95%. It is also recommended to keep the plateau pressure, which measures the pressure applied to the small airways and alveoli by mechanical ventilation, less than 30 cm H_2O (National Heart Lung and Blood Institute, 2014). Other supportive measures in ARDS include use of sedation for comfort and for improving ventilator compliance, hemodynamic monitoring, and both DVT and GI prophylaxis. You may also consider the use of systemic glucocorticoids in patients who are early in the disease course and who have refractory hypoxemia despite the standard supportive measures stated above (Siegel, 2020). The most important point is to give supportive care while treating the underlying cause of ARDS.

Case Study

You continue to monitor her response to the antibiotics and mechanical ventilation over the next week, with attention to reducing the risk for other complications, such as thromboembolism, muscle wasting, and delirium, or ICU psychosis. She is able to slowly turn the corner with careful administration and monitoring of her antibiotic regimen, nutrition and fluid intake, and gastrointestinal management. After 2 weeks, she is extubated and discharged to the general floor with plans for rehabilitation to improve her strength and ADLs before being discharged home.

REVIEW QUESTIONS

1. Which of the following signs in acute asthma exacerbation is ominous?
   a. Wheezing throughout
   b. Tachycardia and tachypnea with an SpO_2 of 98%
   c. Presence of pulses paradoxus
   d. Acute exacerbation that responds after inhaled SABA and IV glucocorticoid

2. SABA is most effective when administered how?
   a. Via nebulizer
   b. Via MDI with a spacer
   c. Long-acting beta-agonist (LABA) is more appropriate for acute asthma exacerbation
   d. Both A and B

3. You have a patient with developing ARDS secondary to severe sepsis. Their VS are as follows: Temp, 102 °F; HR, 110 bpm; RR, 36 breaths per min; BP, 132/67 mm Hg; and SpO_2, 88% on 60% high flow. Which of the following ABGs signifies impending respiratory failure for this patient and would most likely precipitate intubation?
   a. pH, 7.35; PCO_2, 35; PO_2, 100; HCO_3, 22
   b. pH, 7.4; PCO_2, 28; PO_2, 88; HCO_3, 16
   c. pH, 7.25; PCO_2, 55; PO_2, 60; HCO_3, 24
   d. pH, 7.33; PCO_2, 30; PO_2, 76; HCO_3, 20

Answers: 1, c; 2, d; 3, c

REFERENCES

Global Initiative for Asthma (GINA). (2019). *Global strategy for asthma management and prevention.* https://ginas-thma.org/wp-content/uploads/2019/06/GINA-2019-main-report-June-2019-wms.pdf

González-Pérez, A., Aponte, Z., Vidaurre, C. F., & Rodríguez, L. A. (2010). Anaphylaxis epidemiology in patients with and patients without asthma: A United Kingdom database review. *The Journal of allergy and clinical immunology,* 125(5), 1098–1104.

Hamzaoui, O., Monnet, X., & Teboul, J. L. (2013). Pulsus paradoxus. *The European Respiratory Journal,* 42(6), 1696–1705. https://doi.org/10.1183/09031936.00138912

Harman, E. (2020). Acute respiratory distress syndrome. In Pinsky, M. (Ed.), *Medscape.* Retrieved May 2, 2020. https://emedicine.medscape.com/article/165139-overview

Kalil, A. C., Metersky, M. L., Klompas, M., Muscedere, J., Sweeney, D. A., Palmer, L. B., Napolitano, L. M., O'Grady, N. P., Bartlett, J. G., Carratalà, J., El Solh, A. A., Ewig, S., Fey, P. D., File, T. M., Jr, Restrepo, M. I., Roberts, J. A., Waterer, G. W., Cruse, P., Knight, S. L., & Brozek, J. L. (2016). Management of Adults With Hospital-acquired and Ventilator-associated Pneumonia: 2016 Clinical Practice Guidelines by the Infectious Diseases Society of America and the American Thoracic Society. *Clinical Infectious Diseases,* 63(5), e61 -e111. https://doi.org/10.1093/cid/ciw353.

Kaysin, A., & Viera, A. (2016). Community acquired pneumonia in adults: Diagnosis and managment. *American Family Physician,* 94(9), 698–706.

Kew, K., Kirtchuk, L., & Michell, C. (2014). Intravenous magnesium sulfate for treating adults with acute asthma in the emergency department. *Cochrane Database of Systematic Reviews,* 5, CD010909. https://doi.org/10.1002/14651858.CD010909.pub2

Lim, W. S., Van der Eerden, M. M., Laing, R., Boersma, W. G., Karalus, N., Town, G. I., Lewis, S. A., & Macfarlane, J. T. (2003). Defining community acquired pneumonia severity on presentation to hospital: An international derivation and validation study. *Thorax,* 58, 377–382.

Mandell, L., Wunderink, R., Anzueto, A., Bartlett, J. G., Campbell, G. D., Dean, N. C., Dowell, S. F., File, T. M., Jr, Musher, D. M. Niederman, M. S., Torres, A., Whitney, C. G., Infectious Diseases Society of America, & American Thoracic Society. (2007). Infectious disease society of America/American Thoracic Society consensus guidelines on the management of community-acquired pneumonia in adults. *Clinical Infectious Diseases,* 44(S2), S27–S72.

National Asthma Education and Prevention Program. (2007). *Expert panel report 3: Guidelines for the diagnosis and management of asthma.* National Heart, Lung and Blood Institute.

National Heart, Lung and Blood Institute. (2014). *National heart, lung and blood Institute (NHLBI) ARDS network.* Ardsnet.org. Retrieved May 2, 2020. http://www.ardsnet.org

Siegel, M. (2020). Acute respiratory distress syndrome: Clinical features, diagnosis, and complications in adults. In Parsons, P. (Ed.), *UpToDate.* UpToDate. Retrieved May 2, 2020. https://www.uptodate.com/contents/acute-respiratory-distress-syndrome-clinical-features-diagnosis-and-complications-in-adults/print

Simons, F. E. (2010). Anaphylaxis. *The Journal of Allergy and Clinical Immunology,* 125(Suppl. 2), S161–S181.

Thomson, N. C., Chaudhuri, R., & Livingston, E. (2004). Asthma and cigarette smoking. *Eur Respir J.* 2004, 24, 822–833.

14

Gastrointestinal Management

Karen Marie Petrok • Gloriann Albini

THE MANAGEMENT OF ABDOMINAL PAIN

The evaluation of abdominal pain can be both fascinating and frustrating. It can be straight-forward, such as when the pain corresponds to the underlying organ. It can also be a mystery when the pain has absolutely no relation to its location. Abdominal pain represents 5%–10% of ED visits in the United States (Kamin et al., 2003). Mastery of the evaluation of the patient with abdominal pain is a skill that a practitioner will use routinely and a chief complaint that should not be taken lightly.

Case Study 1

You are a nurse practitioner working in a community hospital when Ms. K comes into the emergency department. Ms. K is a 68-year-old female with a past medical history of HTN, diabetes, and obesity. She presented to the emergency department with complaints of palpitations. She was found to have atrial fibrillation with rapid ventricular response. She is to remain in the hospital on telemetry monitoring. Cardiology has been consulted and a plan has been developed for her to have a TEE in the morning followed by electrocardioversion. Her blood pressure has been stable with the systolic in the 130–150 range. Her heart rate has been elevated but has been controlled with a combination of diltiazem intravenous and orally. Overnight she complained of a crampy pain in the periumbilical area. Despite being given an antacid, after 2 hr the pain worsened, and she became nauseated with bilious vomiting. You are called to the bedside by the staff nurse and find her listless and confused. Her BP is now 96/50 mm Hg, her heart rate is in the 110s–160s, and she remains in atrial fibrillation. Her nurse informs you that she has had two stools that were positive for occult blood.

You begin IV fluid resuscitation with a 500-ml bolus of lactated Ringer (LR) solution and then continue at 100 ml/hr. You order laboratory work consisting of a CBC, complete metabolic profile (CMP), lactic acid, and lipase level. You also order a CT abdomen/pelvis with IV contrast only, and a GI consult.

Upon physical examination, she is pale, ill appearing, and diaphoretic. The examination by systems reveals the following:

- Neurological: She is awake and alert with confused conversation. Her pupils are equal and reactive to light and accommodation. She thinks she is at home and cannot remember the day or the year.
- Skin: Cool and clammy
- Cardiac: Irregular rate and rhythm; SM2/6 heard best @LSB; neck veins are flat; radial and pedal pulses are positive.
- Pulmonary: Clear to auscultation bilaterally.
- GI: Abdomen softly distended, tympanic to percussion, no hepatosplenomegaly (HSM), no masses palpated, no rigidity; she is positive for guarding; rectal was refused; pain appears out of proportion to examination.
- Genitourinary: No suprapubic pain or costovertebral angle tenderness with palpation.
- Extremities: No edema, cyanosis, or clubbing.
- Psych: Thought process intact.

While you are waiting for laboratory test results you order an abdominal x-ray.

The laboratory test results return and are as follows: WBC, $14 \times 10^9/L$; Hgb, 11 g/dl; lactic acid, 4 mg/dl.

Hypotension, tachycardia, elevated WBC, and lactic acidosis indicate a sepsis pattern. You continue with aggressive fluid resuscitation and initiate empiric broad-spectrum antibiotic coverage (to cover both aerobic and anaerobic microorganisms) with cefepime 2 g IV every 12 hr and Flagyl (metronidazole) 500 mg IV every 6 hr.

What are your top differentials and what will you do next?

Differential Diagnosis

The differential for diagnosis of abdominal pain is broad. It can be as benign as irritable bowel syndrome or as life threatening as a ruptured abdominal aortic aneurysm. The clinician must learn to develop a systematic method of examination guided by a careful history, remembering that pathology outside of the abdomen can also cause abdominal pain including pulmonary, cardiac, rectal, and genital disorders. Although many patients with abdominal pain will not have life-threatening/-altering disease, the older clientele can be at more risk. Older patients with abdominal pain have a six- to eightfold increase in mortality compared to younger patients (Hustey et al., 2005; Lewis et al., 2005).

Assessment

A detailed history of present illness (HPI) is vital to help determine the etiology of the pain. Here are some questions to ask the patient:

- What are the onset, the timing, the location, the intensity, and the duration of the pain?
- Are there any accompanying symptoms?
- When did the pain start?
- Did it start slowly and become more severe over time?
- Did it start suddenly and become severe quickly?

- Has the pain been going on for weeks, intermittently, waxing and waning?
- What is the quality of the pain? Is it sharp and stabbing, dull and aching, crampy, twisting?
- Do you have fever, chills, hematuria, dysuria, or back pain?
- Do you have nausea, vomiting, constipation, or diarrhea?
- Have you had dark, bloody, clay-colored, or mucus-filled stool?
- Does the pain increase or decrease with movement?
- Does it improve or worsen with food?
- Do OTC medicines such as acetaminophen, ibuprofen, laxatives, or antacids make a difference in the severity of the pain?

Key Points

Pain that is sudden and severe in onset may be indicative of a more serious, acute etiology. Pain that is gradual in onset may be indicative of inflammation, infection, or obstruction.

Referred pain occurs when the nerve pathways are shared among the organs.

A key to the origin of the pain is the location of the pain. Many times, but not always, the location of pain will correspond with the underlying organ. Table 14.1 includes common etiology based on location.

TABLE 14.1 LOCATION OF PAIN TO DISEASE PROCESS

LOCATION	BODY SYSTEM DISEASE PROCESS
Right Upper Quadrant	Biliary Cardiac
Right Lower Quadrant	Appendix Ovary PID
Epigastric	Cardiac MI PUD Pancreatitis Biliary
Umbilicus	IBD Bowel Obstruction Ischemia IBS Appendicitis DKA Gastric Enteritis
Left Upper Quadrant	Splenic Renal Colic Diverticulitis
Left Lower quadrant	Ovary Ectopic Pregnancy

DKA, diabetic ketoacidosis; IBD, inflammatory bowel disease; IBS, irritable bowel syndrome; MI, myocardial infarction; PID, pelvic inflammatory disease; PUD, peptic ulcer disease.

Careful history taking may uncover preexisting conditions that will help to guide your differential diagnosis. For example, a person with cardiovascular disease or peripheral vascular disease is at increased risk of mesenteric ischemia. Someone with previous bowel surgery is at increased risk of developing a small bowel obstruction due to the formation of adhesions. A person who has diarrhea and recent antibiotic use may have a *Clostridium difficile* infection. A history of frequent alcohol use may point toward pancreatitis. It is important to allow differential diagnoses to aid in the decision process and to use them to explore all possibilities leading to a diagnosis.

Case Study

The abdominal x-ray was read by the radiologist as normal. Your patient remains ill appearing despite aggressive fluid resuscitation and administration of antibiotics. She has persistent severe abdominal pain in combination with new onset atrial fibrillation, hypotension, lactic acidosis, and a normal abdominal x-ray. You are beginning to think that an acute intra-abdominal process is occurring. You need more information and decide to order a stat CT of the abdomen/pelvis with IV contrast only.

The abdominal CT reveals segmental bowel wall thickening, and a surgical consult is advised.

You are now becoming suspicious that your patient may have acute mesenteric ischemia.

Acute Mesenteric Ischemia

Acute mesenteric ischemia is an acute condition of inadequate blood flow through the mesenteric vessels. Ischemia that affects the small intestine is generally referred to as mesenteric ischemia, whereas ischemia that affects the large intestine is referred to as colonic ischemia. It can occur in either the arterial or venous blood vessels and can constitute a surgical or medical emergency. If untreated, it can lead to bowel gangrene, sepsis, and/or death (Dang, 2020). Arterial ischemia can be either occlusive or nonocclusive. Arterial occlusive disease is most commonly caused by an arterial embolism and less commonly by thrombus. If the ischemia is secondary to venous causes, venous thrombus has the highest mortality. Symptoms of mesenteric ischemia may be nonspecific; therefore, the clinician must maintain a high level of clinical suspicion for this elusive disease. Acute mesenteric ischemia is considered a disease of the older population.

Initial presenting symptoms of mesenteric ischemia include abdominal tenderness and distention. There may be accompanying symptoms of nausea, vomiting, and/or anorexia. Stool may be positive for occult blood. As bowel ischemia progresses and transmural infarction develops, the abdomen becomes more grossly distended, bowel sounds disappear, and peritoneal signs start to develop.

The timing of the pain may give an indication to the underlying diagnosis. With an acute onset, the pain begins rapidly, is severe, is usually out of proportion to the physical examination, and can be accompanied by nausea and vomiting. Furthermore, the patient normally has one or more risk factors. With a venous thrombosis, the pain may have a more indolent course. There is a lower mortality, and it normally occurs in persons of advanced age.

| BOX 14.1 | Major Causes of Mesenteric Ischemia |

- Mesenteric arterial embolism: 50%
- Mesenteric arterial thrombus: 15%–25%
- Mesenteric venous thrombus: 5%
- Nonocclusive mesenteric ischemia secondary to intestinal hypoperfusion: 20%–30%

Data from Reinus, J. F., Brandt, L. J., & Boley, S. J. (1990). Ischemic diseases of the bowel. *Gastroenterology Clinics of North America, 19*, 319–343.

Anatomy

The arterial blood supply to the intestine consists principally of the superior mesenteric artery (SMA) and the inferior mesenteric artery (IMA). The SMA supplies the entire small intestine except for the proximal duodenum. The SMA and IMA supply the colon. The celiac artery along with others provide a system of collateral blood flow to the intestines. Reviewing the anatomy allows one to realize how the reduction of blood flow to/within the SMA or IMA can lead to intestinal ischemia.

Risk Factors

Risk factors include any condition that reduces perfusion to the intestine or that predisposes it to mesenteric artery embolism, arterial thrombosis, venous thrombosis, or vasoconstriction. Among these are advanced age, atrial fibrillation, cardiovascular disease, CHF, hypovolemia, myocardial infarction, and peripheral vascular disease. Major causes of mesenteric ischemia are listed in Box 14.1.

Types of Mesenteric Ischemia

Mesenteric Arterial Embolism

SMA thrombus associated with cardiac problems is the most common type of arterial occlusion representing approximately 50% of the causes of acute mesenteric occlusion (Wolf, 1994). The majority of arterial emboli originate from the heart from a thrombus that has dislodged from the left atrium, left ventricle, cardiac valves, or proximal aorta. Excessive bowel distention from a bowel obstruction can lead to hypoperfusion to the bowel due to increased venous pressure from formation of thrombus of the involved segment of bowel.

Arterial Thrombus of Mesenteric Circulation

Arterial thrombus of mesenteric circulation usually occurs in patients with a history of chronic intestinal ischemia from atherosclerotic disease. It can also occur in response to abdominal trauma or infection.

Venous Thrombosis

Venous thrombosis may be idiopathic from hypercoagulopathy or from secondary causes such as malignancy. A personal or family history of DVT or PE is present in approximately one half of patients with acute mesenteric venous thrombosis (Harward et al., 1989).

Nonocclusive Mesenteric Ischemia

Nonocclusive ischemia is usually caused by any condition that can drop the cardiac output reducing blood flow to and from the intestine and hypoperfusing the intestine with oxygen. This includes but is not limited to sepsis, shock, hemorrhage, and medication.

Imaging and Laboratory Studies

If a patient presents with abdominal pain and any of the above conditions, you must have suspicion for mesenteric ischemia. A CT of the abdomen with IV contrast should be performed.

In the evaluation of mesenteric ischemia, laboratory work may be of some assistance in narrowing the differential diagnosis, but most of the laboratory test results may be non-specific. Nonetheless, a CBC with differential, CMP, amylase, lactic acid level, and coagulation studies including PT, PTT, INR, and a D-Dimer should be among the laboratory tests ordered. Frequently, the laboratory test results will be normal. They may result in a leukocytosis or signs of hemoconcentration, and there may be an elevation in liver function studies or elevation in amylase. The D-Dimer may be positive in conditions where there is a thrombus present.

In mesenteric ischemia, an abdominal x-ray may be nonspecific and in fact may be normal in more than 25% of patients (McKinsey & Gewertz, 1997). The film may show ileus with distended loops of bowel, bowel wall thickening, pneumatosis intestinalis (gas within the wall of the small or large intestine), or free air. The latter signs are found with advanced ischemia. One of the primary reasons for obtaining an abdominal x-ray is to exclude other cause for the symptoms.

Angiography has been considered the gold standard for diagnosis, as it has 100% specificity for acute arterial occlusion (Boley et al., 1973). Unfortunately, it may not be readily available when needed on an emergency basis. A CT of the abdomen has become a screening tool for abdominal pain, as it can be quickly and easily obtained. CTA of the abdomen may reveal focal or segmental bowel wall thickening, intestinal pneumatosis with portal vein gas, bowel dilatation, mesenteric stranding, portal vein thrombosis, or solid organ infarction (Kernagis et al., 2003; Taourel et al., 1996). As with abdominal x-ray, an abdominal CT is also used to eliminate other causes of abdominal pain.

Management

As with any patient, management of hemodynamic stability is a priority, along with monitoring for decompensation. Acute treatment includes fluid resuscitation with the appropriate IV fluids, bowel decompression with a nasogastric tube (when indicated), pain control, broad-spectrum antibiotics, anticoagulation when indicated for those patients with thrombus, early surgical intervention, and management of the causative agent. Management is individualized to each condition and patient and is beyond the scope of this chapter.

Case Study

Ms. K's condition stabilized after receiving fluid resuscitation and IV antibiotics. Serial abdominal examination showed an abdomen that was increasingly tender. She developed abdominal rigidity and an emergent surgical consult was obtained. She was taken to the operating room for exploratory laparotomy and resection of ischemic bowel. Postoperatively, she was sent to the ICU for serial hemodynamic monitoring. Cardiology was called to assist with managing her atrial fibrillation. Due to early recognition of her mesenteric ischemia, she did well and was downgraded to the surgical floor on day 2. Her diet was advanced and tolerated well. She received appropriate perioperative prophylaxis and, on day 4, was discharged home on Eliquis with close follow-up by surgery and cardiology.

CLINICAL PEARLS

- If a patient has nausea, vomiting, and diarrhea accompanied by severe sudden periumbilical abdominal pain that is out of proportion to the physical examination, suspect arterial embolism.
- A history of a prior embolic event is present in approximately one-third of patients with acute embolic mesenteric ischemia.
- Any patient with acute abdominal pain and metabolic acidosis has intestinal ischemia until proven otherwise.
- Normal laboratory values do not exclude acute mesenteric ischemia and should not delay radiological evaluation when clinical suspicion exists.
- Abdominal computed axial tomography (CAT) scan should be performed without oral contrast because the contrast can obscure the mesenteric vessels, obscure bowel wall enhancement, and delay the diagnosis

LIVER DYSFUNCTION

Case Study 2

You are an APRN working as a hospitalist in a large teaching hospital. Your assignment includes Mr. K, a 52-year-old male admitted to a general medical unit with a chief concern of abdominal pain. His past medical history includes HTN and inflammatory bowel disease (IBD) most consistent with ulcerative colitis (UC). He reports that he has not had a flare up of UC in over 2 years. He has no past surgical history. His current medications include lisinopril 20 mg daily and HCTZ 12.5 mg daily. He admits to taking ibuprofen OTC as needed for mild pain. He denies taking vitamins or herbal supplements. He has an allergy to penicillin, which causes a rash, but this was told to him by his mother, and he never takes it "just in case." His social history reveals that he is married with two children and works in medical equipment sales, which he describes as "very stressful." He has never smoked, vaped, or used smokeless tobacco. He admits to drinking one to two beers per week. He denies illicit drug use. He has no tattoos and has recently been tested negative for HIV. His family history was positive for HTN in both parents. He is an only child.

His review of systems reveals the following: He endorses fatigue, itching, and weight loss of approximately 5 pounds over the past 2 weeks. He has no fever, chills, nausea, or vomiting. He has no constipation, diarrhea, or dark or bloody stool. His stool is formed and brown. He admits to RUQ abdominal pain, which he describes as sharp stabbing and nonradiating. There is no headache, dizziness, chest pain, cough, or shortness of breath. He has no leg swelling or skin discoloration and no cyanosis of skin or nail beds.

His physical examination reveals the following:

- General: He is a well-appearing male in no acute distress. He looks his stated age.
- HEENT (Head, Eyes, Ears, Nose, Throat): Normocephalic, atraumatic, no scleral jaundice, no cervical lymphadenopathy.
- Cardiac: S1, S2 regular rate and rhythm without murmur, gallop, or rub.
- Chest: Clear anterior and posterior bilaterally with easy work of breathing.
- Abdomen: Soft, normoactive bowel sounds in all four quadrants. RUQ tenderness to palpation without rebound guarding or rigidity. Negative Murphy sign. Liver edge is palpated approximately two fingers breadth below the costal margin. No nodularity noted.
- Extremities: Without edema, cyanosis, or clubbing.
- Skin: Warm, dry, and intact.
- Neurological: Awake, alert, oriented to person, place, day, and date; neurological examination is non focal.

As you start your workup, you order laboratory studies consisting of a CBC, CMP, and a lipase level. You also order a CXR. Laboratory work results reveal a CBC that is WNL. There is no leukocytosis or anemia. Electrolytes, glucose BUN, Cr., and lipase are also WNL. LFTs are part of a CMP. You notice that the LFTs are highlighted as abnormal, what do you do next?

Liver Pathophysiology

When a patient's LFTs are abnormal, a repeat LFT panel or a clarifying test is warranted in order to confirm that the liver chemistry is abnormal. In order to decide what to do next, you need to understand how to evaluate the patient with abnormal liver studies. To do this, you first need to understand the basic pathophysiology of the liver.

The liver is the largest internal organ in the body. It weighs about 3 lbs and is located in the right side of the abdomen sitting just below the diaphragm. The gallbladder sits underneath it on its right. The spleen and the stomach are on the left, and all of these organs are covered by the peritoneum, which protects it and holds it in place in the abdomen. The primary job of the liver is to detoxify various metabolites, synthesize proteins, and produce enzymes necessary for digestion. It plays a role in metabolism, regulation of RBCs, and glucose synthesis and storage (Lala, 2020). The magnitude of functions the liver performs are too numerous to discuss in the scope of this chapter.

Liver Function Studies

Liver chemistries are markers of liver injury, not function, and should be called liver chemistries or tests, not LFTs (Kwo et al., 2017). The goal of these tests is to detect the release of products that are characteristic of the liver into the bloodstream, thereby indicating liver injury. Laboratory value results differ from laboratory to laboratory, all considered within a range of normal. Therefore, they will not be discussed in this chapter.

Basic liver function studies include ALT, AST, bilirubin, alkaline phosphatase (ALP), albumin, INR, and PT. Other tests include ammonia level, albumin level, and GGT. Among the most ordered tests are ALT, AST, and ALP. The serum aminotransferases ALT and AST are sensitive indicators of liver injury (Lindenmeyer, 2019).

ALT is found in large concentrations in hepatocytes (liver cells). It enters the bloodstream in response to hepatocellular injury and therefore is more specific to liver injury. ALP is produced in the liver, bones, intestine, placenta, and kidneys. The production of ALP is often increased secondary to cholestasis. Cholestasis occurs when the flow of bile from the liver is obstructed or blocked. AST is found in the liver, heart, and kidneys and to a smaller amount in muscles. AST is released in response to injury of liver cells, but it is less specific for liver disease secondary to its production by other tissues. The amount of ALT measured in the blood is related to the extent of liver damage.

One of the many functions of the liver is to conjugate and eliminate bilirubin. Bilirubin is a breakdown product of Hgb, formed from the destruction of RBCs within the reticular endothelial system. Bilirubin can be either conjugated or unconjugated. Unconjugated bilirubin is transported to the liver loosely bound to albumin. Since unconjugated bilirubin is lipid soluble, in other words, water insoluble, it cannot be excreted in the urine. Once transported into the liver, it then becomes conjugated, making it water soluble. Once it becomes conjugated, it can be excreted as bile and it is cleared in urine and in stool. Unconjugated bilirubin is water insoluble and does not color urine. Unconjugated bilirubin is represented on laboratory studies as indirect bilirubin not as in a direct bilirubin. Conjugated or direct bilirubin can pass into the urine as urobilinogen and turns the urine a darker color. Serum bilirubin equals the sum of conjugated bilirubin plus the sum of unconjugated bilirubin (Rothenberg, 2005).

An elevation of GGT is suggestive of biliary epithelial damage and bile flow obstruction. It can be increased in response to drugs or alcohol. When ALP is greatly elevated with an increase in GGT, it is suggestive of a cholestasis injury. When ALP is increased without an increase in GGT, it is an indication of nonhepatic biliary pathology. This pathology includes any process that increases bone breakdown, such as the presence of a tumor and vitamin-D deficiency.

The liver also synthesizes clotting factors and is responsible for gluconeogenesis, which is the making of glucose from noncarbohydrate and carbon substrates. PT measures blood clotting abilities, specifically the cardioversion of prothrombin to thrombin. All coagulation processes except for factor XIII are made in the liver.

Ammonia is produced by the body during normal protein metabolism and by intestinal material.

Albumin is made exclusively by hepatocytes. Normal liver function studies with a low albumin may indicate diminished intake of protein or loss of protein through other processes (Pratt, 2000).

5′-nucleotidase is found in the liver, intestine, brain, heart, blood vessels, and endocrine pancreas. It is only released into circulation by hepatocellular tissue (Friedman, 2019).

Key Points

ALT, AST, ALP, and bilirubin are biomarkers of liver injury. Albumin, bilirubin, and PT are markers of hepatocellular function.

Once you have reviewed your laboratory study results, you need to determine the pattern of the abnormality. Interpreting LFTs may be challenging. The pattern of liver laboratory test abnormalities may suggest the underlying cause of the patient's disease, namely, whether there is a hepatocellular injury, cholestasis, or a mixed patten of injury. Once you determine the pattern of elevation, you can use it to elicit the differential diagnosis while considering the patient's risk factors, presentation, and physical examination. The two most common patterns are hepatocellular and cholestatic. There is also a mixed pattern of injury (cholestasis and hepatocellular with elevation in AST, ALT, and ALP) and the less common pattern of isolated hyperbilirubinemia, both of which are beyond the scope of this chapter.

Hepatocellular Injury

In a hepatocellular injury pattern, serum aminotransferase (AST and ALT) are elevated out of proportion to ALP. There are many possible causes of acute and chronic hepatocellular injury, including medication, alcoholic liver disease, poisoning, infection, chronic viral hepatitis, and liver ischemia (Ross, 2020). Most causes of hepatocellular injury are associated with a serum AST level that is lower than the ALT. An AST-to-ALT ratio of 2:1 or greater is suggestive of alcoholic liver disease, particularly when the GGT is also elevated (Moussavian et al., 1985).

Cholestatic Injury

In a cholestatic pattern, the opposite is present: the ALP elevation is greater than the elevation of AST and ALT. Cholestasis may develop in the setting of extrahepatic or intrahepatic biliary obstruction. There are many possible causes of a cholestatic injury, including biliary obstruction, drugs, primary biliary cholangitis, primary sclerosing cholangitis (PSC), amyloid, granuloma, and infiltrative disease such as tumors. Patterns of liver injury are included in Table 14.2.

TABLE 14.2 PATTERNS OF HEPATIC INJURY

	ACUTE HEPATOCELLULAR INJURY	CHRONIC HEPATOCELLULAR INJURY	CHOLESTASIS
ALT	↑↑	Normal or ↑	Normal or ↑
ALP	Normal or ↑	Normal or ↑	↑↑
GGT	Normal or ↑	Normal or ↑	↑↑
Bilirubin	↑ or ↑↑	Normal or ↑	↑↑

ALP, alkaline phosphatase; ALT, alanine transaminase; GGT, gamma-glutamyl transpeptidase; ↑, increased; ↑↑, very increased.

Case Study

Mr. K's LFT results are as follows: ALP, 280 U/L (normal range, 45–115 U/L); ALT, 73 U/L (normal range for an adult male, 29–33 U/L); AST, 47 U/L (normal range for an adult male, 10–40 U/L) (Lindenmeyer, 2019). Since abnormal LFTs should be repeated, you repeat the tests and obtain similar results. You confirm the results by ordering a GGT. The GGT result is 93 U/L (normal range, 8–61 U/L).

These results reveal a cholestatic pattern. The next step is to determine whether this is an intrahepatic cholestasis (absence of biliary dilatation) or extrahepatic cholestasis (presence of ductal dilatation).

To help determine this, you order a limited RUQ abdominal ultrasound to assess the hepatic parenchyma and bile ducts. The ultrasound shows bile duct wall thickening without bile duct dilation, cholecystitis, or gallstones. This is a nonspecific finding. What is next? As Mr. K is still describing persistent abdominal pain, you request a consult from a gastroenterologist. The gastroenterologist recommends that a magnetic resonance cholangiopancreatography (MRCP) be performed along with bloodwork consisting of an antinuclear antibodies and perinuclear antineutrophil cytoplasmic antibodies.

MRCP results show annular structuring within the intrahepatic and/or extrahepatic bile ducts with alternating normal or slightly dilated segments (MacCarty et al., 1983). The gastroenterologist informs you that he feels that Mr. K is suffering from PSC.

Primary Sclerosing Cholangitis

PSC is a chronic, cholestatic liver disease characterized by both inflammation and fibrosis of both intra- and extrahepatic bile ducts, leading to the formation of multifocal bile duct strictures (Kaplan et al., 2007). PSC is a progressive disease that may develop over time in many patients into cirrhosis, portal HTN, and liver decompensation (Molodecky et al., 2011).

Demographics and Diagnostic Imaging

The occurrence of PSC differs in various regions of the world (Lindor et al., 2015). It ranges from 0 to 1.3 cases per 100,000 per year (Boonstra et al., 2012). PSC is more common in males than in females. Typically, it is diagnosed in the third to fourth decade of life. Seventy percent of patients with PSC have irritable bowel disease (IBD), most often chronic ulcerative colitis (Chapman et al., 2010). Approximately 50% of those patients diagnosed have no symptoms, but elevated LFTs are found on routine laboratory studies (Chapman et al., 2010; Tischendorf et al., 2007). Endoscopic retrograde cholangiopancreatography (ERCP) had long been the gold standard for diagnosis of PSC. However, ERCP is an invasive procedure that can have serious complications such as pancreatitis infection. MRCP is noninvasive and without radiation exposure, and it has been shown to provide good to excellent diagnostic performance compared with ERCP for detection of PSC (Dave et al., 2010). Assessment of the extrahepatic and intrahepatic biliary tree is required to establish a diagnosis of PSC (Lee & Kaplan, 1995; MacCarty et al., 1983). MRCP will show stricture alternating with dilatation of the common bile duct, a beading effect, which is the classic finding of PSC. Lymphadenopathy in the abdomen is common in PSC and should not be interpreted as metastasis or as a lymphoproliferative disorder (Johnson et al., 1998).

Management

PSC is a lifelong disease. The goal of treatment is to retard disease progression. The uncertainty over the disease pathogenesis and factors responsible for its progression has limited the success of treatment. Immunosuppression has been tried along with immune modulating agents, but they have not been shown to be effective (Cullen & Chapman 2005). Liver transplantation may be an option in those patients whose disease progression has led to liver failure and who meet the criteria for transplant. The 5-year survival rate is approximately 85% (Graziadei et al., 1999).

Case Study

Mr. K's symptoms improved without further intervention. He was discharged to home to follow-up with the gastroenterologist. He was lost to medical follow-up, but your care of him was not. You now feel more confident investigating and treating liver dysfunction.

CLINICAL PEARLS

- Always repeat the initial abnormal LFT to confirm an abnormal result.
- In patients with UC, you must consider the possibility of PSC.
- An AST-to-ALT ratio of 2:1 or greater may be indicative of alcoholic liver disease.
- Patients with PSC may be asymptomatic. Although it is rare, it should remain in the differential diagnosis.

REVIEW QUESTIONS

1. What is the most common presenting symptom in patients with acute mesenteric ischemia?
    a. Hypotension
    b. Abdominal pain
    c. Fever
    d. Tachycardia

2. What is the most common cause of acute mesenteric ischemia?
    a. Neoplasm
    b. Decreased cardiac out put
    c. SMA embolism
    d. Venous thrombosis

3. What common medical condition puts a patient at increased risk for acute mesenteric ischemia?
   a. Cardiovascular disease
   b. COPD
   c. Hypothyroidism
   d. Diabetes

4. In a cholestatic liver pattern
   a. AST/ALT is greater than ALP
   b. ALP is greater than AST/ALT
   c. Bilirubin/AST is greater than ALP
   d. ALP is greater than bilirubin/AST

5. To help determine the etiology of an elevated ALP level you would order
   a. GGT
   b. Albumin
   c. AST
   d. Alk Phos

6. What pattern of liver injury would you expect to see in alcoholic liver disease?
   a. AST to ALT ratio is 1:2
   b. AST to ALT ratio is 2:1
   c. AST to GGT ratio is 2:1
   d. GGT to AST is 2:1

Answers: 1, a; 2, c; 3, a; 4, b; 5, a; 6, b

REFERENCES

Boley, J. J., Sprayregen, S., Veith, T. J., & Siegelman, S. S. (1973). An aggressive roentgenologic and surgical approach to acute mesenteric ischemia. *Surgery Annual*, 5, 355–378.

Boonstra, K., Beuers, U., & Ponsion, C. Y. (2012). Epidemiology of primary sclerosing cholangitis and biliary cirrhosis: A systematic review. *Journal of Hepatology*, 56(5), 1181–1188.

Chapman, R., Fevery, J., Kalloo, A., Nagorney, D. M., Boberg, K. M., Shneider, B., Gores, G. J., & American Association for the Study of Liver Diseases. (2010). Diagnosis and management of primary sclerosing cholangitis. *Hepatology*, 51(2), 660–678.

Cullen, S. N., & Chapman, R. W. (2005). Review article: Current management of primary sclerosing cholangitis. *Alimentary Pharmacology & Therapeutics*, 21, 933–948.

Dang, C. V., Su, M., & Nishljlma, D. K. (2020). *Acute mesenteric ischemia differential diagnosis*. Medscape.

Dave, M., Elmunzer, B. J., Dwamena, B. A., & Higgins, P. D. (2010). Primary sclerosing cholangitis: meta-analysis of diagnostic performance of MR cholangiopancreatography. *Radiology*, 256, 387–396.

Friedman, L. S. (2019). Approach to the patient with abnormal liver biochemical and function tests. *UpToDate*. from https://www.uptodate.com/contents/approach-to-the-patient-with-abnorma-liver-biochemical

Graziadei, I. W., Wiesner, R. H., Marotta, P. J., Porayko, M. K., Hay, J. E., Charlton, M. R., Poterucha, J J., Rosen, C. B., Gores, G. J., LaRusso, N. F., & Krom, R. A. (1999). Long term results of patients undergoing liver transplant for primary sclerosing cholangitis. *Hepatology*, 30, 1121–1127.

Harward, T. R., Green, D., Bergman, J. J., Rizzo, R. J., & Yao, J. S. (1989). Mesenteric venous thrombosis. *Journal of Vascular Surgery*, 9, 328–333.

Hustey, F. M., Meldon, S. W., Manet, G. A., Gerson, L. W., Blanda, M., & Lewis, L. M. (2005). The use of abdominal computed tomography in older ED patients with acute abdominal pain. *The American Journal of Emergency Medicine*, 23(3), 259–265.

Johnson, K. J., Olliff, J. F., & Olliff, S. P. (1998). The presence and significance of lymphadenopathy detected by CT in primary sclerosing cholangitis. *The British Journal of Radiology*, 71, 1279–1282.

Kamin, R. A., Nowicki, T. A., Courtney, D. S., & Powers, R. D. (2003). Pearls and pitfalls in the emergency department evaluation of abdominal pain. *Emergency Medicine Clinics of North America*, 21(1), 61–72.

Kaplan, G. G., Laupland, K. B., Butzer, D., Urbanski, S. J., & Lee, S. S. (2007). The burden of small and large duct primary sclerosing cholangitis in adults and children: A population based analysis. *The American Journal of Gastroenterology*, 102, 1042–1049.

Kernagis, L. Y., Levine, M. S., & Jacobs, J. E. (2003). Pneumatosis intestinalis in patients with ischemia: Correlation of CT findings with viability of the bowel. *AJR American Journal of Roentgenology*, 180(3), 733–736.

Kwo, P. Y., Cohen, S. M., & Lim, J. K. (2017). ACG clinical guideline: Evaluation of abnormal liver chemistries. *The American Journal of Gastroenterology*, 112, 18–35.

Lala, V., Goyal, A., Bansal, P., & Minter, D. A. (2020). *Liver function tests*. StatPearls Publishing. https://www.ncbi.nlm.nih.gov/books/NBK482489/

Lee, Y. M., & Kaplan, M. M. (1995). Primary sclerosing cholangitis. *The New England Journal of Medicine*, 32, 924–933.

Lewis, L. M., Banet, G. A., Blanda, M., Hustey, F. M., Meldon, S. W., & Gerson, L. W. (2005). Etiology and clinical course of abdominal pain in senior patients: A prospective, multicultural study. *The Journals of Gerontology. Series A, Biological Sciences and Medical Sciences*, 60(8), 1071–1076.

Lindenmeyer, C. C. (2019). *Laboratory tests of the liver and gallbladder*. Merck Manual Professional Version.https://www.merckmanuals.com/professional/hepatic-and-biliary-disorders/testing-for-hepatic-and-biliary-disorders/laboratory-tests-of-the-liver-and-gallbladder

Lindor, K. D., Kowdley, K. V., Harrison, M. E, & American College of Gastroenterology. (2015). ACG clinical guideline: Primary sclerosing cholangitis. *The American Journal of Gastroenterology*, 110(5), 646–659, quiz 660.

MacCarty, R. L., LaRusso, N. F., Weisner, R. H, & Ludwig, J. (1983). Primary sclerosing cholangitis: Findings on cholangiography and pancreatography. *Radiology*, 140, 39–44.

McKinsey, J. F., & Gewertz, B. L. (1997). Acute mesenteric ischemia. *The Surgical Clinics of North America*, 77, 307–318.

Molodecky, N. A., Kareemi, H., Parab, R., Barkema, H. W., Quan, H., Myers, R. P., & Kaplan, G. G. (2011). Incidence of primary sclerosing cholangitis: A systematic review and meta-analysis. *Hepatology*, 53, 1590–1599.

Moussavian, S. N., Becker, R. C., Piepmeyer, J. L., Mezey, E., & Bozian, R. C. (1985). Serum gamma-glutamyl transpeptidase and chronic alcoholism. Influence of alcohol ingestion and liver disease. *Digestive Diseases and Sciences*, 30, 211.

Pratt, D. S., & Kaplan, M. N. (2000). Evaluation of abnormal liver-enzyme results in asymptomatic patients. *New England Journal of Medicine*, 342, 1266.

Reinus, J. F, Brandt, L. J, & Boley, S. J. (1990). Ischemic diseases of the bowel. *Gastroenterology Clinics of North America*, 19, 319–343.

Ross, C. (2020). *Interpretation of liver function tests (LFTs)*. Geeky Medics. geekymedics.com/interpretation-of-liver-function-tests-lfts/

Rothenberg, M. A. (2005). *Laboratory tests made easy*. Pesi Healthcare.

Taourel, P. G, Deneuville, M., Pradel, J. A., Regent, D., & Bruel, J. M (1996). Acute mesenteric ischemia: Diagnosis with contrast-enhanced CT. *Radiology*, 199, 632–636.

Tischendorf, J. J., Hecker, H., Kruger, M., Manns, M. P., & Meier, P. N. (2007). Characterization, outcome and prognosis in 273 patients with primary sclerosing cholangitis: A single study center. *The American Journal of Gastroenterology*, 102, 107–114.

Wolf, E. L. (1994). Ischemic disease of the gut. In R. M. Gore, M. S. Levine, & I. Laufer, (Eds.), *Textbook of gastrointestinal radiology* (pp. 2694–2706). Saunders.

15

Renal Management

Megan E. Speich

ACUTE KIDNEY INJURY

Case Study

Ms. S is a 67-year-old 70-kg woman admitted to the ICU where you are the covering APRN. She initially presented to the ED earlier that morning after being sent in by her PCP with complaints of dizziness and a 7-day history of persistent fever, cough with production, diarrhea, poor oral intake, and generalized body aches. She has a long-standing history of HTN and breast cancer, which was treated 20 years ago with mastectomy. She reports that she was only able to tolerate a few sips of water each day to take her medications (lisinopril 40 mg daily, metformin 1,000 mg twice daily, amlodipine 5 mg daily) and occasionally a dose of ibuprofen for treatment of her subjective fever. She got laboratory tests done by her PCP. Her blood pressure in the ED was found to be 90/54 mm Hg and after 2 L of IV fluid did not improve, so a norepinephrine infusion was initiated. Preliminary laboratory work done in the ED revealed the following: positive influenza screen; Hgb, 10.1 g/dl; Hct, 30%; BUN, 45 mg/dl; creatinine, 1.2 mg/dl; sodium, 143 mEq/L; and potassium, 5.1 mEq/L.

In further review of systems, Ms. S mentions that she felt nauseous but had no vomiting. She denies any chest pain, shortness of breath, headache, or rash. She intermittently does get swelling in her ankles, especially after eating out at restaurants. Her stools have been watery, but she denies any blood in her stool.

On physical examination, Ms. S is awake but lethargic. She has pallor; normal S1; single S2; no murmur, rub, or gallop; scattered rhonchi in all lung fields; and no edema noted in her extremities.

The RN comes to tell you that her urine output is about 25 ml/hr (her weight was 70 kg at admission) and her BP continues to be labile, and she has had to up-titrate the norepinephrine twice/hour.

You order a STAT chemistry panel and urine electrolytes. The creatinine comes back and is 2.9 mg/dl. What happened?

Introduction

AKI is present in nearly 10%–30% of ICU admissions (Hall et al., 2015).

> **Key Points**
>
> AKI is defined by the Kidney Disease: International Global Outcomes (KDIGO) group as a change in serum creatinine of 0.3 mg/dl or more within 48 hr or creatinine increase of 1.5 or more times the baseline value (within 7 days) or a decrease in urine output to less than 0.5 ml/kg/hr for 6–12 hr.

KDIGO divides worsening kidney failure into three stages, the first being a change in serum creatinine of 0.3 mg/dl or more within 48 hr or creatinine increase of 1.5 or more times the baseline value (within 7 days) or a decrease in urine output to less than 0.5 ml/kg/hr for 6–12 hr, followed by stage two, which is an increase in creatinine 2–2.9 times the baseline value or urine output less than 0.5 ml/kg/hr for 12 hr or more. Stage three is an increase in creatinine 3 times the baseline value, creatinine of 4 mg/dl or more, or urine output less than 0.3 ml/kg/hr for 24 hr/anuria for 12 hr or requiring RRT (Kellum et al., 2012). There are other classification systems available, for example, the RIFLE (Risk, injury, Failure, Loss, and End-Stage Kidney) criteria that include GFR and the Acute Kidney Injury Network (AKIN) classification. The AKIN system was released after RIFLE (updated version) (Gilbert & Weiner, 2018; Lopes & Jorge, 2013). GFR is difficult to identify when not in a steady state. See Tables 15.1–15.3 for AKI definitions.

TABLE 15.1 KDIGO ACUTE KIDNEY INJURY DEFINITIONS AND STAGING

DEFINITION	STAGING	
	Creatinine	Urine Output
Increase in serum creatinine (SCr) by ≥ 0.3 mg/dl within 48 hr OR increase in serum creatinine ≥ 1.5 times baseline (known or presumed within prior 7 days) OR urine output <0.5 ml/kg/hr for 6 hr	1. 1.5–1.9 × baseline OR ≥ 0.3 mg/dl increase	1. <0.5 ml/kg/hr for 6–12 hr
	2. 2–2.9 × baseline	2. <0.5 ml/kg/hr for ≥12 hr
	3. 3 × baseline OR increase >4 mg/dl OR RRT (adults >18 years old), eGFR decrease to <35 ml/min/1.73 m²	3. <0.3 ml/kg/hr for ≥24 hr OR anuria for ≥ 12 hr

eGFR, estimated glomerular filtration rate; KDIGO, Kidney Disease: International Global Outcomes; RRT, renal replacement therapy.

Data from Kellum, J. A., Lameire, N., Aspelin, P., Barsoum, R. S., Burdmann, E. A., Goldstein, S. L., Herzog, C. A., Joannidis, M., Kribben, A., Levey, A. S., MacLeod, A. M., Mehta, R. L., Murray, P. T., Naicker, S., Opal, S. M., Schaefer, F., Schetz, M., Uchino, S. (2012). Kidney disease: Improving global outcomes (KDIGO) acute kidney injury work group. KDIGO clinical practice guideline for acute kidney injury. *Kidney International Supplements*, *2*(1), 1–138.

TABLE 15.2 RIFLE ACUTE KIDNEY INJURY CRITERIA		
RIFLE	**GFR CRITERIA**	**URINE OUTPUT CRITERIA**
Risk	Increase in serum creatinine × 1.5 OR GFR decrease >25%	Urine output <0.5 ml/kg/hr for 6 hr
Injury	Increase in serum creatinine × 2 OR GFR decrease >50%	Urine output <0.5 ml/kg/hr for 12 hr
Failure	Increase in serum creatinine × 3, GFR decrease >75% OR serum creatinine ≥4 mg/dl	Urine output <0.3 ml/kg/hr for 24 hr OR anuria for 12 hr
Loss	Persistent renal failure >4 weeks	Persistent renal failure >4 weeks
ESKD	End-stage kidney disease >3 months	End-stage kidney disease >3 months

GFR, glomerular filtration rate.
Data from Lopes, J. A., & Jorge, S. (2013). The RIFLE and AKIN classifications for acute kidney injury: A critical and comprehensive review. *Clinical Kidney Journal, 6*(1), 8–14.

Classification

The etiologies of AKI are usually grouped into three categories: prerenal, intrarenal, and postrenal. Identification of the type of AKI includes a comprehensive survey of both past medical history and history of the present illness in conjunction with objective data.

Prerenal AKI

Prerenal-derived AKI (also called prerenal azotemia) includes conditions where there is diminished renal perfusion, similar to etiologies of shock. These conditions include the following:

- Hypovolemia
- Poor cardiac output (e.g., heart failure)
- Low systemic vascular resistance (e.g., liver cirrhosis and splanchnic vasodilation)
- Vasoconstriction of renal vasculature

TABLE 15.3 AKIN ACUTE KIDNEY INJURY CRITERIA		
	SERUM CREATININE	**URINE OUTPUT**
Modification of RIFLE:	Stage 1: Increase ≥0.3 mg/dl OR increase 1.5×	Stage 1: <0.5 ml/kg/hr for >6 hr
• Diagnosis made after volume resuscitation/obstruction ruled out	Stage 2: Increase 2×	Stage 2: <0.5 ml/kg/hr for <12 hr
• No GFR change used • No baseline SCr needed • Need 2 SCr within 48-hr time frame	Stage 3: Increase 3× or ≥4 mg/dl (acute rise of 0.5 mg/dl) OR requiring RRT independent of staging	Stage 3: <0.3 mg/kg/hr for 24 hr OR anuria for 12 hr

AKIN, Acute Kidney Injury Network; RIFLE, Risk, Injury, Failure, Loss, and End-stage kidney failure; RRT, renal replacement therapy.
Data from Lopes, J. A., & Jorge, S. (2013). The RIFLE and AKIN classifications for acute kidney injury: A critical and comprehensive review. *Clinical Kidney Journal, 6*(1), 8–14

Twenty-five percent of cardiac output is received by the kidneys, so disruption in renal perfusion can have deleterious effects. The physiologic response to a prerenal environment is for the kidney to create maximally concentrated urine and sodium reabsorption. This is done to volume expand and attempt to restore adequate perfusion to the kidneys (Basile et al., 2012).

> **Key Points**
>
> Prerenal AKI accounts for 55%–60% of AKI occurrences (Hall et al., 2015).

Intrarenal AKI

Intrarenal etiologies of AKI are identified by structural locations within the kidney, including tubules, glomeruli, interstitium, and vasculature. Prerenal AKI that evolves into tubular damage occurring as a result of prolonged and severe perfusion (ischemia) is often called acute tubular necrosis (ATN). ATN accounts for 85%–90% of intrarenal AKI (Hou et al., 1983; Zager, 1992). ATN can be mild, with tubular injury only, or more severe. Additionally, tubular injury can be a result of both endogenous (e.g., myoglobulins) and exogenous (e.g., radiocontrast material) nephrotoxic substances (Hall et al., 2015). Just as severity can range, so too can recovery.

Tubulointerstitial damage, called acute interstitial nephritis, arises not only in allergic reaction pictures but also secondary to autoimmune conditions, infectious processes, and infiltrative disorders such as amyloidosis. New parenchymal glomerular damage can present as rapidly worsening renal function with urine sediment on analysis and can be considered a medical emergency. These conditions often require urgent escalation of diagnostic workup including renal biopsy and prompt treatment with high-dose steroids and often immunosuppressant therapy (Hall et al., 2015). Vascular injuries include damage to small, medium, and large vessels within the kidney. Table 15.4 reviews intrarenal etiologies of AKI.

TABLE 15.4 EXAMPLES OF INTRARENAL ETIOLOGIES OF ACUTE KIDNEY INJURY

STRUCTURAL ETIOLOGY	EXAMPLES
Vascular	• Dissection • Thrombus: atheroembolic, thrombolytic thrombocytopenia purpura, hemolytic uremic syndrome • Vasculitis • Severe HTN (e.g., eclampsia)
Glomerular	• Acute glomerular nephritis lupus nephritis, IgA nephropathy, poststreptococcal infection, vasculitis
Interstitial	• Acute interstitial nephritis: medication mediated (allergic response), infectious
Acute tubular necrosis	• Ischemic (e.g., shock) • Toxic (e.g., IV contrast, rhabdomyolysis)

Data from Basile, D. P., Anderson, M. D., & Sutton, T. A. (2012) Pathophysiology of acute kidney injury. *Comprehensive Physiology*, *2*(2), 1303–1353 and Reilly, R. F., & Perazella, M. A. (2014). *Nephrology in 30 days*. McGraw-Hill.

Postrenal AKI

Postrenal injuries of the kidney occur when an obstruction prevents flow of urine either from both kidneys or from one kidney in the setting of impaired function of the other kidney and inability to properly compensate for diminished filtration of the obstructed kidney. Postrenal etiologies are often reversible and account for 5%–10% of AKI episodes (Papadakis et al., 2019). When the urine flow is obstructed, it refluxes back into the renal parenchymal tissue subsequently causing perfusion abnormalities and tubular damage and thus decreased filtration rate (Papadakis et al., 2019). Bladder obstruction can quickly be ruled out with a bedside bladder scan.

Evaluation of AKI

After obtaining the history necessary to set the stage for the patient's AKI and preforming a physical examination including evaluation of volume status, laboratory and other diagnostic studies are necessary to further stage and evaluate. Serum creatinine is the predominant laboratory test used to evaluate kidney function. It is easy to obtain but not entirely reliable given that its value is determined not only by kidney function but also by other variants such as gender, muscle mass, age, and rate of protein catabolism (Gilbert & Weiner, 2018). Additionally, the bump in creatinine can lag behind the actual injury.

As the serum creatinine is produced in the body, the kidney filters it away, so alterations in renal function result in increased serum creatinine levels. The amount of creatinine production, the filtration rate of the glomeruli, and volume status affect serum creatinine.

Key Points

Caution must be used in those who have normally functioning kidneys prior to the acute injury. The initial acute event may cause the remaining intact nephrons to increase filtration, so initial creatinine levels may not adequately reflect actual tubular damage. Additionally, in the fluid resuscitated patient, the serum creatinine change may not adequately reflect the severity of the acute injury, given that the increase in total body water can dilute the concentration (Gilbert & Weiner, 2018).

An essential component of using serum creatinine for diagnostic purposes and severity indexing of the AKI is knowledge of what the creatinine was prior to the current situation. Historical data with the electronic medical record can assist in finding data points in a patient's history. A preinjury baseline can help to identify how close to resolution the acute injury is.

BUN is also another commonly obtained serum test, evaluating clearance of urea. This, too, can vary by situation, for example, volume status, catabolic activity, and dietary intake (protein). Generally, the BUN/Cr ratio is 15:1, so in absolute renal failure, the BUN would increase by 10–15 for every 1–1.5 mg/dl increase in creatinine. Some exceptions exist, for example, heart failure (BUN may increase with steady creatinine) or decreased intravascular volume status (BUN may increase out of proportion with creatinine) (Gilbert & Weiner, 2018).

Cystatin-C can also be measured in some laboratory tests. Like creatinine, cystatin-C increases as GFR decreases. It is not affected by secretion (not reabsorbed), and thus, the GFR equals excretion only. It is helpful in circumstances where the creatinine may increase, but the GFR remains the same.

TABLE 15.5 URINE SEDIMENT FINDINGS IN ACUTE KIDNEY INJURY

	PRERENAL	INTRARENAL	POSTRENAL
Specific gravity	>1.020	~1.010	~1.010
Urine sediment	Bland or hyaline cast	Glomerular nephritis: erythrocyte casts, proteinuria, and dysmorphic RBC casts Drug-induced AIN: leukocytes, leukocyte casts, eosinophils (in absence of infection) ATN: muddy brown casts, renal tubular cells and casts	Bland or hyaline cast
Additional findings		GN: significant proteinuria Proximal tubular injury (Fanconi syndrome): glycosuria Hematuria: infection, nephrolithiasis, acute glomerular damage, acute tubular damage[a]	

AIN, acute interstitial nephritis; ATN, acute tubular necrosis; GN, glomerulonephritis; RBC, red blood cell.
[a]If UA is positive but microscopy is negative for red blood cells, consider hemoglobinuria or myoglobinuria.
Data from Papadakis, M. A., McPhee, S. J., & Rabow, M. W. (2019). *2019 Current medical diagnosis & treatment*. McGraw-Hill Education.

In addition to serum testing, urine studies are a necessary and helpful part of the diagnostic process. A urinalysis with microscopic evaluation, including specific gravity, any protein, hematuria, leukocyte esterases, or nitrites as well as identification of any urine sediment, can assist in differential diagnosis of etiologies (Table 15.5).

Key Points

It may be necessary should testing reveal suspicious findings that a 24-hr urine collection may need to be completed, for example, to quantify proteinuria.

Urine volume measurement is helpful in identifying AKI as well as stratifying severity. Given the body's compensatory mechanism in a hypovolemic/hypoperfused state to increase the reabsorption of sodium and concentrate the urine, urine output volume can be a component in differentiating etiology of AKI (Gilbert & Weiner, 2018). Urine volume, however, can ineffectively identify the cause given the multiple influences on its output. Examples include medications and intravascular volume resuscitation. A patient who is volume expanded can have a robust urine output, despite elevated creatinine and AKI from tubular necrosis, for example. Anuria is defined as daily urine output of <100 ml, oliguria is 100–400 ml/day, and nonoliguria is >400 ml/day. Table 15.6 describes AKI etiologies and associated urine volume outputs (Gilbert & Weiner, 2018). Using urine output as the sole piece of evidence to identify AKI etiology is erroneous, as there are often multiple urine volume outputs possible for different stages of the diagnosis, such as in ATN.

Urine electrolytes and the fractional excretion of sodium (FeNa) and urea (FeUrea) provide additional information regarding differentiation between prerenal azotemia and intrarenal injury. These values, obtained using a spot urine sample, have a widely variable sensitivity and specificity and do not reliably capture the actual state of renal dysfunction in what is often a highly fluctuating environment.

TABLE 15.6 URINE VOLUME AND ACUTE KIDNEY INJURY

URINE VOLUME	ASSOCIATED ACUTE KIDNEY INJURY
Anuria (<100 ml/day)	Severe acute GN, profound ATN, total urinary tract obstruction, bilateral vascular occlusion
Oliguria (100–400 ml/day)	Prerenal azotemia, interstitial nephritis, ATN, GN
Nonoliguria (>400 ml/day)	ATN, AIN, intermittent obstruction (partial)

AIN, acute interstitial nephritis; ATN, acute tubular necrosis; GN, glomerulonephritis.
Data from Hall, J. B., Schmidt, G. A., & Kress, J. P. (2015). *Principles of critical care*. McGraw-Hill Education.

Key Points

FeNa is only useful if the patient is oliguric.

FeNa <1% is traditionally thought to be indicative of prerenal azotemia, and FeNa >1% indicates ATN when in oliguria phase. FeNa is affected by the use of diuretics as well as volume resuscitation (intravenous fluid; IVF), so an alternate index is the fractional excretion of urea. An intact kidney should have a low FeUrea (<35% for prerenal) given that urea is reabsorbed from urine, and a kidney with tubular damage would have an FeUrea >50% (Gilbert & Weiner, 2018).

Diagnostic Imaging

Visualization of the kidney and urinary tract can identify any structural alterations to suggest either etiologies of AKI or possible sequela of the injury. Ultrasound is often the initial study and should include visualization of the size, contour, and echogenicity of the kidneys, bladder, ureters, and prostate in men. These images can be most helpful in identifying any hydronephrosis and may suggest an obstructive process giving rise to uropathy. Further imaging with CT scan or MRI may be necessary. In the setting of AKI and chronic kidney disease, care must be taken in obtaining any images with intravenous contrast material, especially gadolinium-based agents used in MRI. Gadolinium-based agents in the MRI setting can cause nephrogenic system fibrosis (NSF), an irreversible systemic fibrosing condition that can be detrimental (Gilbert & Weiner, 2018). Oral contrast agent materials used for CT scans are generally accepted in these scenarios.

Additional Considerations

In addition to history/review of systems, vital signs, renal-centric laboratory testing, and images, other testing may be necessary to further identify acute injury etiology or further support the diagnosis. Additional laboratory testing may be necessary, especially in identifying etiology of intrarenal kidney injury. In the setting of positive serologic testing or if there is no evidence to suggest an etiology, a kidney biopsy may be necessary (Gilbert & Weiner, 2018).

Case Study

As the APRN covering the ICU where Ms. S is a patient, what is the next step for the diagnostic component of her care? You redraw laboratory tests, collect a urine sample, and obtain a renal ultrasound. Results are as follows:

- BUN, 55 mg/dl; creatinine, 2.9 mg/dl; sodium, 141 mEq/L; potassium, 4.9 mEq/L; chloride, 104 mEq/L
- Urine sodium, 30 mEq/L; urine urea, 250 mg/dl; urine creatinine, 80 mg/dl
- Calculated FeNa: 0.77%; calculated FeUrea, 16.48%
- Renal ultrasound: right kidney, 10.7 cm; left kidney, 11.3 cm; normal echogenicity, contour; no hydronephrosis

What diagnosis can you confirm?

At this point, the likely diagnosis is prerenal azotemia, in the setting of poor oral intake in the time frame preceding hospital arrival, as well as hypoperfusion with likely septic shock requiring vasoactive drugs.

Management

Once the etiology of AKI has been identified, the first key factor in management is stopping the insulting event and supportive care aimed at reversing the situation and providing assistance in renal functions that are diminished. Supportive care can include intravenous fluid as well as monitoring and correction of electrolyte disturbances (hyperphosphatemia, hyperkalemia, metabolic acidosis). Additionally, it is essential to avoid further damaging insults including avoiding known medications or nephrotoxic agents that can cause renal injury (nonsteroidal anti-inflammatories, IV contrast), dosing medications appropriately for reduced creatinine clearance (which can include an increase or decrease in dosing, depending on the drug).

Key Points

Frequent renal function monitoring should be done to assess for recovery, plateauing, or worsening renal function. When renal failure is detected, early recognition and intervention is key, as is obtaining a nephrology consultation if initial attempts to gain recovery are unmet and RRT is indicated (Gilbert & Weiner, 2018).

Case Study

Despite giving Ms. S IV fluid, she developed bacteremia and further septic shock. She had continued episodes of hypotension and eventually required a second vasoactive medication to support her blood pressure. During the night, she had an episode of acute delirium and her central line (where the vasoactive meds were infusing) was pulled out. She had blood pressures in the 60/40 mm Hg range for approximately 12 min, while the new central line was emergently placed. Her urine output for the last 24 hr was 300 ml total. Repeat creatinine now is 5.9 mg/dl, her BUN is 112 md/dl, and her potassium is 6.2 mEq/L. You call for a nephrology consultation. They ask you to obtain urine electrolytes before they arrive on the unit, and now your FeUrea is 55%.

Ms. S's AKI has now evolved into ATN. Etiology of the ATN is likely related to the profound hypotension in the already injured state and resultant ischemia. Additional findings suggestive of ATN include muddy brown casts (granular) and renal tubular epithelial casts within urine sediment, urine osmolality of 250–300 mOsm/kg, and urine sodium >20 mEq/L (Papadakis et al., 2019).

The nephrology inpatient service evaluates the patient, and in addition to the current supportive measures, they suggest that, given the hyperkalemia and new findings of anasarca, oliguria, and elevated BUN/Cr, RRT is the next step.

Renal Replacement Therapy

RRT is the artificial process of blood purification. In the ICU, the common modalities used are intermittent hemodialysis (IHD) and continuous renal replacement therapy (CRRT). IHD operates using a faster blood flow and thus has a shorter duration. CRRT, however, is a slower blood flow rate and done over the course of 24 hr. IHD has often been considered to be more suitable for the hemodynamically stable patient; however, there is suggestion that there is no difference between IHD and CRRT in episodes of overall outcomes including mortality, hospital stay length, and postdischarge RRT dependency, but CRRT requires less titration of vasoactive drugs (Gilbert & Weiner, 2018).

Regardless of modality option, vascular access must be obtained. The initial catheter is typically a nontunneled type, placed in the internal jugular vein (right side preferably, given the anatomy). As with any central line, precautions for both insertion and postinsertion care must be taken in an effort to avoid central line–associated complications such as lung puncture, clot, and infection. Ideally, avoiding the femoral (due to the high infection risk) and subclavian (due to the high venous stenosis risk) locations is preferred (Gilbert & Weiner, 2018). If RRT is predicted to be more than 30 days, a tunneled dialysis catheter should be considered.

Making the decision to start a patient on RRT is often not based on one factor but rather on the entire clinical picture. There are some significant clinical events that require CRRT, such as profound hyperkalemia, which are not improved with conventional medical management. Other indications include severe acidosis or hypervolemia with further organ failure such as respiratory compromise that too is refractory to medical management (Gilbert & Weiner, 2018).

Case Study

Ms. S is dialyzed via CRRT, transitioned to IHD, and eventually discharged to an SNF where she continues to require hemodialysis three times a week.

RENAL FAILURE WITH AN OBSTRUCTIVE ETIOLOGY

Case Study

Mr. P is a 74-year-old man with past medical history significant for HTN and a 70 pack-year history (2 packs per day for 35 years) who presented to the emergency room this evening after he noticed a generalized feeling of malaise accompanied by a noted decrease in urine output and a feeling of fullness in his lower umbilical region. The initial workup reveals the following: creatinine, 2.1 mg/dl; BUN, 80 mg/dl; and bicarbonate, 12 mEq/L. You have laboratory test results from about 2 months ago, and Mr. P's creatinine was 0.7 mg/dl.

What are your initial suspicions?

With the knowledge of Mr. P's renal function in the months prior to his presentation, he now has a worsening of his renal function by nearly 67% with a worsening creatinine of 1.4 mg/dl, suggestive of an AKI. Before further laboratory data are obtained, parts of his history such as nicotine use, his subjective feeling of fullness in his lower umbilical region, and the decrease in urine output suggest that this could potentially be an obstructive process.

Obstructive Processes Causing AKI

Obstructive processes that cause AKI occur along the urinary tract from the collecting ducts outward in both males and females. The process can occur either within the tract or outside, causing an external compression of the renal pelvis, ureter, or bladder. Within the tract anatomically, the injury can be in the urethra, bladder, ureters, renal pelvis, or renal parenchyma, the most common being at the level of the bladder neck (Hall et al., 2015). Obstruction increases pressure (hydrostatic) that then reduces the GFR (Gilbert & Weiner, 2018).

Obstruction at the ureteral level can be bilateral or unilateral. Bilateral ureteral obstruction (BUO) can be distinguished from unilateral obstruction in that the efferent artery is consistently vasoconstricted and the afferent is dilated. Sodium reabsorption and the ability of the kidney to properly concentrate the urine are impaired (Gilbert & Weiner, 2018). The tubular damage occurs because of the loss of GFR and sequelae of damaging events from vasoconstriction in addition to damage from the hydrostatic pressure (Hall et al., 2015).

Diagnosis

Diagnostic imaging is necessary to further visualize the kidney and identify any concerning pathology that may be causing the AKI.

Key Points

Renal ultrasound offers quick and noninvasive (with no radiation) evaluation and should be ordered urgently if obstruction is high on the differential list.

Hydronephrosis is the classic finding, but this may not be present in certain situations, such as in the very acute obstruction (where dilation has yet to occur) or hypovolemic patient. Ultrasound for identification of obstruction has a 90% sensitivity and specificity rate (Reilly & Perazella, 2014). If further visualization is needed or if the ultrasound shows no evidence of obstruction yet suspicion remains, then a CT scan may be necessary. CT offers more visualization of surrounding organs and structures, which is helpful in situations where an external pathology is suspected as causing the obstruction (for example, a peritoneal tumor).

Case Study

You were considering obtaining a renal ultrasound, but decided to go forward with a noncontrast CT of the abdomen and pelvis given his additional complaints of lower umbilical fullness. You obtain the CT and the radiologist notes a right-central retroperitoneal mass that encases the abdominal aorta and IVC as well as the right ureter, causing severe right hydroureteronephrosis.

You call for an urgent urology consultation. They evaluate him and take him for urgent surgery to stent the ureter and remove the tumor. He returns postoperatively, hemodynamically stable and with a Foley catheter draining yellow, clear urine. The RN calls you to tell you that Mr. P's blood pressure has continually been dropping and now it is about 90/60 mm Hg. You go to his bedside and notice 750 ml of urine in his Foley catheter and, upon closer examination, realize it is continuing to fill rapidly. What is happening?

Postobstruction Repair

Postobstructive diuresis occurs secondary to osmotic diuresis from the now improved filtration rate, clearing the fluids and osmoles that were not filtered during the acute injury. Given that the urine output can be polyuric (3.5 L/24 hr), it is essential to ensure that there are no excessive renal losses without replacement to avoid a hypovolemic state. It should be noted, however, that fluid resuscitation for each 1 ml of urine output is not necessary and can continue or worsen the diuresis process. Ideally, fluid replacement should be 1/2 normal saline stat, with 50% of the output replaced if the patient is hemodynamically stable to avoid volume depletion. Laboratory tests should be checked frequently, especially monitoring for electrolyte imbalances.

Case Study

You administer 500 cc of LR, and start replacement of 1/2 normal saline based on his urine output. Mr. P's blood pressure stabilizes. You observe him overnight. His urine output normalizes, his metabolic panel and renal function show improvement, and he remains hemodynamically stable. He is transferred to the medical floor for further monitoring.

CLINICAL PEARLS

- Knowing the baseline creatinine prior to the acute event is helpful in distinguishing how severe the injury is.
  - Serum creatinine and BUN are the traditional markers for kidney injury and help guide GFR, but their values can vary based on clinical situation and result in unreliable GFR.
- 10%–30% of critically ill patients in the ICU have a diagnosis of AKI, with severe AKI having a 50% mortality rate (Hall et al., 2015).
- AKI is traditionally thought to be prerenal, intrarenal, or postrenal in classification, with prerenal being most common.
- Prerenal AKI occurs when there is impaired blood flow or hypoperfusion to the kidney and can include volume depletion, liver disease, or heart failure.
- Intrarenal AKI occurs within one of the structural components of the kidney, including vasculature, glomeruli, tubules, or interstitium.
- ATN is the most common cause of intrarenal AKI (Reilly & Perazella, 2014).
- AKI management focuses on relieving the inciting event if possible and supportive care while renal recovery is awaited.
- If renal function does not improve, RRT may be required.

REVIEW QUESTIONS

1. A 78-year-old man walks into the ED with complaints of anuria for 12 hr. What is the first diagnostic test you should perform?
   a. A CT scan with contrast
   b. A bedside ultrasound looking for bladder volume
   c. Serum electrolytes
   d. Place a urinary catheter

2. What is the physiologic response to a prerenal environment?
   a. Maximal dilution of urine and sodium excretion
   b. No change in urine-concentrating mechanisms
   c. Maximal concentration of urine and sodium reabsorption
   d. No change in serum sodium

3. Initial laboratory testing when suspecting AKI should include:
   a. Serum electrolytes, urine sodium, urine urea, urine creatinine
   b. BUN, sodium, and urine sodium
   c. BUN, creatinine, sodium, and glucose
   d. Lactic acid

   Answers: 1, b; 2, c; 3, a

REFERENCES

Basile, D. P., Anderson, M. D., & Sutton, T. A. (2012) Pathophysiology of acute kidney injury. *Comprehensive Physiology*, 2(2), 1303-1353.

Gilbert, S. J., & Weiner, D. E. (2018). In Bomback A. S., Perazella M. A., & Tonelli M. (Eds.), *National kidney foundation's primer on kidney diseases* (7th ed.). Elsevier.

Hall, J. B., Schmidt, G. A., & Kress, J. P. (2015). *Principles of critical care*. McGraw-Hill Education.

Hou, S. H., Bushinksky, D. A., Wish, J. B., Cohen, J. J., & Harrington, J. T. (1983). Hospital-acquired renal insufficiency: A prospective study. *The American Journal of Medicine*, 74(2), 243–248.

Kellum, J. A., Lameire, N., Aspelin, P., Barsoum, R. S., Burdmann, E. A., Goldstein, S. L., Herzog, C. A., Joannidis, M., Kribben, A., Levey, A. S., MacLeod, A. M., Mehta, R. L., Murray, P. T., Naicker, S., Opal, S. M., Schaefer, F., Schetz, M., & Uchino, S. (2012). Kidney disease: Improving global outcomes (KDIGO) acute kidney injury work group. KDIGO clinical practice guideline for acute kidney injury. *Kidney International Supplements*, 2(1), 1–138.

Lopes, J. A., & Jorge, S. (2013). The RIFLE and AKIN classifications for acute kidney injury: A critical and comprehensive review. *Clinical Kidney Journal*, 6(1), 8–14.

Papadakis, M. A., McPhee, S. J., & Rabow, M. W. (2019). *2019 Current medical diagnosis & treatment*. McGraw-Hill Education.

Reilly, R. F., & Perazella, M. A. (2014). *Nephrology in 30 days*. McGraw-Hill.

Zager, R. A. (1992). Endotoxemia, renal hypoperfusion, and fever: Interactive risk factors for aminoglycoside and sepsis-associated acute renal failure. *American Journal of Kidney Diseases*, 20(3), 223–230.

16 Trauma

Paula McCauley · Julie D. Culmone

INTRODUCTION

Trauma is the leading cause of death in the United States among individuals between 1 and 46 years of age and the fourth leading cause of death for all ages (Oyeniyi et al., 2017). Trauma-related injuries account for 27 million ED visits and 3 million hospital admissions annually adding over $671 billion to the cost of healthcare in the United States (Centers for Disease Control and Prevention, 2020). Trauma-related injuries have proven detrimental to the current healthcare system in terms of morbidity, mortality, and dollars spent. This chapter will explore the diagnosis, management, and prevention of traumatic injuries and the occurrences that impact the elderly population who fall victim of trauma.

TRAUMA SYSTEMS AND GUIDELINES

Case Study

You are an APRN student with several years' nursing experience on a medical surgical unit in a level 3 designated trauma facility. Your primary unit is largely devoted to cardiac diagnoses. Your program director calls to let you know that she has a potential clinical site for you, assigned to a preceptor in the ED of a level 1 trauma facility. Your first day of clinical is tomorrow, and it will be your first exposure to trauma both as an RN and now as a provider. To better prepare for the rotation, you contact your preceptor and ask her what you might review prior to starting clinical. She gives you some resources to consider and you jump onto your university library site to further explore. You discover that trauma is a much broader topic than you expected and work to develop a better understanding of related concepts and diagnoses. Let us review what you have found that will be valuable in preparation for your experience in this new area.

Classifications of Trauma

According to Burlew & Moore (2019), trauma is defined as "cellular disruption caused by environmental energy that is beyond the body's resilience, which is compounded by cell death due to ischemia/reperfusion." Trauma is broadly classified into three groups: penetrating, blunt, and deceleration. Penetrating trauma occurs when an object pierces the body and creates an open wound, resulting in acute blood loss and the potential for hypovolemic shock (Dumovich & Singh, 2020). Blunt trauma is the result of a force striking the body, resulting in injury dependent on the location of the trauma. Deceleration trauma is an injury caused by a sudden stop in motion such as from a motor vehicle crash or shaken-baby syndrome (Dumovich & Singh, 2020).

Trauma Systems

In 1990, Congress passed the Trauma Care Systems Planning and Development Act in an effort to improve EMS and trauma care delivered in the United States. Subsequently, the American College of Surgeons Committee on Trauma partnered with the American College of Emergency Physicians and published Guidelines for Trauma Care Systems to improve care delivery for trauma victims (Cameron et al., 2020). In the United States, trauma center levels are identified according to both a designation process, outlined and developed at a state and local level, and a verification process, completed by the American College of Surgeons (American Trauma Society, 2020).

Level 1

A level 1 trauma center is a comprehensive regional center that is capable of providing total care for every aspect of injury from trauma prevention through rehabilitation. A level 1 trauma center has 24-hr in-house coverage by general surgeons and prompt availability of care in specialties including neurosurgery, anesthesiology, emergency medicine, orthopedic surgery, oral and maxillofacial surgery, radiology, internal medicine, plastic surgery, pediatric medicine, and critical care.

Level 2

A level 2 trauma center initiates definitive care for all injured patients. A level 2 trauma center has 24-hr immediate coverage by general surgeons as well as coverage by specialties of orthopedic surgery, neurosurgery, anesthesiology, emergency medicine, radiology, and critical care.

Level 3

A level 3 trauma center provides prompt assessment and stabilization of injured patients and emergency operations with established transfer agreements for patients requiring more comprehensive care at a level 1 or level 2 trauma center. A level 3 trauma center has 24-hr immediate coverage by emergency medicine and the prompt availability of general surgeons and anesthesiology.

Level 4

A level 4 trauma center provides advanced trauma life support (ATLS), evaluation, stabilization, and diagnostic studies prior to transfer of the patient to a higher level trauma center. A level 4 trauma center has available trauma nurse(s) and emergency medicine upon arrival.

Level 5

A level 5 trauma center provides initial evaluation, stabilization, and diagnostic studies and prepares the patient for transfer to a higher level trauma center. A level 5 trauma center has available trauma nurse(s) and physicians upon arrival (American Trauma Society, 2020).

> ### Key Points
>
> A facility cannot market itself as a trauma center unless they have been designated by their state trauma system after successful verification by the ACS.

The Center for Disease Control and Prevention Field Triage Guidelines for Injured patients directs EMS providers to transport all patients with a GCS <13 or those with any level of TBI and GCS ≤15 and extracranial injuries Abbreviated Injury Scale (AIS) ≥3 to the highest level trauma center (American College of Surgeons, 2014). Activation of the trauma team at a designated trauma facility includes the following criteria for classification of major trauma (Box 16.1) and minor trauma (Box 16.2).

Advanced Trauma Life Support

The American College of Surgeons Committee on Trauma developed the ATLS program in an effort to improve the outcome of the injured patient. First introduced in 1980, ATLS provides a structured approach for management of the trauma patient with standard algorithms of care and emphasis on the first hour after a traumatic injury, considered to be the most critical, commonly referred to as the "golden hour" (Burlew & Moore, 2019). Assessment of the trauma patient involves a primary, secondary, and tertiary survey to identify and treat life-threatening injuries. The primary survey encompasses the components using an ABCDE format (Box 16.3).

BOX 16.1 Criteria for Classification of Major Trauma

- GCS <13 or GCS ≤15 in the presence of extracranial injuries
- SBP <90
- Respiratory rate <10 or >29
- Flail chest
- Patient intubated in the field
- Airway compromise
- Respiratory compromise in need of an emergent airway
- Two or more proximal long bone fractures
- All penetrating injuries to the head, neck, torso, or extremities proximal to the elbow/knee
- Combative
- Transfer of patients actively receiving blood to maintain vital signs

---

BOX 16.2 **Criteria for Classification of Minor Trauma**

- Ejection from/of a vehicle
- Vehicle rollover with unrestrained patient
- Death in the same passenger compartment
- Motor vehicle vs. bicyclist/pedestrian with impact >20 mph
- Fall >3 times the patient's height or >15 feet
- Exposure to blast or explosion
- Motorcycle crash >20 mph
- Amputations proximal to the wrist/ankle
- Suspected pelvic fractures
- Limb paralysis
- Crush injury; degloved or mangled extremity
- Vascular deficit
- Combination of trauma with thermal injury
- Child abuse with known or suspected significant injury

Conditions identified as life-threatening are addressed emergently at the time of the primary survey and include management of airway, pneumothorax, flail chest, hemorrhagic shock, pelvic fracture, cardiac tamponade, neurogenic shock, ICH, or cervical spine injury (Hemmila, 2020). The secondary survey begins immediately after the primary survey has been completed and any life-threatening injuries have been addressed to provide stabilization. The secondary survey includes obtaining a comprehensive health history and performance of a head-to-toe physical examination with inspection to the axillae, perineum, and posterior surface by logrolling the patient. A digital rectal examination should be performed on all seriously injured patients to assess sphincter tone, rectal perforation, presence of blood, or a high-riding prostate (Burlew & Moore, 2019). This is especially critical in patients with suspected spinal cord injury or pelvic fracture. Adjuncts to the secondary survey include reassessment of all vital signs, cardiac monitoring, nasogastric tube placement, indwelling urinary catheter placement, radiologic imaging, focused abdominal sonography for trauma (FAST) examination, and laboratory studies including Hgb, base deficit measurements, and urinalysis. Approximately 24 hr after admission, the trauma team completes a tertiary surgery which involves performing the primary and secondary assessment once again to assess for missed injuries from the initially performed primary and secondary survey (Hemmila, 2020).

BOX 16.3 **Primary Survey**

A—Airway and alertness
B—Breathing
C—Circulation
D—Disability
E—Exposure and environment

Case Study

You spent the afternoon reviewing the trauma guidelines and arrive at the clinic the next morning. Initially, it is quiet in the ED and you have time to review the environment and protocols for trauma with your preceptors. You no sooner finish reviewing the trauma activation protocols when the alert is sounded. A 35-year-old man presents to the ED with multiple gunshot wounds to the abdomen and a single gunshot wound to the right upper extremity. Upon presentation, he is breathing spontaneously. His vital signs on the EMS monitor reveal the following: blood pressure, 90/52 mm Hg; heart rate, 118 bpm; sinus tachycardia; respiratory rate, 10 breaths/min; pulse oximetry, 99% on 2LPM nasal cannula. The left upper extremity contains two 16-gauge peripheral IVs with lactated ringers running wide open. The trauma team is present in the trauma room upon arrival and together slide the patient onto the trauma table. The chief surgical resident is identified as the team lead and quickly performs the primary survey while the ED attending tends to the airway. On primary survey, the chief surgical resident identifies

A. Airway: intact
B. Breathing: spontaneous
C. Circulation: intact; BP, 88/50; HR, 126; sinus tachycardia
D. Disability: GCS, 9
E. Exposure: clothes are cut off with trauma shears; three penetrating gunshot wounds to the abdomen are identified with minimal external blood loss; a single perforating gunshot wound to the right upper extremity has a compression dressing in place with moderate sanguineous drainage.

He is then logrolled and his back is assessed by the chief surgical resident for trauma. There are no exit wounds to the back and no further trauma identified. The primary survey is complete, and the patient is rolled onto his back and covered with a warm blanket. According to the ATLS guidelines, the patient is intubated by the ED attending for a GCS of 9 and a compromised airway. Vital signs are reassessed and unchanged. The chief surgical resident proceeds to the secondary survey.

The secondary survey is completed from head to toe. The patient is intubated and sedated. His heart is regular without murmur or gallop. His lungs are clear to auscultation without adventitious sounds. His abdomen is firm and distended. His femoral pulses are palpable bilaterally. His skin is warm and diaphoretic without mottling. His popliteal and pedal pulses are palpable. The trauma nurse obtains a full trauma panel and inserts an indwelling urinary catheter per protocol. The trauma attending performs a FAST examination which reveals free air and free intraperitoneal fluid. His laboratory studies show WBC, 7,000/L; Hgb, 12 g/dl; Hct, 34%; platelets, 246,000/L; ETOH, 112 mg/dl; cocaine, positive. What will you do next? Are there modalities you will employ to evaluate his injuries in the resuscitation room?

Provided with the identified penetrating trauma to the abdomen, he is taken emergently to the operating room for an exploratory laparotomy. Intraoperative findings reveal multiple gunshot wounds to the abdomen with small bowel perforation for which he undergoes a small bowel resection with abdominal washout. The gunshot wound to his right upper extremity is assessed for vascular injury with benign findings. The wound is irrigated and loosely packed with ½-in packing strip and a dry, sterile dressing is applied.

Trauma and Shock

Shock is an abnormality of the circulatory system that results in inadequate organ perfusion and tissue oxygenation; shock is further defined in Chapter 17. There are three types of shock most commonly associated with trauma-related injuries: cardiogenic, hemorrhagic, and neurogenic. Septic shock secondary to infection immediately after trauma is rare but can occur from penetrating abdominal injuries and contamination of the peritoneal cavity by intestinal contents.

Cardiogenic Shock

Cardiogenic shock is defined as decreased cardiac output with tissue hypoxia in the presence of adequate intravascular volume secondary to blunt cardiac injury. Cardiogenic shock is common with traumatic injuries including cardiac tamponade, myocardial contusion, or tension pneumothorax.

Cardiac tamponade secondary to a pericardial effusion results in obstructive shock with tachycardia and the classic Beck triad: distended neck veins, muffled heart sounds, and a decrease in arterial pressure with hypotension that is unresponsive to fluid bolus. Pericardiocentesis is a procedure that is 80% effective in decompressing cardiac tamponade. If ineffective, the tamponade may be due to the presence of clotted blood within the pericardium and warrants resuscitative thoracotomy of opening of the pericardium to allow for rapid decompression and control of bleeding.

Tension pneumothorax is characterized by acute respiratory distress, absent breath sounds, hyperresonance to percussion, and trachea deviation away from the affected side. This is a surgical emergency and is initially treated by the insertion of a large caliber needle into the second intercostal space in the midclavicular line of the affected hemothorax followed by placement of a large-bore chest tube (Hemmila, 2020).

Hemorrhagic Shock

Hemorrhagic shock is the most common cause of shock after injury and a serious concern in trauma. Sources of blood loss include injuries to the chest, abdomen, pelvis, retroperitoneum, and extremities. Initial management is focused on controlling external bleeding. If the patient is stable upon arrival, isotonic crystalloids are initiated; if the patient is unstable or has persistent hypotension after 2 L of IV fluids, activation of the massive transfusion protocol is initiated. End organ perfusion indicates a positive response to fluid resuscitation and is indicated by normalization of vital signs, warm extremities, normal capillary refill, and adequate urinary output of 0.5 ml/kg/hr in an adult (Burlew & Moore, 2019).

Neurogenic Shock

Neurogenic shock is a form of distributive shock in which injury to the spinal cord results in systemic pooling of blood caused by the loss of autonomic tone and dilation of the venous system. Clinical presentation includes hypotension without tachycardia and temperature dysregulation (Hemmila, 2020).

Thoracic Trauma

Common and potentially lethal injuries of the chest include simple pneumothorax, hemothorax, pulmonary contusion, tracheobronchial tree injury, traumatic aortic transection, diaphragmatic injury, and blunt esophageal rupture.

Pneumothorax

A simple pneumothorax results from air entering the potential space between the visceral and parietal pleura. Management of a simple pneumothorax is achieved by insertion of a chest tube in the fourth and fifth intercostal space anterior to the midaxillary line. Observation with oxygen therapy may be appropriate for a simple pneumothorax in which the patient is asymptomatic.

Hemothorax

A hemothorax is a collection of blood in the pleural cavity commonly caused by penetrating or blunt trauma. Bleeding is usually self-limited and usually does not require surgical intervention. A hemothorax noted on CXR should be managed with the insertion of a 36 or 40 French chest tube.

Pulmonary Contusion

Pulmonary contusion is the most common potentially lethal chest injury and should be suspected with blunt trauma and presentation with flail chest or multiple rib fractures. A pulmonary contusion, or a "bruise of the lung," is an injury to the lung tissue that causes blood to accumulate in the lung tissue as a result of damage to the capillaries. This accumulation of blood interferes with gas exchange and frequently leads to hypoxia. The work of breathing is increased significantly and many patients who initially appear to be compensating may acutely deteriorate and require intubation. Therefore, it is strongly recommended that this population be monitored in the ICU.

Tracheobronchial Injury

Tracheobronchial injury is an injury to the tracheobronchial tree (trachea and bronchi). Although tracheobronchial injury is uncommon, it must be suspected and managed immediately. Initial management involves stabilization of the airway and then performance of a flexible bronchoscopy by the surgeon credentialed to repair an identified injury (Altinok & Atilla, 2014).

Traumatic Aortic Transection

Traumatic aortic transection is the second most common cause of sudden death in victims of blunt chest trauma from a motor vehicle crash, fall, or crush injury of the chest. Traumatic transection of the aorta typically occurs at the aortic isthmus, which is the transition zone between the relatively mobile aortic arch and the tethered descending aorta. During major blunt trauma to the chest, there is shearing of the aortic wall. Unfortunately, more than 90% of patients who sustain this type of injury die at the scene (Benjamin & Roberts, 2012). Of the remaining 10% who survive, 50% will succumb to this injury within the first 24 hr and 90% die within 4 months (Benjamin & Roberts, 2012).

Traumatic Diaphragmatic Injury

Traumatic diaphragmatic injury is commonly missed on a CXR. If diaphragmatic injury is suspected, a gastric tube should be inserted and an upper GI series should be performed to confirm this diagnosis.

Abdominal Trauma

Physical examination and a FAST examination can identify patients requiring an emergent laparotomy. Although computed tomography (CT) scanning is commonly used to determine the location and magnitude of the injury, penetrating trauma of the abdomen is an indication for an emergent exploratory laparotomy and CT scan may be deferred.

Extremities: Fractures, Compartment Syndrome, and Vascular Injury

A large number of trauma-related injuries involve the extremities and include vascular injury, fractures, and compartment syndrome. Fractures may lead to complications such as hemorrhagic shock, fat embolism, and compartment syndrome. Neuromuscular examinations are critical during the secondary survey to establish a baseline examination. Concern for compartment syndrome should be evaluated if there is pain out of proportion to the injury in the setting of neurovascular compromise. Frequent evaluation of compartment pressures is essential, and an emergent fasciotomy should be performed with elevated pressures (Ebraheim et al., 2019).

Deeply impaled objects in the chest and abdomen should be left in place and emergently removed in the operating room under direct visualization to ensure hemostasis and vascular control. The impaled object may be cut or shortened outside of the skin to facilitate transport (Cameron et al., 2020).

Burns

Burns are commonly classified as thermal, electrical, or chemical. Thermal burns include contact, flame, or scald burns. Wounds resulting from burns are classified as first degree (superficial), second degree (partial thickness), third degree (full thickness), or fourth degree (skin and underlying soft tissue as well as deeper tissue, possibly involving muscle and bone). Care of the burn victim is complex and should involve designated burn specialty centers throughout the United States (Anderson et al., 2019).

Key Points

The American Burn Association (ABA) recommends transfer to a specialized burn center after early stabilization.

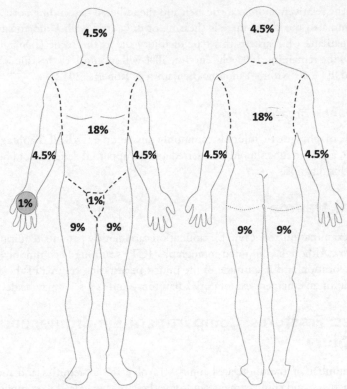

Figure 16.1 Rule of nines. (From Wiener-Kronish J. P. (2016). *Critical care handbook of the Massachusetts general hospital*. Lippincott Williams & Wilkins.)

The rule of nines (Figure 16.1) is used to quickly estimate the size of a burn by dividing the body's surface area into percentages to determine total body surface area (TBSA) affected by the burn. Advanced Burn Life Support (ABLS, 2018) Provider Manual criteria for transfer to a burn center are included in Box 16.4.

BOX 16.4 **Criteria for Transfer to a Designated Burn Center**

- Second- and third-degree burns greater than 10% TBSA for those under the age of 10 or over the age of 50
- Second- and third-degree burns to greater than 20% TBSA in all other ages
- Third-degree burns to greater than 5% TBSA in all ages
- All second- and third-degree burns with the threat of functional or cosmetic impairment to the face, hands, feet, genitalia, perineum, or major joints
- All electrical burns, including lightning burns
- Chemical burns
- Burns involving chemical inhalation
- Circumferential burns of the extremities and/or chest
- Burns involving concomitant trauma among which the burn injury poses the greatest risk of morbidity or mortality
- Burns to those with preexisting conditions that may complicate management and/or prolong recovery, such as CAD, lung disease, or diabetes

Assessment

> **Key Points**
>
> There are four critical points of assessment for burn victims: airway management, evaluation of other injuries, estimation of burn size, and diagnosis of carbon monoxide and cyanide poisoning (Anderson et al., 2019).

Anticipating the need for intubation and prompt establishment of an airway is critical in the evaluation of burn victims. Findings such as singed nasal, facial, and perioral hairs; nasal burns; hoarseness; or dyspnea should prompt the trauma team to consider early intubation. Hypothermia in burn victims is a common complication that contributes to resuscitation failure. Warmed IV fluids and warmed blankets can be used to address hypothermia (Anderson et al., 2019).

Resuscitation

Initial fluid resuscitation of a burn victim with moderate or severe burns consists of intravenous crystalloid solution, typically lactated ringers. Fluid replacement requirements for burn victims are calculated using the following formula: 2 ml/kg/% burn, administered over the first 24 hr (Anderson et al., 2019).

Case Study 1

Your preceptor encourages you to follow up on the patient who is admitted post op to the ICU. Postoperatively, he remains intubated and is transferred to the surgical ICU for further monitoring. Shortly after his arrival to the ICU, he is brought to CT scan for a PanScan to identify any missed injuries. CBC is obtained 6 hr after presentation to the ED and demonstrates Hgb of 7.8 and Hct of 24.1. Two units of PRBCs were ordered and transfused, and the patient is started on Zosyn and Diflucan × 5 days. On postoperative day 1, the patient is successfully extubated, and the trauma tertiary survey is able to be completed. On postoperative day 3, he is transferred out of the surgical ICU to the medical/surgical floor where he continues to be followed up by the trauma service for daily RUE dressing changes and inpatient care. He is started on a clear liquid diet, which he tolerates. He is evaluated by chemical dependency, physical therapy, occupational therapy, speech therapy, and case management per trauma protocol. On postoperative day 4, the patient is A/O × 4, pleasant, and cooperative. His lungs are clear to auscultation without adventitious breath sounds. His heart is regular without murmur or gallop and he is presently in sinus rhythm. His abdomen is soft, nontender, and nondistended. His abdominal surgical incision is clean, dry, and intact with staples that are open to air. There is no erythema, induration, or drainage noted to the periwound of his surgical incision. He is passing flatus and reports a small, soft bowel movement earlier this morning. He is tolerating a regular diet without complaints of nausea or emesis and he rates his pain as a 2 on a 0–10 pain scale. The packing is removed from his RUE wound and a dry, clean dressing is placed. This wound is beginning to granulate without signs or symptoms of infection; therefore, daily dressing changes with packing will be discontinued. The patient has been evaluated by all of the recommended consulting services and has been cleared for discharge to home without visiting nurse services. An appointment has been made for him to follow up in the trauma clinic in 7 days.

HEAD INJURIES

Case Study 2

You come in for your second day of clinical in the ED and your preceptor meets you at the door and directs you into a room to join the team in evaluation of a patient who has just arrived by ambulance. You walk in to hear the EMS handoff. They have brought in an 80-year-old woman with PMH of mild dementia, HTN, and atrial fibrillation who had a mechanical fall at home witnessed by her live-in nursing assistant. She was walking across the living room with her walker when she reportedly bumped it into the wall and fell over on her side, striking her head against the wall. She was initially unresponsive for about 30 s but quickly recovered and returned to her baseline mental status. EMS found her sitting on the floor, awake and slow to respond but able to articulate where she was and what had happened. She complained of some mild hip pain and they elected to immobilize her and transport her. Additional ROS is positive for frequent falls, "dropping things," and worsening short-term memory loss.

Your primary assessment for ABCDE is stable for A and B; she has no evidence of airway or respiratory compromise; her HR is 92 and irregular; her RR is 20; her BP is 174/96; and she is afebrile. Her GCS is 15, and she has an expanding area of soft-tissue edema on her left frontal scalp area with no laceration or bleeding. Your exposure reveals only edema to her left knee and nothing on her posterior examination. You cover her with warm blankets and begin your secondary survey keeping her flat on the stretcher for now as her cervical spine has not yet been cleared.

Her son has arrived and through further investigation of her AMPLE history you confirm that she is on Coumadin and a beta-blocker for her atrial fibrillation. Her blood pressure is well controlled with her BB at home, although she has "white coat syndrome" with elevated pressures documented on her routine office visits. She has had multiple falls over the past several weeks, which she reported were due to her unstable gait, saying that it is "because I'm old." None has had LOC prior to today, although her aide endorses that there was one time about 2 weeks ago when she did "bump" her head. She has had issues with fine motor function recently, "dropping things," which she attributed to her arthritis. When questioned about the events leading up to her admission today, she does endorse that she remembers feeling a "bit lightheaded" right before she fell. She uses the walker for stability, is able to do her normal ADLs such as bathing and toileting, and has her live-in aide to help with her nutrition and housework but more specifically because she is forgetful and the family worries about her safety.

Her secondary assessment is obtained with no focal neurologic deficits, 4/5 motor strength to LE, and 5/5 to UE. Her sensation is intact, she does have trouble with repetitive movements of her right side, and her LE is uncoordinated with heel to shin attempts. Her cardiovascular examination reveals that she is irregularly irregular with a soft SM and no rub or gallop. Her lungs are clear, her abdomen is benign, and she is warm with 2+ pulses throughout and no peripheral edema.

You leave the room to find your preceptor and discuss your differentials. Your top three include the following:

- The mechanical fall
- Stroke. You are concerned that she may have had a stroke with the history and her fine motor skills. It could be hemorrhagic with HTN and her anticoagulation.
- Atrial fibrillation. You consider that she could have tachy-brady syndrome causing her recent symptoms.

Your preceptor agrees and you sit down to place some orders when the nurse calls you urgently into the room. You find your patient unresponsive with agonal breathing. A code is called, and the ED physician quickly intubates the patient. Her vital signs stabilize except for persistent HTN. She is rushed to CT scan for a dry CT of her head. You request a stat consult from neurology and neurosurgery. Stat labs including a coagulation panel are sent.

Have your differentials changed?

Traumatic Brain Injuries

Approximately 1.7 million TBIs occur in the United States annually with an estimated 90,000 people experiencing long-term disability from head injury. The primary injuries include contusion, hematoma, hemorrhage, diffuse axonal injury, direct cellular damage, loss of the blood-brain barrier, and disruption of the neurochemical homeostasis (Ramayya et al., 2019). Further damage is caused by the impact that results in a series of cellular events known as the secondary neurotoxic cascade. This cascade causes ongoing damage to the brain resulting in outcomes more severe than what may have occurred from the primary injury (Oropello et al., 2014). Traumatic brain lesions are classified as diffuse or focal. Diffuse brain injuries range from mild concussions to severe hypoxic ischemic injuries. Focal brain injuries include epidural hematomas, subdural hematomas, intracerebral hematomas, and cerebral contusions (Ramayya et al., 2019).

Epidural Hematoma

Commonly located in the temporal or temporoparietal region, an epidural hematoma results from trauma to the middle meningeal artery. Clinical presentation is a lucid interval between the time of injury and neurological deterioration. The resulting hematoma is described as biconvex or lenticular shape on CT scan and requires emergent surgical intervention. Delayed surgery may result in permanent brain damage or death. Without surgical intervention, death typically occurs secondary to brain herniation caused by hematoma enlargement.

Subdural Hematoma

A subdural hematoma results from shearing of small surfaces or bridging blood vessels of the cerebral cortex. Clinical presentation involves a persistent headache, confusion, lethargy, nausea and vomiting, slurred speech, changes in vision, weakness on one side, loss of balance, and/or difficulty with ambulation. Large or symptomatic subdural hematomas may require surgical intervention, whereas small or asymptomatic subdural hematomas may only require monitoring.

Cerebral Contusion

Cerebral contusions are another fairly common TBI and may evolve to form an intracerebral hematoma or a contusion within a period of hours to days. Emergent surgical intervention is required if a shift develops. Patients with contusions generally undergo serial CT scans to evaluate for changes (Wright & Merck, 2020).

Key Points

The primary goal of treatment for patients with suspected TBI is to prevent secondary brain injury.

Cerebral Perfusion Pressure

CPP is the product of mean arterial pressure (MAP) and ICP. ICP is determined by the volume of the three intracranial compartments: brain parenchyma (<1,300 ml in the adult), CSF (100–150 ml), and intravascular blood (100–150 ml). When one compartment expands, there is a compensatory reduction in the volume of another, and/or the baseline ICP will increase.

Key Points

Elevations in ICP are life-threatening and may lead to a phenomenon known as Cushing reflex (HTN, bradycardia, and respiratory irregularity).

With a TBI, autoregulation is lost and attempts to regulate by addressing one of the three components—CSF, intracranial blood volume, or brain parenchyma—which are the goals of your treatment (Ramayya et al., 2019; Wright & Merck, 2020). With brain injury, autoregulation may be impaired, so even modest drops in blood pressure can decrease brain perfusion and result in cellular hypoxia. A goal CPP of <60 mm Hg is considered as the lower limit of autoregulation in humans. Traumatic hypotension leads to ischemia within low-flow regions of the injured brain, so aggressive fluid resuscitation may be required to prevent hypotension and secondary brain injury. It is important to maintain a MAP of ≥80 mm Hg because low blood pressure in the setting of elevated ICP will result in a low CPP and brain injury (Wright & Merck, 2020). Clinical findings of elevated ICP include altered mental status, pupillary irregularities, focal neurologic deficits, and decerebrate or decorticate posturing. Traumatic hypotension leads to ischemia within low-flow regions of the injured brain. Ischemia amplifies the neurotoxic cascade and increases cerebral edema. Normal saline is recommended for volume resuscitation with a goal of systolic blood pressure ≥100 mm Hg for patients 50–69 years of age and SBP ≥110 mm Hg for patients 15–49 years of age or ≥70 years old. Other measures to improve ICP and minimize secondary injury include glucose, pain and temperature control, and seizure prophylaxis. Mannitol and/or hypertonic saline can lower ICP and help reduce edema (Wright & Merck, 2020).

Key Points

Hypotension, hypoxemia, and hyperglycemia accelerate neurotoxic damage and worsen long-term outcomes.

Case Study

You observe your patient's CT scan. She is found to have an acute epidural bleed as well as a chronic subdural hematoma. The neurosurgical team arrives and evaluates her. The lab calls to let you know her INR is 2.5. The neurosurgeon calls her family to discuss the emergent need for surgery along with the risks and benefits, including the possibility of high mortality due to additional bleeding with her anticoagulation. They support the decision to take her to surgery. She is given vitamin K and Kcentra, a type and cross is sent, 2 units of FFP are ordered, and she is taken urgently to the OR. She undergoes successful evacuation of the hematoma and control of the epidural bleed. Postoperatively, she remains intubated and is transferred to the ICU. Are there any concerns that you have regarding her age and comorbidities?

Trauma in the Elderly

Trauma in the elderly is the leading cause of disability and institutionalization, resulting in morbidity and mortality (Gioffre-Florio et al., 2018). The elderly trauma patients, defined as those over the age of 65, account for 25% of all major traumas annually in the United States, with falls remaining the leading cause of injury-related death (Peterson et al., 2015). Advanced age is a well-recognized risk factor for adverse outcomes following trauma. Current literature demonstrates increased morbidity and mortality in elderly trauma patients when compared with those under the age of 65 years. Although the reason for this phenomenon remains unclear, many suggest this outcome difference is the result of the physiologic changes associated with aging and a higher incidence of preexisting medical conditions (Jacobs et al., 2003). Positive outcomes can be achieved in this patient population when appropriately aggressive trauma care is provided to the geriatric patient with survivable injuries (Jacobs et al., 2003).

The elderly are more susceptible to serious injury from low-energy mechanisms and are more likely to suffer complications during treatment and recovery. When providing care for the elderly trauma patient, it is essential to treat both trauma-related injuries and preexisting medical conditions. When obtaining a comprehensive history, ask the patient, caregivers, and established community providers about potential events leading up to the injury. Obtain a detailed past medical history, past surgical history, and current medication list (Fleischman & John Ma, 2020).

Hypovolemia can easily result in shock because the aging myocardium has a decreased chronotropic response to catecholamines and is dependent on preload. Medications, including digoxin, beta-blockers, and calcium channel blockers, impair the tachycardic response to catecholamines, making the heart rate an unreliable predictor of hypovolemia. Deterioration of the cardiac conduction system leads to atrial fibrillation and bundle branch blocks (Callaway & Wolfe, 2007). Older trauma victims with underlying cardiovascular disease actively being treated with anticoagulants or antiplatelet agents have an increased mortality risk that is many times higher than that in patients without such risk factors.

Pulmonary

The elderly have decreased respiratory muscle strength, chest wall compliance, and capacity for oxygen exchange. Response to hypoxia may decline due to loss of alveolar surface area with diminished gas exchange, and the elderly may not exhibit symptoms of respiratory distress despite impending respiratory failure. Other respiratory changes include reduced functional residual capacity, diminished respiratory reserve, and ineffective cough reflex. These physiologic changes predispose the injured elder adult to ARDS, pneumonia, and respiratory failure (Sheetz, 2011).

Renal

Renal function declines with age, predisposing geriatric patients to dehydration and nephropathy (Fleischman & John Ma, 2020).

Musculoskeletal

A loss of muscle strength and bone density decreases the stability of the musculoskeletal system. These physiologic changes make the elderly more prone to mechanical falls and at an increased risk for fractures, most commonly of the ribs, pelvis, and sternum (Fleischman & John Ma, 2020).

Neurological

Brain atrophy that occurs with aging predisposes older adults to intracranial bleeding. With more intracranial space, there is also the potential for increased movement of the brain and a risk for tearing of the vasculature during sudden impact. Neurosensory impairments increase the risk for fall and pose a challenge for assessing the elderly trauma patient, especially in terms of rehabilitation and prevention of complications. Such impairments that occur with aging include diminished hearing, vision, taste, and smell; decline in proprioception of lower limbs; and cognitive delay (Fleischman & John Ma, 2020).

Case Study

Your patient's comorbidities may impact her course and outcome. She is on beta blockade and she may not have a typical response of tachycardia to volume loss (Burlew & Moore, 2019). She did stabilize after evacuation of the clot and hematoma, and her CPP maintained above 80 mm Hg. She required ventilator support for 3 days postoperatively and tolerated weaning before extubation on day 3. Her anticoagulation was held for the immediate postoperative course, and after discussion with cardiology, the trauma service, and her family, it was determined that her risk was higher than the benefit of continuing her DOAC upon discharge. A rehabilitation consult was ordered, and PT/OT began. She was able to regain significant motor function, requiring a walker and assistance for ambulation but had significant cognitive dysfunction including aphasia and worsening memory issues. Case management secured a bed for her at a rehabilitation facility. Her code status was addressed with her family and DNR/DNI status was agreed upon by all due to her decline in cognitive function. She was discharged to rehab on day 10.

CONCLUSION

Trauma is a leading cause of injury and mortality and involves all age groups. In your practice as an ACNP, you will likely encounter patients with traumatic injuries. Having a solid foundation of knowledge and skills needed to address the various aspects of care, types of trauma, mechanisms of injury, triage, resuscitation, and common sequela encountered with these patients is the minimum necessary. Awareness of your local and regional trauma system along with your facility capabilities for trauma patient care is valuable in optimal care of the injured patient.

CLINICAL PEARLS

Early identification and treatment of trauma patients is crucial for positive outcomes. Trauma systems were developed to ensure that the injured patient is delivered to the best equipped facility.
- The primary survey identifies the life-threatening injuries that require immediate treatment using an ABCDE algorithm.
- A GCS of 8 or less is indication for intubation and major trauma activation.
- Recognizing the etiology of shock and providing appropriate treatment are paramount in care of the trauma patient. Hemorrhagic shock is the most commonly encountered shock.
- Trauma care is multidisciplinary care from the moment the patient is encountered, and potential rehabilitation is addressed upon admission.
- The lethal triad of hypothermia, acidosis, and coagulopathy must be addressed to prevent further deterioration.
- Investigating the cause of a fall may uncover serious underlying medical issues and/or prevent future trauma.

- Thermoregulation is less effective, increasing susceptibility to hypothermia in older trauma patients.
- Avoid feeling reassured by "normal" vital signs (Fleischman & John Ma, 2020).
- In blunt trauma patients ≥65 years old, there is an association between hypotension and mortality when systolic blood pressure is below 110 mm Hg and heart rates above 90 beats/min.
- Older trauma patients with underlying cardiovascular disease who take warfarin, clopidogrel, and beta-blockers have an increased mortality risk that is many times higher than that in patients without such risk factors (Sheetz, 2011).
- Recent studies suggest that the SBP cut-off point for predicted mortality in injured older adults is approximately 110 mm Hg (Scheetz, 2011).

REVIEW QUESTIONS

1. Which of the following is the suggested systolic blood pressure goal for injured older patients?
   a. 95 mm Hg
   b. 100 mm Hg
   c. 105 mm H
   d. 110 mm Hg

2. Which of the following is a respiratory change that occurs with aging that predisposes older adults to respiratory complications?
   a. Decreased reserve volume
   b. Increased alveolar surface area
   c. Increased chest wall compliance
   d. Increased maximum expiratory force

3. Reduced thermal regulation predisposes geriatric trauma patients to an increased risk of developing which of the following complications?
   a. Coagulopathies and MODS (multiple organ dysfunction syndrome)
   b. Infection and SIRS (systemic inflammatory response syndrome)
   c. SIRS and ARDS
   d. MODS and infection

4. When resuscitating the geriatric trauma patient, which of the following guidelines should be considered?
   a. Administration of intravenous fluids based on urinary output
   b. Aggressive administration of intravenous fluids and blood
   c. Administration of blood, blood products, and inotropes, and limited administration of intravenous fluids
   d. Judicious administration of intravenous fluids

5. Hypotension without tachycardia is a classic sign of:
   a. Pericardial tamponade
   b. Neurogenic shock
   c. Hypovolemic shock
   d. Tension pneumothorax

6. Beck triad (dilated neck veins, muffled heart tones, and a decline in arterial pressure with hypotension that is resistant to fluid bolus) is classic presentation of:
   a. Pericardial tamponade
   b. Tension pneumothorax
   c. Aortic dissection
   d. Pulmonary contusion

7. Your patient is admitted with a TBI. She had an LOC at the scene, followed by return to lucidity. She presents to the ED with GCS of 8. Your primary concern is for:
   a. Subdural hematoma
   b. Epidural hematoma
   c. Subarachnoid hemorrhage
   d. Cerebral contusion

8. Which of the following is a common prehospital complication that contributes to resuscitation failure in burn patients?
   a. Inadequate volume resuscitation
   b. Hypothermia
   c. GCS of 13
   d. TBS burn area of more than 20%

Answer: 1, d; 2, a; 3, a; 4, a; 5, b; 6, a; 7, b; 8, b

REFERENCES

Advanced Burn Life Support Group. (2018). *Advanced burn life support course provider manual.* American Burn Association. Retrieved July 15, 2020. http://ameriburn.org/wp-content/uploads/2019/08/2018-abls-providermanual.pdf.

Altinok, T., & Can, A. (2014). Management of tracheobronchial injuries. *The Eurasian Journal of Medicine,* 46(3), 209–215. https://doi.org/10.5152/eajm.2014.42

American College of Surgeons – Committee on Trauma. (2014). *Resources for optimal care of the injured patient.* American College of Surgeons.

American Trauma Society. (2020). Accessed October 7, 2020. https://www.amtrauma.org/page/TraumaLevels.

Anderson, J. H., Mandell, S. P., & Gibran, N. S. (2019). Burns. In Brunicardi, F, Andersen, D. K., Billiar, T. R., Dunn, D. L., Kao, L. S., Hunter, J. G., Matthews, J. B., & Pollock, R. E. (Eds.), *Schwartz's principles of surgery* (11th ed.). McGraw-Hill.

Benjamin, M. M., & Roberts, W. C. (2012). Fatal aortic rupture from nonpenetrating chest trauma. *Proceedings (Baylor University. Medical Center),* 25(2), 121–123. https://doi.org/10.1080/08998280.2012.11928805

Burlew, C. C, & Moore, E. E. (2019). Trauma. In Brunicardi, F., Andersen, D. K., Billiar, T. R., Dunn, D. L., Kao, L. S., Hunter, J. G., Matthews, J. B., & Pollock, R. E. (Eds.), *Schwartz's principles of surgery* (11th ed.). McGraw-Hill.

Callaway, D. W., & Wolfe, R. (2007). Geriatric trauma. *Emergency Medicine Clinics of North America,* 25(3), 837–860.

Cameron, P. A., Knapp, B. J., & Teeter, W. (2020). Trauma in adults. In Tintinalli, J. E., John Ma, O., Yealy, D. M., Meckler, G. D., Stephan Stapczynski, J., Cline, D., & Thomas, S. H. (Eds.), *Tintinalli's emergency medicine: A comprehensive Study guide* (9th ed.). McGraw-Hill.

Centers for Disease Control and Prevention. *CDC Yellow Book 2020: Health Information for International Travel.* New York: Oxford University Press.

Dumovich, J, & Singh, P. (2020). *Physiology, trauma.* In *StatPearls.* StatPearls Publishing. https://www.ncbi.nlm.nih.gov/books/NBK538478/. [Updated 2019 Feb 12].

Ebraheim, N. A., Thomas, B. J., Fu, F. H., Muller, B., Vyas, D., Niesen, M, Pribaz, J, & Draenert, K. (2019). Orthopedic surgery. In Brunicardi, F., Andersen, D. K., Billiar, T. R., Dunn, D. L., Kao, L. S., Hunter, J. G., Matthews, J. B., & Pollock, R. E. (Eds.), *Schwartz's principles of surgery* (11th ed.). McGraw-Hill.

Fleischman, R. J., & John Ma, O. (2020). Trauma in the elderly. In Tintinalli, J. E., John Ma, O., Yealy, D. M., Meckler, G. D., Stephan Stapczynski, J., Cline, D., & Thomas, S. H. (Eds.), *Tintinalli's emergency medicine: A comprehensive study guide* (9th ed.). McGraw-Hill.

Gioffre-Florio, M., Murabitol, M., Visalli, C., Pergolizzi, F. P., & Fama, F. (2018). Trauma in elderly patients: A study of prevalence, comorbidities and gender differences. *Il Giornale di Chirurgia*, 39(1), 35–40.

Hemmila, M. R. (2020). Management of the injured patient. In Doherty, G. M. (Ed.), *Current diagnosis & treatment: Surgery* (15th ed.). McGraw-Hill.

Jacobs, D., Plaisier, B. R., Barie, P. S., Hammond, J. S., Holevar, M. R., Sinclair, K. E., Scalea, T. M., Wahl, W., & for the EAST Practice Management Guidelines Work Group. (2003). Geriatric trauma: Parameters for resuscitation. *The Journal of Trauma and Acute Care Surgery*, 54(2), 391–416.

Oropello, J. M., Mistry, N., & Ullman, J. S. (2014). Head injury. In Hall, J. B., Schmidt, G. A., & Kress, J. P. (Eds.), *Principles of critical care* (4th ed.). McGraw-Hill.

Oyeniyi, B., Fox, E., Scerbo, M., Tomasek, J., Wade, C., & Holcomb, J. (2017) Trends in 1029 trauma deaths at a level 1 trauma center. *Injury*, 48(1), 5–12. https://doi.org/10.1016/j.injury.2016.10.037

Peterson, B. E., Jiwanlal, A., Della Rocca, G. J., & Crist, B. D. (2015). Orthopedic trauma and aging: It isn't just about mortality. *Geriatric Orthopedic Surgery & Rehabilitation*, 6(1), 33–36.

Ramayya, A. G., Sinha, S., & Grady, M. (2019). Neurosurgery. In Brunicardi, F., Andersen, D. K., Billiar, T. R., Dunn, D. L., Kao, L. S., Hunter, J. G., Matthews, J. B., & Pollock, R. E. (Eds.), *Schwartz's principles of surgery* (11th ed.). McGraw-Hill.

Sheetz, L. (2011). Life-threatening injuries in older adults. *AACN Advanced Critical Care*, 22(2), 128–139.

Wright, D. W., & Merck, L. H. (2020). Head trauma. In Tintinalli, J. E., John Ma, O., Yealy, D. M., Meckler, G. D., Stephan Stapczynski, J., Cline, D., & Thomas, S. H. (Eds.), *Tintinalli's emergency medicine: A comprehensive study guide* (9th ed.). McGraw-Hill.

17

Multisystem Disorders

Paula McCauley

INTRODUCTION

Multisystem is a broad concept and includes too many topics to capture in our limited space, so we will use a "multisystem" case study. Within this case, we will incorporate shock, sepsis, acid-base disorders, nutritional needs of the critically ill patient, fever, and infectious workup. These are all complex problems that we can only begin to address in limited format but we will attempt to provide a launching pad for further individual or group exploration of the topics or provide the foundation for a comprehensive, complex, unfolding case.

Case Study

You are the APRN on the critical care service and respond to the medical floor for a rapid response. There you find Mrs. P, a 64-year-old female with a history of COPD and obstructive sleep apnea. She presented to the ED yesterday with suspected cellulitis of her right lower extremity. She had stable vital signs, received appropriate antibiotics including vancomycin due to concerns for MRSA, and was admitted to the floor. Overnight, she refused to use the hospital CPAP machine because it was uncomfortable and created "too much pressure." At 6:00 a.m., the phlebotomist found the patient unresponsive and the rapid response team was called. She is currently being ventilated by the respiratory therapist with a bag valve mask with an O_2 saturation of 85%. Further examination reveals a morbidly obese white female, lying in bed, obtunded. She attempts to push you away with noxious stimuli but does not respond verbally or appropriately to commands. She is pale and cool, and she has a rapid, palpable radial pulse and a blood pressure (BP) of 90/45. The ECG monitor displays atrial fibrillation with rapid ventricular response of 134. Her saturation rises to 90% on high flow. A stat metabolic panel and CBC have been obtained and sent, and a point-of-care ABG has been drawn.

She remains largely unresponsive to your attempts to wake her with noxious stimuli. She is normocephalic and atraumatic, with no evidence of facial asymmetry. Her pupils are pinpoints; her cardiac examination includes normal S1, S2, no MRG (murmurs, rubs, or gallops), and no noted JVP; her lung sounds are diminished bilaterally; and she has scattered expiratory wheezes and crackles to both bases. Her abdomen is distended and tympanic to percussion with hypoactive Bowel Sounds. Her right lower extremity appears larger than the left and has an inflamed area from the knee down, which is warm to touch and indurated, with no open wounds or drainage. Her ABG results are obtained as follows: pH of 7.01, PO_2 of 55, PCO_2 of 90, and HCO_3 of 20.

You call anesthesia for intubation and notify the ICU that she will be transferred once her airway is secure. You confirm that she has adequate access and ask for a liter of normal saline to be hung and available for intubation. You query the nurses about additional PMH and ROS (review of systems). They inform you that she is diabetic; has chronic kidney disease stage 3, paroxysmal atrial fibrillation, and chronic LBP; comes from a skill nursing facility; and is largely bed-bound, requiring a lift to the commode. Her home medications include metoprolol 50 mg daily, apixaban 5 mg bid, Symbicort and albuterol for her COPD, oxycodone for chronic pain, and recent use of naproxen for acute back and leg pain. She has not been febrile and denied chills or rigors on admission. She did complain of shortness of breath and a nonproductive cough, positive orthopnea, and PND, but no chest pain. Her labs on admission include a mild leukocytosis of 13% on her initial CBC with a normal H/H. Her procalcitonin was 0.25, and her BUN/creatinine was 43/1.5 (baseline of 1.0). She received her second dose of cefepime this morning at 4 a.m. and was taking po (by mouth) overnight. Anesthesia arrives and she is successfully intubated. Her blood pressure drops with the intubation meds but responds to a fluid bolus. Respiratory therapist continues to bag, and you transport her to the ICU.

Based on the information you have, you formulate possible differentials:

- Hypercarbic respiratory failure due to exacerbation of her COPD with potential CAP or aspiration pneumonitis compounding this and contributing to the hypoxic respiratory failure
- Sepsis or septic shock with hypotension and tachycardia in the setting of either the pneumonia or suspected cellulitis
- Acute HF with atrial fibrillation with RVR, cardiogenic shock, and acute pulmonary edema
- Opioid toxicity
- Hypoglycemia
- AKI secondary to her NSAID use
- Must-not-miss diagnoses, including PE, ACS, aspiration, stroke, and seizure

Your patient is complex with potential for multisystem dysfunction. Now that her airway is secured and you are safely back in your unit, you can focus on your data to address these differentials. Let us start with analysis and treatment of her acid-base status. This will provide valuable direction in establishing your primary diagnosis and treatment.

ACID-BASE DISORDERS

Acid-base balance is crucial to effective function of body systems. Acidemia is defined as a decrease in the blood pH below 7.35, whereas acidosis is a physiologic process characterized by a primary decrease in HCO_3 level (metabolic acidosis) or a primary increase in

PaCO$_2$ (respiratory acidosis). Conversely, alkalemia is defined as an increase in the blood pH above 7.45, whereas alkalosis is a physiologic process characterized by a primary increase in HCO$_3$⁻ level (metabolic alkalosis) or a primary decrease in the PaCO$_2$ (respiratory alkalosis) (Woodrow, 2010).

Acids are substances that dissociate or lose ions. Bases are substances capable of accepting ions. Buffers are substances that react with acids or bases to maintain neutral environment of stable pH. Elevated hydrogen ions (H⁺) will cause a drop in pH resulting in acidity or academic state. A decrease in H⁺ will cause an increase in the pH resulting in an alkaline or alkalemic state. Volatile acids, such as carbonic acid and H$_2$CO$_3$, can be converted to a gas form for secretion by the lungs. Nonvolatile acids, such as lactate and ketones, cannot be converted to gas and are excreted by the kidneys. Compensation is the counterbalancing of acid-base activities to return pH to normal limits (7.4) (Ayers et al., 2015).

Key Points

As long as the ratio of bicarbonate to Pco$_2$ remains equal 20:1, the pH will remain at 7.4.

Cho (2014).

There are two primary mechanisms of the body that will maintain a normal pH: respiratory compensation and metabolic or renal compensation. Respiratory compensation is rapid. A normal compensatory response to metabolic alkalosis is alveolar hypoventilation, which results in retention of CO$_2$. Conversely, in metabolic acidosis, the result is alveolar hyperventilation in an attempt to exhale or blow off CO$_2$. Metabolic compensation is slow and can take hours to days to effectively resolve an acid-base disorder. The bicarbonate buffer system controls rate of elimination or reabsorption of H⁺ and bicarbonate in the kidneys. Common H⁺ ions include Hgb and potassium phosphates. Attempts to compensate with an acidotic state would be an increase in H⁺ elimination and an increase in HCO$_3$ reabsorption. In an alkalotic state, there will be in an increase in H⁺ reabsorption and increase in HCO$_3$ elimination (Kaufman et al., 2015).

Key Points

It is important to remember that in evaluation of acid-base disorders, your ABG or serum electrolytes are a snapshot of a single point in time. They must be incorporated into the overall clinical picture. You must trend the results and correlate with other values such as your volume status and hemodynamics (Berend et al., 2014).

Interpretation of Acid-Base Disorders

Evaluation of acid-base disorders requires an ABG and serum electrolytes simultaneously. Evaluation should include a systematic process such as the one provided in Box 17.1.

When evaluating acid-base disorders, it is helpful to keep in mind the most common causes. If presented with results that are specific for the various types of disorders, it will help

BOX 17.1 Step-by-Step Evaluation of Acid-Base Disorders

1. Compare the HCO_3^- on ABG and serum electrolytes to verify accuracy.
2. Calculate the anion gap (AG).
3. Compare the AG and HCO_3^-.
4. Compare the change in $[Cl^-]$ with change in $[Na^+]$.
5. Estimate compensatory response.

Data from Kaufman, D. C., Kitching, A. J., & Kellum, J. A. (2015). Acid-base balance. In J. B. Hall, G. A. Schmidt, & J. P. Kress (Eds.), *Principles of critical care* (4th ed.). McGraw-Hill Education and Berend, K., de Vries, A. P. J., & Gans, R. O. B. (2014). Physiological approach to assessment of acid–base disturbances. *New England Journal of Medicine, 371*, 1434–1445.

you to quickly establish the underlying cause vs. looking for the anomalies that occasionally occur. The four most common causes of anion gap (AG) metabolic acidosis (AGMA) are ketoacidosis, lactic acidosis, renal failure, and toxins. Two causes of hyperchloremic or nongap acidosis are bicarbonate loss from the GI tract and renal tubular acidosis. Common causes of respiratory acidosis are conditions in which there is hypoventilation such as altered mental status or pulmonary embolus (PE). Respiratory alkalosis includes etiologies that occur with hyperventilation, such as pain or anxiety, hypoxemia, or pulmonary edema (Ayer et al, 2015; Cho, 2014; Kaufman, et al, 2015).

Key Points

Calculating an AG is an early and easily obtained measure that you must include in your evaluation for all patients. Your patient may have a compensated AGMA with a normal pH but a wide gap. If not calculated, you may overlook it in your evaluation.

To calculate the AG, use the following equation:

$$AG = \left(Na^+\right) - \left(Cl^-\right) + \left(HCO_3^-\right)$$

A normal AG is less than 12 (Ayers et al., 2015; Berend et al., 2014). In a metabolic acidosis caused by the addition or accumulation of acid in the plasma, including lactic acidosis, ketoacidosis, or renal failure, there will be an increase in the AG. If the metabolic acidosis is due to the loss of bicarbonate from causes such as diarrhea or a GI fistula, the AG will remain WNL despite the presence of a metabolic acidosis (Ayers et al., 2015; Berend et al., 2014).

AG is used in interpretation of ABGs, which should also provide information on level of compensation and oxygenation. The ABG includes a PaO_2, which measures the amount of O_2 available in arterial blood for possible tissue use and reflects alveolar ventilation. A normal PaO_2 is 70–100. Alterations in oxygenation are covered in the pulmonary chapter. Box 17.2 outlines the step-by-step approach for evaluating ABGs.

BOX 17.2	Step-by-Step Process for Evaluating Arterial Blood Gases

Step 1: Evaluate the pH. Remember: normal is 7.40 (7.35–7.45), a decrease is acidic, and an increase is alkalotic.

- Is it normal? If not, in which direction is it heading? This indicates acid or base.

Step 2: Evaluate the $Paco_2$ keeping in mind that $Paco_2$ is an acid. The normal range is 35–45. Less than 35 is alkaline, and greater than 45 is acidic.

- Is it normal? If not, in which direction is it heading? Correlate this with your pH.

Step 3: Evaluate the bicarbonate (HCO_3). The normal range is 22–26. Less than 22 is acidic, and greater than 26 is alkaline.

- Is it normal? If not, in which direction is it heading? Correlate this with your pH.

Step 4: Which component matches the pH state? The answer identifies the primary disorder. If both match, the pH state it is a mixed picture.
Step 5: Return to the pH.

- Is it normal or abnormal?
- Does it show a compensated state (normal pH but abnormal $PaCO_2$ or HCO_3) or an uncompensated state (abnormal pH)?

Data from Cho, K. C. (2014). Electrolyte & acid-base disorders. In M. A. Papadakis, S. J. McPhee, & M. W. Rabow (Eds.), Current medical diagnosis & treatment 2015 and Palmer, B. F. (2008). Approach to fluid and electrolyte disorders and acid-base problems. Primary Care, 35(2), 195–213, v.

Case Study

Mrs. P's ABG and electrolytes have also come back from the lab. Her ABG shows the following: pH, 7.01; PaO_2, 55 mmHg; $PaCO_2$, 90 mmHg; HCO_3, 20 mEq/L. Her serum electrolytes are as follows: Na, 136 mEq/L; K, 5.0 mEq/L; Cl, 102 mEq/L; HCO_3, 18 mEq/L; BUN, 44 mEq/L; creatinine, 2.0 mEq/L; Blood Glucose (BG), 394. We can use the stepwise approach first with her electrolytes. Her serum and blood gas bicarb both are low and correlate with an acidemia. We then calculate her AG:

$$AG = (Na^+) - (Cl^-) + (HCO_3^-)$$
$$AG = 136 - 102 + 18 = 16$$

At 16, her AG is elevated, and her serum bicarb correlates with this finding. Her chloride and sodium are consistent. What do you think of her compensatory response? If you have a primary AGMA, you would expect her compensatory response to be decreased in CO_2; hers is elevated. Now incorporating the ABG, (1) her pH is low, or acidotic; (2) her $PaCO_2$ is elevated, which correlates with the pH; (3) her HCO_3 is low, also correlating with her pH; (4) both correlate with the pH, so you have a mixed picture; and (5) her pH is uncompensated. Mrs. P has a mixed picture of both uncompensated respiratory and metabolic acidosis with a dangerously low pH. You need to act fast. What is your best approach to her condition? Exploring the primary disorders will help us decide how to address this.

Primary Disorders

We will briefly review the primary acid-base disorders and the common causes of each derangement.

Respiratory Acidosis

In respiratory acidosis, $PaCO_2$ >45 mm Hg (hypercapnia) and pH <7.35. This reflects alveolar hypoventilation leading to excess carbonic acid secondary to the inability of the lungs to blow off CO_2. The causes may be acute or chronic and can be differentiated into disorders affecting gas exchange, respiratory muscle weakness, and decreased respiratory drive or airway obstruction. Disorders affecting gas exchange include pneumothorax, pulmonary edema, PE or COPD exacerbation, respiratory muscle weakness that can occur with acute spinal cord injury, neuromuscular disorders such as Guillain-Barré, neuromuscular blockade, decreased respiratory drive, narcotics, anesthetics, hypothyroidism or cerebral trauma, and airway obstruction secondary to foreign body, secretions, or laryngospasm (Cho, 2014).

Respiratory Alkalosis

In respiratory alkalosis, $PaCO_2$ <35 mm Hg and pH >7.45. This reflects alveolar hyperventilation leading to CO_2 retention. Common causes can be separated into categories including hypoxemia (which results in tachypnea), cardiopulmonary disease, and direct stimulation of the respiratory center. Specific examples causing hypoxemia include asthma, COPD, high altitude, pneumonia, and severe anemia. Cardiopulmonary causes include HF, mitral valve disease, and pulmonary HTN. Direct stimulation of the respiratory center includes anxiety or pain, hepatic failure, neurologic disorders, pregnancy, salicylate intoxication, and mechanical ventilation (Cho, 2014).

Metabolic Acidosis

In metabolic acidosis, HCO_3 <22 mEq/L and pH <7.35. It is caused by an increase in metabolic acids due to increased production or decreased excretion or excessive loss of base. There are several causes, and determining the AG will help narrow the differential. Mnemonics for AGMA include MUDPILES (methanol, uremia, DKA, paraldehyde, isoniazid and iron, lactic acid, ethylene glycol and ethanol, and salicylates) and KUSSMAUL (ketoacidosis, uremia, salicylates, starvation ketosis, methanol, alcoholic ketosis, unmeasured osmoles, lactate). The most common causes of AGMA are increased lactate, ketones, uremia, or toxins. The most common cause of nonanion gap metabolic acidosis is GI bicarbonate losses with diarrhea (Ayer et al., 2015; Cho, 2014; Vichot & Rastegar, 2014).

Metabolic Alkalosis

In metabolic alkalosis, HCO_3 >26 mEq/L and pH >7.45. It is due to an increased amount of alkali or excessive loss of acid usually combined with chloride loss. In the hospitalized patient, it is most commonly caused by diuretics, prolonged gastric suctioning, or vomiting, causing volume depletion and hypochloremia (Cho, 2014).

Winters Formula

$$PaCO_2 = 1.5 \times (serum\ HCO_3) + 8 \pm 2$$

The $PaCO_2$ should increase by 1.2 mm Hg for every 1 mEq/L decrease in HCO_3. If the $PaCO_2$ is not at an appropriate compensatory level, the patient has more than one disorder.

Data from Cho, K. C. (2014). Electrolyte & acid-base disorders. In M. A. Papadakis, S. J. McPhee, & M. W. Rabow (Eds.), Current medical diagnosis & treatment 2015.

Mixed Conditions

A mixed acid-base disorder develops when two or more primary acid-base disorders occur simultaneously. These disorders may mask each other and can be diagnosed only with a thorough evaluation of acid-base status. To determine the expected compensatory responses to primary disorders, there are several calculations you can employ.

With metabolic acidosis, the primary change should be a decreased HCO_3. The compensatory response is respiratory or a change in $PaCO_2$. You can evaluate for a mixed picture by first calculating the AG. If there is an AG, use Winters formula to determine if there is appropriate compensation. Box 17.3 reviews calculations of Winters formula (Jameson et al., 2020).

Key Points

In fully compensated metabolic acidosis, the $PaCO_2$ closely approximates the last two digits of the blood pH within the range of 7.10–7.40. This rule of thumb does not apply for a pH outside of this range. If the $PaCO_2$ does not approximate the last two digits of the pH, a mixed acid-base disturbance should be considered (Appel & Downs, 2008).

Compensations in respiratory disorders are defined and calculated as acute or chronic conditions. In respiratory acidosis, the primary change is an increase in Pco_2. Box 17.4 includes calculations for the respiratory compensation in acute situations (Jameson et al., 2020).

In respiratory alkalosis, the primary change is decreased $PaCO_2$. The compensatory response is separated into acute or chronic situations. Box 17.5 outlines calculations for compensation for respiratory alkalosis (Jameson et al., 2020).

An alternative approach is to calculate what is referred to as the delta-delta. This approach gives you a sense of whether the body is holding onto or losing more bicarbonate than you would expect simply based on the pH, AG, and the bicarbonate values. Box 17.6 describes how to calculate the delta-delta change (Berend et al., 2014).

Respiratory Compensation in Acute Situations

The HCO_3^- concentration increases by up to 1 mEq for every 10 mm Hg increase in $PaCO_2$.
In chronic respiratory acidosis, the HCO_3^- concentration increases by up to 3.5 mEq for every 10 mm Hg increase in $PaCO_2$.

Data from Cho, K. C. (2014). Electrolyte & acid-base disorders. In M. A. Papadakis, S. J. McPhee, & M. W. Rabow (Eds.), Current medical diagnosis & treatment 2015.

BOX 17.5 | Compensation for Respiratory Alkalosis

Acute respiratory alkalosis:

HCO_3^- concentration decreases by up to 2 mEq for every 10 mm Hg decrease in $PaCO_2$.

Chronic respiratory alkalosis:

HCO_3^- concentration decreases by up to 5 mEq for every 10 mm Hg decrease in $PaCO_2$.

If the measured values do not approximate the predicted values using the formulas and rules in Box 17.2, step 2, a mixed acid-base balance is present.

Data from Cho, K. C. (2014). Electrolyte & acid-base disorders. In M. A. Papadakis, S. J. McPhee, & M. W. Rabow (Eds.), Current medical diagnosis & treatment 2015.

BOX 17.6 | Calculating the Delta-Delta

1. Calculate the delta gap: Measured serum anion gap (SAG) − Normal SAG (12 mEq/L)
2. Calculate the delta-delta: Add the delta gap to the measured bicarbonate (from the chemistry panel)
3. Compare the delta-delta to a normal bicarbonate (22–26 mEq/L):
   - If the delta-delta <22, the patient is losing bicarbonate somewhere and there is a nongap acidosis.
   - If the delta-delta >26, the patient is holding onto bicarbonate and there is an additional metabolic alkalosis.

Data from Berend, K., de Vries, A. P. J., & Gans, R. O.B. (2014). Physiological approach to assessment of acid–base disturbances. *New England Journal of Medicine*, *371*, 1434–1445.

Case Study

Mrs. P has a severe acidosis with the pH of 7.01 with derangements in both $PaCO_2$ and HCO_3 that reflect acidosis so your assessment and plan will focus on life-threatening causes first. She is profoundly altered, and you need to secure her airway and ventilate for her, which should address the respiratory acidosis. She has an AG acidosis and your differential includes sepsis due to her lower extremity infection; she also has uremia and elevated glucose. That puts lactic acidosis, uremia, and ketoacidosis on your list of differentials. You send off further diagnostics including serum lactate, serum and urine ketones, and additional cultures to rule out other sources of infection. You initiate antibiotics for coverage of her presumed infection and review additional infectious disease concepts as well. This should support your treatment for AKI, which is reviewed in the renal chapter. We also need to address her hyperglycemia and possible DKA. Specifics related to this topic are covered in the endocrine chapter. Her clinical findings are indicative of shock. A discussion of shock and sepsis can help determine next steps.

CLINICAL PEARLS

- Develop a systematic approach.
- Obtain simultaneous ABG and serum electrolytes.
- Always calculate the anion gap.
- Memorize the most common causes of each disorder.
- Remember to calculate compensation: The body cannot overcompensate, so you may have a mixed disorder.

SHOCK AND SEPSIS

Shock is a pathophysiologic abnormality resulting from a life-threatening response to alterations in circulation that results in inadequate blood flow to vital organs and inability of the tissues or cells to metabolize nutrients normally. Shock is a syndrome; it is not low blood pressure. Shock is the clinical manifestation of inadequate oxygen delivery compared to cellular needs. It begins when the cardiovascular system fails. Disturbances to key determinants of oxygen delivery form the basis of the major shock types, which are based on the underlying alteration, hypovolemic, cardiogenic, or distributive shock. Cardiogenic shock includes obstructive etiologies; distributive shock includes sepsis, anaphylaxis, and neurogenic shock. Each includes an alteration in at least one of the following: blood volume and/or flow, myocardial contractility, and vascular resistance (Massaro, 2018).

The cardiovascular system is a closed system that includes the heart, blood volume, vascular bed, and microcirculation. It functions to deliver oxygen and nutrients and remove waste products. The system regulates blood volume through the vascular response that involves constriction or dilatation of the vascular bed to regulate blood flow. Variables that affect the pressure of the system include vessel length, blood viscosity, and vessel diameter (Massaro, 2018).

Whalley (2014) encourages the use of questions when establishing a differential with shock, reminding us that mean blood pressure is the product of cardiac output and systemic vascular resistance (SVR). Hypotension may be caused by reduced cardiac output or reduced SVR. The initial examination of the hypotensive patient seeks to answer the question, *Is cardiac output increased or decreased?*

Whalley also outlines the SHOCK mnemonic, which is defined by asking four questions:

- Is cardiac output increased (septic shock) or decreased (other forms)?
- Are central veins empty (hypovolemic shock) or full (other forms)?
- Are breath sounds clear (obstructive shock) or are crackles heard (cardiogenic shock)?
- What does not fit?

Additional physical findings, laboratory tests, and echocardiographic and other examinations will help to further define these questions.

Key Points

Early recognition of shock is important. If recognized and addressed during the early stages, morbidity and mortality may be prevented.

Stages of Shock

Stage One

Stage one is described and categorized as early, reversible, or compensatory. Compensatory mechanisms include neural, endocrine, and chemical responses. The physiologic goal is to restore homeostasis. If recognized and reversed, there is minimal morbidity (Massaro, 2018).

Neural compensation encompasses baroreceptors, which are sensitive to pressure changes, and chemoreceptors, which are sensitive to chemical changes. When activated, they cause increased respiratory rate and depth and stimulate the autonomic system, which in turn causes increased heart rate and contractility, along with vasodilation of coronary arteries and compensatory systemic vasoconstriction.

Endocrine compensation is triggered in response to low blood pressure causing activation of the anterior and posterior pituitary glands, resulting in stimulation of renin-angiotensin response, release of antidiuretic hormone, glucose regulation, and increased intravascular blood volume.

Chemical compensation includes chemoreceptors in the aorta and carotids, which react to low oxygen tension. This, in turn, activates the respiratory rate and depth to increase, resulting in hyperventilation. Respiratory alkalosis occurs with resulting vasoconstriction of cerebral blood vessels in an attempt to increase oxygen supply. This does cause a negative effect on cerebral perfusion, which may manifest as an alteration in mental status.

Stage Two

Stage two is the intermediate, or progressive, stage. Here, compensatory mechanisms begin to work independently, and pathological symptoms occur. Classic signs and symptoms include tachycardia, tachypnea, and hypotension. The periphery is cool and clammy or warm and mottled, depending on the underlying syndrome. Systemic vasoconstriction promotes ischemia and hypoxia and leads to metabolic acidosis. The microcirculation dilates and capillary pressure increases, which in turn pushes fluid into interstitial space. Intravascular volume decreases and cardiac perfusion is impaired, leading to decreased contractility, cardiac output, and blood pressure (Massaro, 2018).

Stage Three

Stage three is refractory or irreversible. There is profound inadequate tissue perfusion, which is unresponsive to therapy and may progress rapidly to multiple organ dysfunction and death.

Classification and Etiology

Hypovolemic Shock

Hypovolemic shock results from inadequate circulating blood volume. It may be secondary to external losses, such as acute hemorrhage, burns, and losses from the GI tract, or internal losses, such as fluid shifts that occur with acute pancreatitis. The severity of hypovolemic shock depends on the volume of loss and the rate of loss and is compounded by the extremes of age and preexisting conditions. The clinical examination will reveal manifestations of blood loss (hematemesis, tarry stools, or trauma) or manifestations of dehydration (reduced tissue turgor, vomiting or diarrhea, or negative fluid balance) (Whalley 2014). Treatment is aimed at reducing or eliminating the causative factors and restoring vascular volume (Massaro, 2018). Treatments can include direct interventions such as surgical repair in situations such as trauma, endoscopic interventions for acute GI bleed, or supportive care in cases with causes such as pancreatitis or dehydration from GI losses or poor intake. Several examples can be found throughout this text in chapters that address these conditions.

Cardiogenic Shock

Cardiogenic shock is best classified as pump failure. Causes include myocardial infarction, dysrhythmias, cardiomyopathy, and structural disorders such as valvular disease. Damage to the myocardium leads to reduced contractility and reduced stroke volume. Ventricular pressure is increased, leading to decreased cardiac output. There is compensatory peripheral vasoconstriction (Massaro, 2018). Clinical findings that correlate with cardiogenic shock that also help to distinguish obstructive shock etiologies include dependent crackles on lung auscultation, extra heart sounds (S3, S4), peripheral edema, chest pain, ischemic changes on the ECG, and pulmonary edema (Whalley 2014). Treatment of cardiogenic shock is aimed at restoring or preserving myocardial function and includes surgical interventions through open heart and endovascular approaches for coronary bypass and valvular and pericardial disorders and percutaneous attempts to perform coronary artery interventions. Preservation of function is medically managed for cardiomyopathies and heart failure.

Obstructive Shock

Obstructive shock is often classified as a subsection of cardiogenic shock or as the fourth category of shock. It is caused by physical impairment to blood flow or obstruction of blood return to the heart, which leads to decreased cardiac output, decreased blood pressure with reduced tissue perfusion, and reduced cellular metabolism. On clinical examination, elevated jugular veins along with hypotension are suggestive of obstruction (e.g., pulmonary embolism, cardiac tamponade) or cardiogenic shock (Whalley 2014). Causes of obstructive shock include pericardial tamponade, pulmonary embolus, and tension pneumothorax. Treatment is aimed at removing or reducing the impact of the obstructive process (Massaro, 2018). These topics are further discussed in the cardiology and trauma chapters.

Distributive Shock

Distributive shock, or high-output shock, is due to widespread vasodilation. There are three major classifications of distributive shock: neurogenic, anaphylactic, and septic shock (Massaro, 2018).

Neurogenic Shock

Neurogenic shock is secondary to a disturbance within the nervous system that interrupts sympathetic nerve impulse and leads to vasodilation, bradycardia, and hypovolemia. This may be secondary to injury or disease to the upper spinal cord, from spinal anesthesia or ganglionic or adrenergic-blocking agents. Treatment is aimed at removing or reducing the underlying cause and supporting the HR and vasodilation with chronotropic agents and vasopressors.

Anaphylactic Shock

Anaphylactic shock is due to a severe allergic reaction which initiates the antigen-antibody response. Basophils and mast cells contain histamine, which is a potent vasodilator and causes increased capillary permeability, relative hypovolemia, and fluid shifts leading to decreased perfusion. Treatment includes rapid administration of epinephrine to combat the vasodilation and anti-inflammatory and antihistamine agents such as steroids (Massaro, 2018).

Septic Shock

Septic shock is a high cardiac output state most often signaled by a high pulse pressure, a low diastolic pressure, warm extremities with good nail bed return, fever or hypothermia, leukocytosis or leukopenia, and other evidence of infection (Whalley 2014). These clinical findings strongly suggest a systemic inflammatory response that leads to sepsis, septic shock, and MODS.

Hemodynamic Parameters

A solid understanding of hemodynamic parameters is necessary for establishing a differential diagnosis in the setting of shock. The two major components of oxygen delivery (DO_2) are cardiac output (CO) and arterial oxygen content (CaO_2). The product of the two is the oxygen delivery: $DO_2 = CO \times CaO_2$. The two components of CO are heart rate (HR) and stroke volume (SV), which can be substituted in the above equation as $DO_2 = (HR \times SV) \times CaO_2$ (Massaro, 2018).

We can determine the cause of the alteration in SV or cardiac index by assessing its determinants: preload, afterload, and contractility. SV is an independent variable for cardiac output and evaluates the heart's pumping ability. A normal SV indicates that there is no immediate threat to cardiac output. A low SV is associated with a failing heart secondary to cardiogenic shock. A high SV indicates little or no resistance and is seen with distributive shock (Adams, 2004). Keeping this in mind will help you determine the etiology of your patient's shock state. These parameters are established first by physical examination and directly measured with a pulmonary artery catheter.

The relationship of SV to preload, afterload (systemic vascular resistance or SVR), and cardiac contractility is represented by the following equation: SV = α (preload × contractility)/SVR. Normal CO is 4–9 L/min. Cardiac index is the calculated CO based on the patient's body surface area and is more specific to the individual. The normal range for cardiac index is 2.5–4 L/min/m² (Adams, 2004; Massaro, 2018).

Preload

Preload is the amount of stretch on the ventricle at the end of diastole. Preload is influenced by the amount of intravascular volume as well as venous tone. It is decreased with volume loss such as hemorrhage or dehydration and increased with cardiogenic shock, volume overload, or renal failure. Clinical findings that reflect preload are JVD, hepatomegaly or peripheral edema, skin turgor, and dry mucous membranes. Preload indicators include RAP and pulmonary artery wedge pressure (PAWP), both which are directly measured with a pulmonary artery catheter. JVP is reflective of RAP (Adams, 2004; Massaro, 2018).

Afterload

Afterload is the amount of resistance the heart has to overcome to eject blood out of the ventricle. Afterload is influenced by the volume and mass of blood ejected, the size and wall thickness of the ventricle, and the vascular impedance. Afterload is decreased by vasodilators and anemia and increased with vasoconstriction, as a compensatory mechanism with low cardiac output from cardiogenic shock or hypovolemic shock or from pulmonary or systemic HTN. Clinical signs and symptoms include alterations such as thready peripheral pulses and widened pulse pressure in distributive shock or narrow pulse pressure in cardiogenic shock. SVR reflects afterload and is calculated by the equation (MAP–RAP)/CO × 80, with a normal range being 800–1200 dynes s/cm^5. Pulmonary vascular resistance is calculated using the pulmonary arterial mean (PAM): (PAM − PAWP)/CO × 80 with a normal range of 100–250 dynes s/cm^5 (Adams, 2004; Massaro, 2018).

Contractility

Contractility refers to the pumping strength of the myocardium and is impacted by both preload and afterload. During preload, optimal volume stretches the ventricles, and greater stretch produces greater contractility. If the ventricle is understretched, contraction will be suboptimal; conversely, when the ventricle is overdistended, there will be no improvement or augmentation in contraction. During afterload, as resistance to outflow increases, contractility decreases. Decreased contractility is associated with myocardial ischemia, cardiac tamponade, acidosis, hypocalcemia, hypoxia, and some cytokines. Vasodilators, inotropes, and decreased afterload are associated with an increase in contractility. Contractility is reflected in direct measurement of the ejection fraction (EF) and ventricular stroke index (Adams, 2004; Massaro, 2018):

$$\text{Left ventricular EF} = \left(\text{MAP} - \text{PAWP}\right) \times \text{SVI} \times 0.0136$$

$$\text{Right ventricular EF} = \left(\text{PAM} - \text{RAP}\right) \times \text{SVI} \times 0.0136.$$

Mixed venous oxygenation (SvO$_2$) provides immediate information as to the adequacy of tissue oxygenation. A decrease in SvO$_2$ can be the result of oxygen supply-demand imbalance.

Table 17.1 describes variations in hemodynamic parameters with specific shock states.

TABLE 17.1 HEMODYNAMIC PARAMETERS IN VARIOUS SHOCK STATES					
CLASSIFICATION	CO/CI	RAP	PAWP	SVR	SVO$_2$
Hypovolemic	Decreased	Reduced	Decreased	Increased	Decreased
Cardiogenic	Decreased	Elevated	Increased	Increased	Decreased
Obstructive	Decreased	Elevated	Increased	Increased	Decreased
Distributive	Increased	Reduced	Decreased	Decreased	Increased

CI, cardiac index; CO, cardiac output; PAWP, pulmonary artery wedge pressure; RAP, right arterial pressure; SvO$_2$, mixed venous oxygenation; SVR, systemic vascular resistance.

Treatment

The *ABCDE* tenets of shock resuscitation include establishing airway, controlling the work of breathing, optimizing the circulation, ensuring adequate oxygen delivery, and achieving end points of resuscitation (Balas et al., 2012). Treatments of shock include assessment of the hemodynamic parameters with specific treatment of the underlying cause and selective pharmacologic treatment incorporating inotropes for contractility with low cardiac output, vasopressors for conditions requiring vasoconstriction, and vasodilators for conditions with increased vascular resistance.

Case Study

Mrs. P is exhibiting signs of shock, and her symptoms include a mixed picture of sepsis and cardiogenic shock. She has hypotension, tachycardia, tachypnea, hypoxia, and leukocytosis. Physical findings that support cardiogenic shock are tachycardia and crackles on the lung examination, which may indicate pulmonary edema. Her c/o orthopnea and PND in her ROS also may be of concern for cardiogenic dysfunction. Sepsis is also high on your list as she has metabolic acidosis, fever, leukocytosis, and a probable source of infection with her extremity wound. She responds to a fluid bolus, which indicates she is vasodilated, but this could be secondary to the medications she received for intubation. Her crackles may be secondary to atelectasis or noncardiogenic pulmonary edema. Now that you have her intubated and positive pressure applied, you are less concerned about the possibility of pulmonary edema causing further hypoxia. But you need to work through your differential. Do you need inotropes or vasopressors to support her cardiac output? Should you diurese or give volume? Are there any CDRs you can apply to aid in your decision? You are more concerned with sepsis and pull out the guidelines for reference.

The Surviving Sepsis Campaign

The Surviving Sepsis Campaign designed evidence-based guidelines for the identification and treatment of sepsis (Bone et. al, 1992). Septic shock is defined as a subset of sepsis in which particularly profound circulatory, cellular, and metabolic abnormalities are associated with a greater risk of mortality than with sepsis alone. Recommendations from the most recent updates to the sepsis guidelines in 2016 include the definition of sepsis as life-threatening organ dysfunction caused by a dysregulated host response to infection (Howell & Davis, 2017; Singer et al., 2016). Organ dysfunction can be represented by an increase in the Sequential Organ Failure Assessment (SOFA) score of 2 points or more. The content in this section is based on these guidelines, which have undergone multiple revisions. In 2005, the campaign revised and converted its guidelines into protocols, with sets of quality indicators that could be implemented by hospitals working to improve outcomes (Ferrer et. al., 2008). The sepsis bundles are a series of therapies that have demonstrated improved outcomes when implemented together (Howell & Davis, 2017; Rhodes et al., 2016; Singer et al., 2017). In 2018, the Surviving Sepsis Campaign published the new Hour-1 Bundle, which emphasizes the importance of beginning resuscitation and management immediately, then escalating care seamlessly on the basis of ongoing clinical parameters rather than waiting or extending resuscitation measures over a longer period.

BOX 17.7   **The Five Elements of the Hour-1 Bundle**

1. Lactate: Measure lactate level upon admission. Remeasure if initial lactate is >2 mmol/L.
2. Blood cultures: They must be obtained prior to administration of antibiotics.
3. Select and administer broad-spectrum antibiotics based on suspected source and your population/facilities antibiogram.
4. If hypotension or lactate ≥4 mmol/L volume resuscitate rapidly with 30 ml/kg crystalloid.
5. If patient is hypotensive during or after fluid resuscitation, administer vasopressors to maintain MAP ≥65 mm Hg.

Data from Society of Critical Care Medicine. *SSC Hour-1 Bundle*. Retrieved August 14, 2020. https://www.sccm.org/getattachment/SurvivingSepsisCampaign/Guidelines/Adult-Patients/Surviving-Sepsis-Campaign-Hour-1-Bundle.pdf?lang=en-US

The Hour-1 Bundle consists of five elements that are intended to be initiated within the first hour from the earliest documentation of all elements of sepsis or septic shock (Box 17.7).

Key Points

Sepsis and septic shock are medical emergencies, and treatment and resuscitation should begin immediately upon recognition.

After implementing the Hour-1 Bundle, the SOFA scoring system can assist with screening and diagnosis of sepsis and with predicting the clinical outcomes of critically ill patients. The total SOFA score is a maximum of 6 points: 1 point each for the respiratory, cardiovascular, hepatic, coagulation, renal, and neurological systems. The higher the score is, the worse the prognosis because of the number of systems involved. For rapid screening, the quick version (qSOFA) initially identifies patients at high risk for poor outcome with an infection. The score ranges from 0 to 3 points and a score of 2 or more near the onset of infection is associated with a greater risk of death or prolonged ICU stay (Singer et al., 2016) and should prompt providers to do a comprehensive examination to evaluate for sepsis. The elements of qSOFA are included in Box 17.8.

BOX 17.8   **Sequential Organ Failure Assessment, Quick Version (qSOFA)**

Quick SOFA score: One point for each of the following that are present:

- Respiratory rate greater than 22 per min
- Alteration in mental status
- Systolic blood pressure less than 100 mm Hg

Data from Singer, M., Deutschman, C. S., Seymour, C. W., Shankar-Hari, M., Annane, D., Bauer, M., Bellomo, R., Bernard, G. R., Chiche, J. D., Coopersmith, C. M., Hotchkiss, R. S., Levy, M. M., Marshall, J. C., Martin, G. S., Opal, S. M., Rubenfeld, G. D., van der Poll, T., Vincent, J. L., & Angus, D. C. (2016). The Third International Consensus Definitions for Sepsis and Septic Shock (Sepsis-3). *Journal of the American Medical Association, 315*(8), 801–810.

Management

In the initial resuscitation of sepsis, restoration of intravascular volume is a priority. At least 30 ml/kg of IV crystalloid fluid should be given within the first 3 hr. Following initial fluid resuscitation, administration of additional fluids is guided by frequent reassessment of hemodynamic status. Reassessment should include a thorough clinical examination and evaluation of available physiologic variables such as heart rate, blood pressure, arterial oxygen saturation, respiratory rate, temperature, urine output, and other noninvasive or invasive monitoring, as available.

Albumin may be used in addition to crystalloids for initial resuscitation and subsequent intravascular volume replacement in patients with sepsis and septic shock when patients require substantial amounts of fluid to restore intravascular volume. Other treatments should include maintaining oxygen carrying capacity and hemodynamic stability with pharmacologic therapies. Initial diagnostics should include trending lactate to help determine if your management is appropriate (Rhodes et al., 2017). A brief review of the other major components of the guidelines follows.

Antimicrobial Therapy

Sepsis guidelines recommend that administration of IV antimicrobials be initiated as soon as possible after recognition and within 1 hr for both sepsis and septic shock. Empiric broad-spectrum therapy is recommended with one or more antimicrobials that will cover all likely pathogens and should be narrowed once a specific pathogen is identified and sensitivities are established. Providers should also consider de-escalation of combination therapy within the first few days in response to clinical improvement and/or evidence of infection resolution. Measurement of procalcitonin levels can be used to support shortening the duration of antimicrobial therapy in sepsis patients to support the discontinuation of empiric antibiotics in patients who initially appeared to have sepsis, but subsequently have limited clinical evidence of infection (Rhodes et al., 2017).

Source Control

Many causes of sepsis and septic shock include invasive devices or a specific anatomic diagnosis of infection requiring emergent source control. These need to be identified or excluded as rapidly as possible in patients with sepsis or septic shock, and prompt removal of possible source of sepsis or septic shock included (Rhodes et al., 2017).

Vasoactive Medications

The guidelines recommend norepinephrine as the first-choice vasopressor with the addition of either vasopressin (up to 0.03 U/min) or epinephrine as needed with a goal of raising the MAP to target of 65 and to decrease norepinephrine dosage. Dopamine is an alternative vasopressor agent to norepinephrine in patients with low risk of tachyarrhythmias and absolute or relative bradycardia. Dobutamine can be considered in patients who show evidence of persistent hypoperfusion despite adequate fluid loading and the use of vasopressor agents (Rhodes et al., 2017).

Mechanical Ventilation

Conservative volume settings have been well-documented as effective in patients with sepsis. A target tidal volume of 6 ml/kg predicted body weight with an upper limit goal for plateau pressures of 30 cm H_2O has less volume-related lung injury vs. higher plateau pressures in adult patients with sepsis-induced severe ARDS (Rhodes et al., 2017).

Glucose Control

A protocolized approach to blood glucose management in ICU patients with sepsis with early introduction with two consecutive blood glucose levels >180 mg/dl has correlated with improved outcomes. The target of an upper blood glucose level ≤180 mg/dl is strongly recommended (Rhodes et al., 2017).

Corticosteroids

The guidelines recommend against using IV hydrocortisone to treat septic shock patients if adequate fluid resuscitation and vasopressor therapy are able to restore hemodynamic stability. If this is not achievable or there is concern for adrenal insufficiency, IV hydrocortisone at a dose of 200 mg/day is recommended (Rhodes et al., 2017).

Key Points

In order to improve outcomes for sepsis, hospital systems must have a performance improvement program and employ specific systematic screening for sepsis, which has been shown to improve early identification and treatment of high-risk patients.

CLINICAL PEARLS

- Shock is a clinical state, not just hypotension.
- Know your hemodynamics.
- Is the patient exhibiting a high output or low output state: warm and wet or cold and clammy?
- qSOFA is a quick reference to screen for sepsis.
- Surviving Sepsis Campaign is a dynamic and important resource. Visit their site often.

Case Study

Mrs. P has significant findings consistent with septic shock. Her qSOFA score is 3. She has a lactic acidosis as well as respiratory acidosis. The initial fluid bolus was administered, but her systolic blood pressure remained low and you initiated Levophed. You have her intubated and initially place her on FiO_2 of 100%, volume-controlled ventilation with rate of 14, vT of 400, and PEEP of 10 cm. A post intubation CXR shows increased interstitial edema, alveolar congestion, and a possible RLL infiltrate. A transthoracic echocardiogram reveals a hyperdynamic picture with an EF of 65% with no wall motion abnormalities. There is no evidence of right heart failure or elevated pulmonary pressures. This helps to support your diagnosis of sepsis and rule out cardiogenic or obstructive shock. Further investigating for the underlying factor exacerbating her sepsis is crucial. You have already determined that she has a possible cellulitis of her RLL, but do you treat her for pneumonia as well?

ANTI-INFECTIVE THERAPY

The spread of infectious disease is prevented by eliminating the conditions necessary for the microorganism to be transmitted from a reservoir to a susceptible host. This can be accomplished by destroying the microorganism, blocking the transmission, protecting individuals from becoming vectors of transmission, and decreasing the susceptibility of potential hosts (Southwick, 2020). When you are concerned that your patient has an infection, consider the questions for guiding antimicrobial treatment in Box 17.9 that will help you make decisions for your patient (Southwick, 2020).

Key Points

Prescribe antibiotics to treat a true bacterial infection rather than to fulfill the patient's expectation. A single antibiotic cannot fulfill all infectious disease needs. Anti-infective therapy is dynamic and requires a basic understanding of microbiology. Southwick (2020).

Stages of Acute Infectious Disease

A typical infectious disease has four stages:

- The **incubation period** is the time between the acquisition of the organism and the beginning of symptoms. This can vary from hours to days to weeks, depending on the organism, and is important to consider with highly contagious diseases and outbreaks.
- The **prodrome period** is the time during which nonspecific symptoms such as fever, malaise, and loss of appetite occur.
- The **specific-disease period** is the time when the overt characteristic signs and symptoms of the disease occur.
- The **recovery period**, also known as the **convalescence period**, is the time during which the illness abates and the patient returns to the healthy state, leaving antibodies to protect the recovered patient from reinfection by the same organism (Levinson et al., 2020).

BOX 17.9   Questions to Consider When Choosing a Specific Anti-infective Agent

Is the antibiotic action inhibitory or bactericidal and how broad is the spectrum?
Is the drug toxic, and if so, how do I measure or monitor it?
If cleared by the kidney or liver, is my patient's renal or liver function compromised and do I need to adjust the dosage?
Can my patient afford the antibiotic ordered?

Data from Southwick, F.S. (2020). Anti-infective therapy. In F. S. Southwick (Ed.), *Infectious diseases: A clinical short course*, (4th ed.). McGraw-Hill.

Diagnosis

The clinical examination is the primary source of diagnosis of infectious diseases. Southwick (2020) recommends using an illness script when diagnosing infectious diseases, including the following components:

- Epidemiology, including demographics, risk factors, and exposure
- Duration: acute or chronic, constant or episodic
- Classic signs and symptoms
- Other past medical history

The population, potential exposure, review of systems, and physical findings need to be comprehensive and exhaustive and should include any travel, infectious contact, ingestion including dietary, and environmental elements. Review of symptoms should identify fever, chills, night sweats, rigors, cough, congestion, dysuria, urinary frequency, and diarrhea, all of which are examples of classic symptoms. Each body system should be thoroughly reviewed. Clusters of symptoms may be more specific of certain diagnoses: for example, headache, nuchal rigidity, and fever with meningitis; dysuria, frequency, and urgency with UTIs; and right lower quadrant abdominal pain with fever and anorexia with appendicitis. These findings will drive the diagnostics ordered, such as a lumbar puncture for meningitis, renal ultrasound, and urine culture with a UTI or abdominal CT scan for appendicitis.

The WBC differential is widely used in diagnosis of infection. With a bacterial infection, there is an increase in neutrophils; with viral infections, there may be an increase in lymphocytes or monocytes; and with parasitic infections, the eosinophils may be elevated.

Procalcitonin has been found to correlate with bacterial infections and is used as a guide for antibiotic vs. symptomatic treatment. Levels of procalcitonin can be used to monitor response to therapy.

The ESR and CRP level are indirect and direct measures of the acute-phase response, respectively, that can be used to assess a patient's general level of inflammation. Moreover, these markers can be followed serially over time to monitor disease progress/resolution. It is noteworthy that the ESR changes relatively slowly, and its measurement more often than weekly usually is not useful; in contrast, CRP concentrations change rapidly, and daily measurements can be useful in the appropriate context. Although these markers are sensitive indicators of inflammation, neither is very specific (Surana & Kasper, 2018).

Cultures including infected tissue or fluid including blood, urine, and sputum can be sent for bacterial, fungal, and viral examination and include specific information that will aid in antibiotic selection.

CSF evaluation is necessary for the diagnosis of meningitis or encephalitis.

Radiologic imaging may provide data that support the physical examination and include assessment of chest and abdominal diagnosis or provide image-guided sampling in specific situations of an abscess or infection.

Antibiotic Sensitivity Testing

The serum levels of drugs are affected by absorption, volume of distribution, metabolism, and excretion. Clinicians need to be familiar with pharmacodynamic characteristics of each anti-infective agent, including their mechanisms of action and their biological effects. Excretion is of significant importance in the acutely ill patient with acute renal or hepatic impairment. Many antibiotics are renally excreted and can cause or worsen AKI if not adjusted appropriately.

Clinical laboratories use minimum inhibitory concentration (MIC) combined with studies examining achievable antibiotic levels to determine whether an organism is sensitive, intermediate, or resistant to a specific antibiotic. Serum levels of the antibiotic need to be maintained above the MIC for a significant period. For each specific pathogen, the MIC is determined by diluting the antibiotic into liquid medium containing bacteria. These inoculated tubes are incubated until broth without added antibiotic has become cloudy or turbid as a result of bacterial growth. The lowest concentration of antibiotic that prevents active bacterial growth constitutes the MIC. At peak serum level, the total time above the MIC and *area under the curve* are plotted to determine the appropriate drug and dose for the treatment of the pathogen (Southwick, 2020).

Geographic settings are important in choice of antibiotic. Knowledge of your community antibiogram is necessary for awareness of the sensitivities and resistance in your system or community.

Common Pathogens

The most common pathogens encountered clinically are categorized by their shape and susceptibility to Gram staining.

- Gram-positive cocci: *Staphylococcus, Streptococcus, Streptococcus pneumoniae*
- Gram-negative rods: *Klebsiella-Enterobacter-Serratia, Pseudomonas, Escherichia coli.* Others to be aware of that are related to more selective etiology include *Salmonella, Shigella, Campylobacter, Helicobacter, Proteus-Providencia-Morganella, Bacteroides, Hemophilus, Legionella, Bordetella.*
- Gram-positive rods: *Bacillus, Clostridium, Corynebacterium diphtheria, Listeria monocytogenes*
- Gram-negative cocci: *Neisseria*
- Atypicals: *Mycobacterium tuberculosis,* atypical mycobacteria, *Mycoplasma, Chlamydia*

The appropriate antibiotic therapy depends on the questions you ask your patient, the data you gather from your examination and diagnostics, and your institution's formulary and antibiogram. You can also refer to the IDSA guidelines for specific recommendations for the body system and source organism you identify (http://www.idsociety.org/IDSA_Practice_Guidelines). With future exposures and encounters, you will develop a knowledge base for infections you frequently encounter in your practice area. Factors that determine anti-infective agent dosing are included in Box 17.10.

When treating any unusual or complex patients, consult an infectious disease provider for guidance. Table 17.2 outlines general categories of antimicrobial agents, their common uses, and adverse issues.

BOX 17.10   Factors That Determine Anti-infective Agent Dosing

Absorption, volume of distribution, metabolism, and excretion
Minimum inhibitory concentration (MIC)
Concentration dependent killing and postantibiotic effect
Serum levels

Data from Southwick, F. S. (2020). Anti-infective therapy. In F. S. Southwick (Ed.), *Infectious diseases: A clinical short course* (4th ed.). McGraw-Hill.

TABLE 17.2 ANTIMICROBIAL AGENTS, CHARACTERISTICS, COMMON USES, AND ADVERSE ISSUES

DRUG CLASS	CHARACTERISTICS	COMMON USES	ADVERSE ISSUES/SPECIAL CONSIDERATIONS
Penicillin (PCN)	Contains β-lactam ring Requires active bacterial growth for bactericidal action Antagonized by bacteriostatic antibiotics Narrow spectrum Short half-life	Group A strep, viridans streptococci, mouth flora	Causes hypersensitivity reactions and seizures
Aminopenicillins	Similar to PCN with slightly broader spectrum	Otitis, sinusitis, *Haemophilus influenzae*, MSSA	Diarrhea
Carboxypenicillins (piperacillin-tazobactam)	Able to resist β-lactamase Broad coverage including effective anaerobic coverage		Causes seizures at high doses Caution with renal failure patients
Cephalosporins	Similar to PCN		
First generation	Excellent GPC Inexpensive	Soft-tissue infections, surgical prophylaxis	Higher sensitivity reactions
Second generation	Anaerobic activity Moderately broad coverage	Mixed soft tissue infections and pelvic inflammatory disease	Limited usefulness Vitamin K prophylaxis is recommended in malnourished patients
Third generation	Improved gram-negative coverage Broad coverage Long half-life, allowing once a day dosing	Nosocomial infections	
Fourth generation	Excellent gram-positive and gram-negative coverage, excellent broad-spectrum empiric coverage	Nosocomial infections	
Monobactams	Different structure from cephalosporins No cross-reactivity with PCN Excellent when combined with a good antibiotic with gram-positive activity Narrow coverage	Excellent activity against aerobic gram-negative rods	
Aminoglycosides	Low therapeutic-to-toxic ratio Synergy with PCN		Nephrotoxicity is common Monitor serum levels Causes ototoxicity

(Continued)

TABLE 17.2 ANTIMICROBIAL AGENTS, CHARACTERISTICS, COMMON USES, AND ADVERSE ISSUES   (CONTINUED)

DRUG CLASS	CHARACTERISTICS	COMMON USES	ADVERSE ISSUES/SPECIAL CONSIDERATIONS
Macrolides		Recommended for CAP, *Legionella pneumonia*, *Mycoplasma*, *Chlamydia*	GI irritation is the major toxicity Also causes hypersensitivity reactions, transient hearing loss, prolonged QT interval
Clindamycin	Excellent anaerobic coverage		Can cause diarrhea and *Clostridium difficile* infections
Quinolones		Cipro: excellent coverage of *Pseudomonas*, *Mycoplasma*, *Chlamydia* Recommended for UTI, traveler's diarrhea, salmonella gastroenteritis Levofloxacin: CAP, skin infections	May damage cartilage May cause arthropathy, tendonitis

CAP, community-acquired pneumonia; GI, gastrointestinal; GPC, gram-positive cocci; MSSA, methicillin-sensitive *Staphylococcus aureus*; UTI, urinary tract infection.
Data from Southwick, F. S. (2020). Anti-infective therapy. In F. S. Southwick (Ed.), *Infectious diseases: A clinical short course* (4th ed.). McGraw-Hill and Surana, N. K., & Kasper, D. L. (2018). Approach to the patient with an infectious disease. In J. Jameson, A. S. Fauci, D. L. Kasper, S. L. Hauser, D. L. Longo, & J. Loscalzo (Eds.), *Harrison's principles of internal medicine* (20th ed.). McGraw-Hill.

Colonization vs. Infection

Colonization will be encountered with acutely ill patients and lead to misinterpretation of culture results. Cultures may be obtained once the patient has started on antibiotics and reveal new and different findings that do not necessarily indicate new or worsening infection. Remember that once a patient starts an antibiotic, the normal flora will change, but treating these findings may not be appropriate. Colonization vs. infection can be differentiated by a new fever or change in fever pattern, a rise in WBC count with an increase of (polymorphonuclear leukocytes) PMNs and bands, or a Gram stain with increased PMNs along with organisms (Southwick, 2020).

Antibiotic Resistance

Bacteria can quickly alter their genetic makeup by mutation or transformation. Their ability to share DNA allows them to quickly adapt to antibiotic exposure. They can also develop biochemical alterations such as degradation or modification of the antibiotic through β-lactamases and reduction in the bacterial antibiotic concentration by inhibiting entry through mutation of the cell wall in many gram-negative bacteria or by efflux pumps with gram-negative bacteria against many antibiotics, including macrolides and aminoglycosides. Modification of the antibiotic target through cell wall precursors, changes in target enzymes, and alterations in ribosomal binding sites are additional mechanisms of antibiotic resistance (Southwick, 2020).

The growing prevalence of antibiotic resistance is a serious problem for hospitals and for public health. Studies show that treatment indication, choice of antibiotic, or duration of therapy can be incorrect in up to 30% of cases in which antibiotics are prescribed. In 2009, the U.S. Department of Health and Human Services developed the National Action Plan to Prevent Healthcare-Associated Infections (HAI). The national effort to promote antibiotic stewardship was developed in efforts to slow the development of resistance, help prevent untreatable infection, and extend the useful lifetime of the most urgently needed antibiotics (Office of Disease Prevention and Health Promotion, 2020).

The plan includes 5-year goals for nine specific measures of improvement in HAI prevention. Phase I of the plan called for reducing the rate of HAIs in acute care hospitals by the implementation of a collaborative 10-point strategy aimed at prevention. Components of the plan include individual and organizational recommendations. The Frontline Clinician is charged with reducing inappropriate/unnecessary use of devices, improving adherence to hand hygiene and barrier precautions, and implementing and improving antimicrobial stewardship.

Evidence-based guidelines are at the heart of strategies to prevent and control HAIs and drug-resistant infections and address a wide range of issues from hospital design to hand hygiene—hand hygiene being the most basic and single most important preventive measure. Decreasing the number of HAIs will require research to better understand the reasons behind lack of compliance with guidelines and to develop education and interventions that target those reasons (Centers for Disease Control and Prevention, 2020).

The principles are the limitation of unnecessary antibiotics, obtaining timely culture and sensitivity data, selecting the most appropriate treatment, and prescribing the appropriate dose. American Thoracic Society/Infectious Diseases Society of America (ATS/IDSA) guidelines for general ward patients are antipseudomonal coverage and anti-MRSA agent (vancomycin or linezolid). ICU coverage should include empiric MRSA and double coverage of *Pseudomonas pneumonia*. Vancomycin has been considered the first choice for treatment of MRSA infections, although the ATS/IDSA guidelines note that linezolid may have advantages over vancomycin for VAP caused by MRSA (Kalil et al., 2016; Horan et al., 2008).

CLINICAL PEARLS

- Decide whether or not the patient is infected.
- Make a reasonable statistical guess as to the possible pathogens.
- Be aware of susceptibility patterns in your facility.
- Take into account previous antibiotic treatment.
- Consider important host factors.
- Use the fewest drugs possible.
- Switch to narrower-spectrum antibiotic coverage within 3 days.
- When all things are equal, pick the cheapest drug!

Southwick (2020).

Case Study

You apply your astute and appropriate use of guidelines for shock/sepsis and antibiotic therapy with Mrs. P. Her sepsis responded to the volume resuscitation and required short-term vasopressor support and broad-spectrum antibiotics. She had positive blood cultures that grew MRSA on day 2. Her sputum culture was negative for any growth. Her cellulitis improved, and the cefepime was discontinued after 7 days. You narrowed her antibiotic therapy to vancomycin, which she will continue for 14 days. Her renal function improved, but you will do additional dosing along with your pharmacy colleagues based on peak levels and trends of her renal function. The final major consideration you need to make at this point is decisions to support her from a nutritional perspective.

NUTRITION

Nutrition should be considered early in the treatment of acute care patients. General considerations should include feeding early and using the gut if possible.

Nutritional Assessment

A comprehensive nutritional assessment will require a thorough history and physical as well as laboratory data. The patient's medical and surgical history and associated comorbidities need to be taken into consideration along with dietary and bowel habits, level of stress, and medications.

Stressed patients first receive nutritional support in the later stage of the stress response. Treatment should generally focus on correcting fluid and electrolyte imbalances in the earlier stages of stress (Baron, 2019; Jensen, 2019).

Key Points

All patients should have evaluation and institution of nutrition within the first 24 hr of admission.

Calculating Nutritional Needs

Kilocalories per kilogram of body weight is the primary factor in calculating nutritional needs. One pound of body weight is equivalent to 3,500 kcal; 1 kg is equivalent to 7,700 kcal. The requirement for an average adult is 30 kcal/kg or 13 kcal/lb of body weight/24 hr in a highly stressed individual. For maintenance of weight, 25 kcal/kg is a general rule; for weight gain, 35 or more kcal/kg is appropriate. If there is an elevated body temperature, there is an approximate 10% increase in kilocalories per 24 hr required for each degree above 98.6 °F. Initiation of feeding for the acutely ill patient should include evaluation of weight loss and previous nutrient intake before admission, level of disease severity, comorbid conditions, and function of the gastrointestinal (GI) tract (Baron, 2019; Jensen, 2019).

Protein Needs

Protein provides 4 kcal/g; excessive protein intake increases the amount of nitrogenous waste—urea—that must be excreted through the urine. Protein is needed for tissue growth and maintenance and should account for approximately 20% of daily kilocalories. Protein required per day ranges from 0.8 to 2 g/kg of body weight. Highly stressed patients (trauma, burns, sepsis) require 1.5–2 g or more per kilogram of body weight (Baron, 2019).

Carbohydrate Needs

Carbohydrates provide 4 kcal/g. They account for largest proportion of kilocalories in most diets and comprise approximately 50% of daily need. More oxygen is required and more carbon dioxide is released in the metabolism of carbohydrates than in the metabolism of protein or fat. Patients with compromised respiratory function benefit from less than average carbohydrate consumption (Baron, 2019).

Fat or Lipid Needs

Fats provide 9 kcal/g. Fat has the lowest respiratory quotient; in other words, it uses the least amount of oxygen and produces the least amount of carbon dioxide as a by-product of metabolism. Substituting fat for carbohydrates can reduce stress on the respiratory system, particularly if the patient has minimal lung capacity (Baron, 2019).

Type of Nutritional Support

Decisions regarding types of nutritional support for patient not taking in oral nutrients rely on the following guidelines:

- If the GI tract is nonfunctional, parenteral nutrition (PN) is appropriate.
- If the GI tract is functional, enteral nutrition (EN) is preferred to prevent transmigration of GI bacteria through the intestinal wall to the bloodstream, which can cause sepsis (Druyan et al., 2012).

PN support may supplement enteral feedings or be used as the sole nutritional support. In the patient who was previously healthy with no evidence of protein-calorie malnutrition, use of PN should be reserved and initiated only after the first 7 days of hospitalization when EN is not available. If there is evidence of protein-calorie malnutrition on admission and EN is not feasible, it is appropriate to initiate PN as soon as possible following admission and adequate resuscitation. If a patient is expected to undergo major upper GI surgery and EN is not feasible, PN should be provided under very specific conditions: If the patient is malnourished, PN should be initiated 5–7 days preoperatively and continued into the postoperative period. If the treatment is unable to meet the patient's energy requirements (100% of target goal calories) after 7–10 days by the enteral route alone, consider supplemental PN. Concentrations of dextrose greater than 10% require a central line (Druyan et al., 2012).

Using the common formularies of enteral nutritional supplements in your facility, you can calculate the volume needed to meet these needs and order it either as bolus feeds or as continuous feeds, monitoring residual volumes frequently as well as stool consistency and frequency. It is important to consider any patient complications or medical history, for example, reducing the percent of carbohydrates with diabetes mellitus or pulmonary diagnosis or restricting protein with AKI and increasing percent of calories overall by increasing fat and increasing carbs. Enteral formulas are designed to address specific diseases or syndromes such as diabetes, kidney disease, and pulmonary disease. Semielemental feeds, which are semidigested, are available for postpyloric feedings, as bypassing the stomach reduces a portion of digestion. There are also various supplements that allow you to increase specific caloric needs such as protein powders or lipids. These provide concentrated additives without additional volume.

Case Study

Mrs. P is admitted for sepsis due to cellulitis and possible pneumonia. She also has AKI with an elevated creatinine. A dobhoff tube has been placed since she was intubated and placement post pylorus was confirmed with a CXR. Her sepsis puts her in a highly stressed category. She is on propofol for sedation while intubated. You calculate her caloric needs, based on her weight of 55 kg: 55 kg × 30 kcal = 1,650 kcal. For protein needs in a highly stressed state, you consider 2 g/kg, but her AKI indicates that you may need to restrict her protein to reduce creatinine production. You decide to give her 1 g of protein initially: 55 kg × 1 g protein = 55 g protein, which you multiply by 4 kcal/g and determine that 220 of her 1,650 calories will come from protein. She will require lipid/fat calories, but with her propofol infusion she is already receiving 1.1 kcal/ml. If propofol is continued at 20 ml/hr, that is roughly 528 calories from fat. Your basic preparation for enteral feeding on the formulary has 1.2 kcal/ml, 18% from protein. You calculate the amount of the preparation she will need: 1,650 total kcal/1.2 kcal/ml = 1,375 ml over 24 hr for her daily volume, which will also provide roughly 70 g of protein. You can divide it into bolus feeds or run continuously at roughly 55 ml/hr to meet her caloric needs. You decide to give it to her continuously, for convenience. You start at 10 ml/hr and increase by 20 ml every 4 hr until she reaches goal, observing for distention, high residuals, or nausea/vomiting.

Complications

Complications of enteral support include diarrhea, constipation, cramping, and gastric retention. The fiber content of the formula can be manipulated for stool consistency. If there is evidence of diarrhea, soluble fiber-containing or small peptide formulations may be used.

Complications of parenteral nutritional support are many and varied. Metabolic complications, such as hyperglycemia and hypercapnia, may result, along with those involving the GI tract and the liver. Patients receiving parenteral nutrition are at a high risk for infection due to the high glycemic content and the use of central lines for infusion. There is also a risk of pancreatitis with lipid infusion (Baron, 2019).

Evaluating Nutritional Support

Trending laboratory values for nutrition is important, especially if the patient has a prolonged stay and ventilator support. Common values include serum albumin or prealbumin and transferrin, which are good markers of the patient's nutritional status but are impacted by volume status and inflammation, thus altering their sensitivity and specificity. Basic metabolic parameters also need to be monitored and trended. Careful monitoring of triglycerides is important when patients are receiving propofol due to the lipid calories it provides. You may need to restrict fat intake if it is maintained for any length of time (Baron, 2019; Druyan et al., 2012).

Considerations when administering parenteral support include monitoring blood glucose every 6 hr, daily electrolytes, CBC, liver function tests, and calcium, phosphate, magnesium, and triglyceride levels. Infuse fat emulsions slowly over 12–24 hr. Trend nutritional laboratory results a minimum of weekly and adjust additives accordingly.

Case Study

Your early recognition and diagnosis of Mrs. P's multisystem issues has provided a rapid response to therapy. Her overall condition, including her acid-base status and hypoxia, improved. She was successfully weaned and extubated on day 4, and she has agreed to wear CPAP as needed along with supplemental oxygen. You discontinued her tube feeds with extubation, and she transitioned to an oral diet. Her vital signs have been stable, and her lower extremity cellulitis is improving. She is afebrile and her leukocytosis has improved. Repeat blood cultures were negative on day 4. Her AKI improved with support of perfusion. You elected to transition her to a concentrated carbohydrate diet with no protein restrictions. She was discharged on day 7 to short-term rehabilitation for additional support with deconditioning requiring intensive physical therapy and skilled nursing care and for her second week of intravenous antibiotics via a PICC (peripherally inserted central catheter) line that was placed on day 5.

CLINICAL PEARLS

- Feed early and use the gut if possible.

CONCLUSION

Multisystem disorders include much more than we included in this case study, which addressed acid-base disturbances, shock/sepsis, infectious disease, and nutrition. However, other patients may have other issues such as coagulopathy, electrolyte disorders, or acute lung injury, leading to multisystem organ dysfunction. You will need more in-depth education and experience to become proficient in dealing with multisystem disorders as an APP, but the case here provides a solid foundation.

REVIEW QUESTIONS

You are working in the ED and a 62-year-old woman with PMH of diabetes and chronic atrial fibrillation arrives with tachypnea, general malaise, decreased mental status, a fever, and no pain or other significant complaints. You find her to be tachycardic, with an irregularly irregular heart rate in the 130 s, febrile at 102 °F, pale, and confused. Her lung examination is clear, she has diffuse abdominal pain, and peripherally she is warm and dry. You order chemistries, a CBC, and a blood gas and receive the following:

Na, 142 mEq/L; Cl, 108 mEq/L; HCO_3, 16 mEq/L
ABG: pH, 7.20; PCO_2, 26 mm Hg; PO_2, 96 mm Hg; HCO_3, 14 mEq/L

Her procalcitonin and WBCs are elevated.

1. What is her primary acid-base disorder?
   a. Metabolic acidosis
   b. Metabolic alkalosis
   c. Respiratory acidosis
   d. Respiratory alkalosis

2. What is her anion gap?
   a. 20
   b. 18
   c. 22
   d. 16

3. Primary concerns or causes for an anion gap acidosis include all of the following, except:
   a. Uremia
   b. Ketosis
   c. Diarrhea
   d. Lactic acidosis

4. You are concerned that she is developing shock. Based on her clinical signs and symptoms, what type of shock is your top differential?
   a. Sepsis
   b. Cardiogenic
   c. Obstructive
   d. Hypovolemic

5. Afterload is defined as:
   a. The resistance the ventricle must overcome to eject blood
   b. The amount of stretch on the myocardial fibers before contraction, measured as end-diastolic volume
   c. The intrinsic ability of the heart to contract
   d. The fraction of end-diastolic volume ejected from the ventricle during each systolic contraction

6. Contractility is defined as:
   a. The amount of resistance or tension the ventricle must overcome to eject blood
   b. The amount of stretch on the myocardial fibers before contraction, measured as end-diastolic volume
   c. The intrinsic ability of the heart to contract
   d. The fraction of end-diastolic volume ejected from the ventricle during each systolic contraction

7. Which of the following terms describes the report of cultures obtained in the ICU for a 1-year period and rates of resistance to each antibiotic?
   a. Resistance coverage
   b. Antibiogram
   c. ICU antibiotic theory graph
   d. Multiresistance antibiotic therapy

8. Antibiotic resistance is due to multiple pathologic factors at the cellular level including:
   a. The ability to alter their genetic makeup by mutation or transformation
   b. They develop biochemical alterations such as degradation or modification
   c. By inhibiting entry through mutation of the cell wall in many gram-negative bacteria or by efflux pumps
   d. All of the above

9. Which of the following clinical findings would help you differentiate colonization from a new or worsening infection?
   a. A new fever or change in fever pattern
   b. A decrease in WBC count
   c. A Gram stain with new organisms with no increase in PNMs
   d. Increase wound drainage

10. It is Saturday evening and you want to start tube feeds on your patient with sepsis and the dietary clinicians do not cover the weekend. You need to do some calculations to address her basic nutritional needs. She is 65 kg; her creatinine is 1.2 with chronic kidney disease 3; she is febrile and has hyperglycemia with blood glucose 180-200. What kcal/kg and amount of protein will you use to establish her caloric needs?
    a. 25 kcal/kg with high protein; 2 g/kg
    b. 30 kcal/kg with high protein; 2 g/kg
    c. 30 kcal/kg with mod protein; 1.2 g/kg
    d. 25 kcal/kg; with restricted protein of 0.8 g/kg

Answers: 1, a; 2, b; 3, c; 4, a; 5, a; 6, c; 7, b; 8, d; 9, c; 10, b

REFERENCES

Adams, K. (2004). Assessment, the physiologic basis for turning data into clinical informsation. *AACN Clinical Issues*, 15(4), 534–546.

Appel, S., & Downs, C. (2008). Understanding acid-base balance. *Nursing*, 38, 9–11. https://doi.org/10.1097/01. NURSE.0000336658.39936.0c

Ayers, P., Dixon, C., & Mays, A. (2015). Acid-base disorders: Learning the basics. *Nutrition in Clinical Practice*, 30(1), 14–20.

Balas, M. C., Vasilevskis, E. E., Burke, W. J., Boehm, L., Pun, B. T., Olsen, K. M., Peitz, G. J., & Ely, E. W. (2012). Critical care nurses' role in implementing the "ABCDE bundle" into practice. *Critical Care Nurse*, 32, 35.

Baron, R. B. (2019). Nutritional disorders. In M. A. Papadakis, S. J. McPhee, M. W. Rabow, & T. G. Berger (Eds.), *CURRENT medical diagnosis & treatment*. Lange Medical Books.

Berend, K., de Vries, A. P. J., & Gans, R. O. B. (2014). Physiological approach to assessment of acid–base disturbances. *The New England Journal of Medicine*, 371, 1434–1445.

Bone, R. C., Balk, R. A., Cerra, F. B., Dellinger, R. P., Fein, A. M., Knaus, W. A., Schein, R. M., & Sibbald, W. J. (1992). Definitions for sepsis and organ failure and guidelines for the use of innovative therapies in sepsis. The ACCP/SCCM Consensus Conference Committee. *Chest*, 101, 1644–1655.

Centers for Disease Control and Prevention (2020). *National Healthcare Safety Network (NHSN)*. Retrieved January 15, 2019. https://www.cdc.gov/nhsn/

Cho, K. C. (2014). Electrolyte & acid-base disorders. In M. A. Papadakis, S. J. McPhee, & M. W. Rabow (Eds.), *Current medical diagnosis & treatment 2015*. McGraw Hill.

Druyan, M. E., Compher, C., Boullata, J. I., Braunschweig, C. L., George, D. E., Simpser, E., & American Society for Parenteral and Enteral Nutrition Board of Directors. (2012). Clinical guidelines for the use of parenteral and enteral nutrition in adult and pediatric patients: Applying the GRADE system to development of A.S.P.E.N. Clinical Guidelines. *Journal of Parenteral and Enteral Nutrition*, 36(1), 77–80.

Ferrer, R., Artigas, A., Levy, M. M., Blanco, J., González-Díaz, G., Garnacho-Montero, J., Ibáñez, J., Palencia, E., Quintana, M., de la Torre-Prados, M. V., & Edusepsis Study Group. (2008). Improvement in process of care and outcome after a multicenter severe sepsis education program. *Journal of the American Medical Association*, 299(19), 2294–2303.

Horan, T. C., Andrus, M., & Dudeck, M. A. (2008). CDC/NHSN surveillance definition of health care associated infection and criteria for specific types of infections in the acute care setting. *American Journal of Infection Control*, 36(5), 309–332.

Howell, M. D., & Davis, A. M. (2017). Management of sepsis and septic shock. *Journal of the American Medical Association*, 317(8):847–848. https://doi.org/10.1001/jama.2017.0131

Jameson, J., Fauci, A. S., Kasper, D. L., Hauser, S. L., Longo, D. L., & Loscalzo, J (Eds.). (2020). Acid-base disorders. In *Harrison's manual of medicine* (20th ed.). McGraw-Hill.

Jensen, G. L. (2019). Malnutrition and nutritional assessment. In J. Jameson, A. S. Fauci, D. L. Kasper, S. L. Hauser, D. L. Longo, & J Loscalzo. (Eds.), *Harrison's principles of internal medicine*. McGraw-Hill.

Kalil, A. C., Metersky, M. L., Klompas, M., Muscedere, J., Sweeney, D. A., Palmer, L. B., Napolitano, L. M., O'Grady, N. P., Bartlett, J. G., Carratalà, J., El Solh, A. A., Ewig, S., Fey, P. D., File, T. M., Jr., Restrepo, M. I., Roberts, J. A., Waterer, G. W., Cruse, P., Knight, S. L., & Brozek, J. L. (2016). Management of adults with hospital-acquired and ventilator-associated pneumonia: 2016 clinical practice guidelines by the infectious diseases society of America and the American thoracic society. *Clinical Infectious Diseases*, 63(5),1–61.

Kaufman, D.C., Kitching, A. J., & Kellum, J. A. (2015). Acid-base balance. In J. B. Hall, G. A. Schmidt, & J. P. Kress (Eds.), *Principles of critical care* (4th ed.). McGraw-Hill Education.

Levinson, W., Chin-Hong, P., Joyce, E. A., Nussbaum, J., & Schwartz, B., (Eds.), (2020). *Review of medical microbiology & immunology: A guide to clinical infectious diseases* (16th ed.). McGraw-Hill.

Massaro, A. F. (2018). Approach to the patient with shock. In J. Jameson, A. S. Fauci, D. L. Kasper, S. L. Hauser, D. L. Longo, & J. Loscalzo (Eds.), *Harrison's principles of internal medicine* (20th ed). McGraw-Hill.

National Guideline Centre. (2016). *Sepsis: Recognition, diagnosis and early management*. National Institute for Health and Care Excellence. Retrieved July 13, 2018. https://www.nice.org.uk/guidance/ng51

Office of Disease Prevention and Health Promotion. (2020). *National action plan to prevent health care-associated infections: Road map to elimination*. Retrieved June 13, 2020. https://health.gov/hcq/prevent-hai-action-plan. asp

Palmer, B. F. (2008). Approach to fluid and electrolyte disorders and acid-base problems. *Primary Care*, 35(2), 195–213, v. https://doi.org/10.1016/j.pop.2008.01.004

Rhodes, A., Evans, L. E., Alhazzani, W., Levy, M. M., Antonelli, M., Ferrer, R., Kumar, A., Sevransky, J. E., Sprung, C. L., Nunnally, M. E., Rochwerg, B., Rubenfeld, G. D., Angus, D. C., Annane, D., Beale, R. J., Bellinghan, G. J., Bernard, G. R., Chiche, J. D., Coopersmith, C., … Dellinger, R. P. (2017). Surviving sepsis campaign. International guidelines for the management of sepsis and septic shock: 2016. *Intensive Care Medicine*, 43(3), 304–377. https://doi.org/10.1007/s00134-017-4683-6

Singer, M., Deutschman, C. S., Seymour, C. W., Shankar-Hari, M., Annane, D., Bauer, M., Bellomo, R., Bernard, G. R., Chiche, J. D., Coopersmith, C. M., Hotchkiss, R. S., Levy, M. M., Marshall, J. C., Martin, G. S., Opal, S. M., Rubenfeld, G. D., van der Poll, T., Vincent, J. L., & Angus, D. C. (2016). The Third International Consensus Definitions for Sepsis and Septic Shock (Sepsis-3). *Journal of the American Medical Association*, 315(8), 801–810.

Society of Critical Care Medicine (2019). *SSC Hour-1 Bundle*. Retrieved August 14, 2020. https://www.sccm. org/getattachment/SurvivingSepsisCampaign/Guidelines/Adult-Patients/Surviving-Sepsis-Campaign-Hour-1-Bundle.pdf?lang=en-US

Southwick, F. S. (2020). Anti-infective therapy. In Southwick F. S. (Ed.), *Infectious diseases: A clinical short course* (4th ed.). McGraw-Hill.

Surana, N. K., & Kasper, D. L. (2018). Approach to the patient with an infectious disease. Jameson J, Fauci A. S., Kasper D. L., Hauser S. L., Longo D. L., & Loscalzo J (Eds.), *Harrison's principles of internal medicine* (20th ed). McGraw-Hill.

Vichot, A., & Rastegar, A. (2014). Use of anion gap in the evaluation of a patient with metabolic acidosis. *American Journal of Kidney Diseases*, 64(4), 653–657.

Walley, K. R. (2014). Shock. In Hall J. B., Schmidt G. A., & Kress J. P. (Eds.), *Principles of critical care* (4th ed.). McGraw-Hill.

Woodrow, P. (2010). Essential principles: Blood gas analysis. *Nursing in Critical Care*, 15(3), 152–156.

18

Disasters and the Advanced Practice Provider

Michael Beach

INTRODUCTION

Hurricanes, tornados, flooding, extreme snows, earthquakes, terrorist attacks, epidemics, and pandemics can and do happen. There are people who rush toward disasters to help, and there are many others who likely believe that a disaster will never happen to them. If you are in a career in which you are one of the helpers, you will likely be faced with some sort of a disaster. When it does happen, will you be prepared? Will you know how to function within the disaster response, and will you know the role you will play as a nurse practitioner?

Case Study

You survived the storm. Your hospital was on lockdown during the storm, but it is over and there seems to be minimal damage. The hospital's plan was for all personnel working during the storm to stay until the storm ended. The next shift will report after the storm is over, so they should be on their way. You and your significant other are AGACNPs working as part of the hospitalist team. Both of you survived without any concerns, but you cannot get through to family who are caring for your 3-year-old child. Most cell towers are down, as are landlines.

You meet your significant other on a break in the cafeteria. The mood is one of relief. People are happy that the worst is over and they are looking forward to leaving to assess the damage to their homes when the next shift arrives. Then, the power goes out. Emergency lighting comes on and you wait for the generators to start, but they do not. You hear over the public address system that all personnel are to report to their units. You exchange worried looks with your significant other and hurry to your office where you gather with your coworkers. The news is not what you expect.

High numbers of injured have started to present to the ED and you begin to wonder how the hospital can possibly care for all of them. Most of the beds throughout the hospital are full. Power remains off to the whole area and the hospital's emergency generator has failed. A few employees living close to the hospital are reporting to work, but there will be no change of shift. Multiple casualties are expected from the storm. Elevators are down and only battery-operated equipment is functioning, which means you can use the equipment only for a short time. You feel the air getting stuffy as you realize the ventilation system is down. It is 100 °F outside with humidity approaching 100%. As you take everything in, the emergency lighting begins to dim and fail. You wonder what is next and you cannot help think about your 3-year-old daughter. How will you be able to contact her to find out if she is okay?

Some of your coworkers begin to ask questions, including: Who is in charge? Where should I report? Will we have enough food and water? How will we be able to care for our patients? Am I going to be okay? Who is going to take care of me? You know that you and the hospital have prepared for this, but you wonder if the preparations were done correctly and whether you really are prepared.

You begin to move to the ED to head up the triage team and your significant other leaves for the unit to care for incoming admissions. The response has begun.

DEFINING A DISASTER

Disasters can be defined as an event that overwhelms available resources. Healthcare resources are necessary during disasters and include time to treat the ill and injured; supplies, including pharmaceuticals, linens, and wound care supplies; space, including ED beds, operating rooms, and holding areas; personnel; and more. In the immediate aftermath of a disaster, there may be large numbers of ill or injured presenting to a hospital and other healthcare facilities for care. In a disaster response, ambulances will bring severely injured victims from victim collection points in the field, while other victims will present on foot or in private vehicles. There are also patients with illnesses or injuries unrelated to the disaster who will present to the ED. Normal operation is not possible. Disaster plans and protocols must be initiated.

ORGANIZING THE CHAOS

Disasters are chaotic by nature. Miscommunication or a complete lack of communication, confusion over command and control, confusion over roles and responsibilities, concerns about liability, and doubts about being able to care for those in need can lead to disorganization and a less than optimal response. Even with planning and having adequate supplies, protocols, and structures in place to deal with these concerns, there will still be chaos and confusion. In this case, less is definitely more. Less chaos and confusion lead to more care for the injured.

Ethical Planning

Key Points

In 2012, the Institute of Medicine (IOM) published guidelines clarifying the ethical basis for the standard of care for disaster planning and care of victims (Academies, 2012b). It states that care must be based on fairness, a duty to care, a duty to steward resources, transparency, consistency, proportionality, and accountability (Academies, 2012b).

While these guidelines influence our actions, they may also set up conflicts.

Disaster care is often based on utilitarian principles. Do the most good for the most people. From a healthcare perspective, this means to treat and care for those who can be saved with the available resources (Abbasi et al., 2018; Admi et al., 2011; Al Thobaity et al., 2017; Lowe & Hummel, 2014). As stated, these resources include time, personnel, supplies, space, and circumstances. On a normal day, all patients are cared for no matter how severe their injuries or illnesses or how extensive the treatment. In a disaster, this may or may not be true, due to many factors. Some victims may not be able to be saved and treatment may only consist of ensuring the victim's comfort (Abbasi et al., 2018; Admi et al., 2011).

Disaster care is extremely complex, involving ethical and legal concerns (Abbasi et al., 2018; Al Thobaity et al., 2017; Lowe & Hummel, 2014). A full discussion of this is far beyond the scope of this chapter, but here are some basic guidelines. There are few legal protections for acting beyond one's SOP. While Good Samaritan Laws do exist in all 50 states, they have significant limitations. They only protect people who are volunteering; there is no protection for people working in their regular job. They only protect people who are acting within their knowledge, ability, and SOP. People who act beyond these restrictions may be liable for their actions. While these laws may protect you as you help your neighbor injured by a disaster, they are of little or no effect within a hospital or clinic.

In an effort to maximize response within legal and ethical limitations, nursing, medicine, pharmacy, and administrators need to establish a clear disaster plan with standing orders, protocols, and triggers for implementation before an event occurs (Abbasi et al., 2018; Academies, 2012b; Lowe & Hummel, 2014). While it is generally assumed that all personnel will work beyond their normal scope in a disaster, establishing what that means is important. These plans may establish holding areas for victims not requiring immediate care staffed only by nurses who provide care that may include medications, fluids, and treatments, all based on standing orders without advanced provider or physician interaction. Some patients may be seen and treated only by nursing staff and then are discharged to return for follow-up at a later date (Academies, 2012b). Victims may be triaged by nurses or nurse practitioners directly to the operating room or to some limited testing. Procedures, interventions, and life-or-death decisions normally reserved for physicians may have to be made by nurses and nurse practitioners due to limited resources and circumstances.

While there are mass casualty incidents (MCIs) that stretch resources, disasters can overwhelm them. While disaster protocols may not be appropriate for MCIs involving a slight alteration of normal operation, disasters require the implementation of a crisis standard of care, which involves seven attributes cited in the IOM report: fairness, duty to care, duty to steward resources, transparency, consistency, proportionality, and accountability. These guidelines provide a clear, though at times conflicting, framework for disaster preparation and response. Table 18.1 summarizes the descriptions of these qualities of a disaster plan based on the 2009 IOM report on disaster preparedness.

Fairness

Fairness means that all parties involved, including the community as a whole, must view all actions, protocols, and policies as fair. Factors such as race, ethnicity, religion, sexual orientation, gender or gender identity, or personal connections cannot be considered. A fair and just allocation of resources is key and must be done prior to the event.

Protocols must also separate triage from treatment. Those who are providing care should only concern themselves with treatment. They should not be the ones making the decision of who will be treated and who will receive only palliative care (Abbasi et al., 2018; Academies, 2012b; Braunack-Mayer et al., 2010; Shafer & Stocks, 2012).

TABLE 18.1 ETHICAL BASIS FOR DISASTER RESPONSE PLANNING

QUALITY OF DISASTER PLAN	COMMENTS
Fairness	All parties involved, including the community as a whole, must view all actions, protocols, and policies as fair. Factors such as race, ethnicity, religion, sexual orientation, or personal connections cannot be considered.
Duty to care	The primary duty of healthcare workers is to the victim. Victims should not be abandoned even if there is some risk to the provider. Employers have responsibility in this as well. Procedures for proper use of personal protective equipment (PPE) and security for staff and victims must be established.
Duty to steward resources	Providers have a duty to use resources responsibly in order to treat as many victims as possible. There are concerns regarding resupply and available equipment. As victims are treated, supplies are used and may become in short supply. The best preparation may leave gaps, and large numbers of victims with specific needs may use up specific supplies. Providers have a duty both to care for the victims and to steward the available resources for the possibility of additional victims. Stewarding medications and equipment with life-and-death consequences is difficult.
Transparency	Transparency involves a public engagement process and ensures that decisions made reflect the community's values and concerns. Involving the community helps to establish trust between the healthcare facility and the people it serves. If difficult decisions need to be made in the middle of an event, this trust may be essential.
Consistency	Whatever decisions are made, they must be applied consistently to all groups across the event. There must be consistency in providing care throughout the incident, even at differing sites, such as hospitals and clinics.
Proportionality	Proportionality speaks to the development of policies, protocols, and decisions that are proportional to the size of the event and the surrounding circumstances. Decisions expected in a disaster may be extremely burdensome and should reflect the size of the event itself and be limited in scale and scope to what is necessary and no more.
Accountability	Those who make relevant decisions and establish policies are accountable for them. All of those involved in any aspect of planning must take responsibility for those decisions.

Duty to Care

Healthcare providers have a duty to care. Their primary duty is to the victim. Victims should not be abandoned even if there is some risk to the provider. "Some risk," however, is not well defined in this and most codes of ethics by major healthcare groups. If violence is threatened against the hospital by riots during a disaster or violence erupts within the hospital, is that some risk or more than some risk? When dealing with a highly contagious disease with or without established and tested protocols, would a provider be right in refusing to care? Does risk beyond the immediate person providing care impact the decision? Friends, family, children, and children of the provider may need to be considered. The loss of the provider would certainly impact their family as would spreading potentially deadly diseases to their loved ones (Academies, 2012b; Grimes & Mendias, 2010; Shafer & Stocks, 2012; Smith et al., 2018).

Employers have responsibility in this as well. Proper personal protective equipment (PPE) must be provided and procedures for donning and doffing it must be established. Donning PPE must be done effectively and under the supervision of another staff to assure no mistakes are made. Equally important, doffing must be done carefully and under supervision to assure that there is no cross-contamination.

Employers are also responsible for security for staff, patients, and families. Violence does occur and, in a disaster, tensions can run high, which may lead to an increased likelihood of violence. Security staff and protocols must be in place to provide protection for staff, victims, and families (Abbasi et al., 2018; Academies, 2012b; Grimes & Mendias, 2010).

Duty to Steward Resources

Providers have a duty to use resources in a responsible manner in order to treat as many victims as possible. This can be complicated. There are always fluctuating conditions in a disaster, with changing numbers of victims and availability of supplies. Many victims present early in the time immediately following the event and the number may be overwhelming. In time, the number of victims will decrease and acute injuries begin to change to more primary care concerns. Although still disaster related, they may become more about chronic conditions or longer-termed wound care (Abbasi et al., 2018; Academies, 2012a, 2012b; Braunack-Mayer et al., 2010; Hale, 2008; Schoch-Spana et al., 2013; Shafer & Stocks, 2012).

There are also concerns regarding resupply and available equipment. As victims are treated, supplies are used and may become in short supply. The best preparation may leave gaps, or large numbers of victims with specific needs may use up specific supplies. For example, during a respiratory-related epidemic or pandemic, the number of patients requiring respiratory support may exceed the number of ventilators available. Or with a large number of victims presenting with wounds, prophylactic tetanus treatment may begin to run out. While these decisions may be easier when dealing with tetanus, making those decisions involving ventilators would be much more difficult because of concerns of age, comorbidities, order of presentation, and severity of illness and how long they are given to improve while on the ventilators.

This is one of the possible conflicts within these guidelines. We have a duty both to care for the victims and to steward the available resources for the possibility of additional victims. Stewarding medications and equipment when dealing with life-and-death consequences is, at the very least, difficult (Abbasi et al., 2018; Academies, 2012b).

Policies and protocols need to be in place prior to the incident to decide who is treated and who may only get lesser care (Abbasi et al., 2018; Academies, 2012b; Braunack-Mayer et al., 2010; Hale, 2008). They should not be made in the middle of an event when practitioners are under stress and likely have limited information of questionable accuracy.

Transparency

Transparency involves a public engagement process, so it must be done long before an event occurs. Transparency ensures that decisions made reflect the community's values and concerns. Also, involving the community helps to establish trust between the healthcare facility and the people that it serves. If difficult decisions need to be made in the heat of an event, this trust may be essential (Abbasi et al., 2018; Academies, 2012b; Braunack-Mayer et al., 2010; Carrier et al., 2012; Daugherty Biddison et al., 2014; Grimm, 2014; Schoch-Spana et al., 2013; Wells et al., 2013a, 2013b).

All aspects of the community must be represented in this process. While experts and other leaders of the community would naturally be involved, the process should also include educated and uneducated people, minorities, those with disabilities, the elderly, and families with children. This engagement must be racially and ethnically diverse (Abbasi et al., 2018; Academies, 2012b; Carrier et al., 2012; Grimm, 2014; Schoch-Spana et al., 2013) and representative of the community. Each of these groups bring with them very different needs and concerns. Furthermore, the decisions and protocols that need to be established are complex and difficult (Adini et al., 2019; Braunack-Mayer et al., 2010; Daugherty Biddison et al., 2014; Daugherty Biddson et al., 2018; Schoch-Spana et al., 2013; Wells et al., 2013a, 2013b).

Consistency

Whatever decisions are made, they must be applied consistently to all groups across the event. There must be consistency in providing care throughout the incident, even at differing sites, such as hospitals and clinics. The decision to move from a normal standard of care to a crisis standard of care must be made consistently across local healthcare institutions (Abbasi et al., 2018; Academies, 2012b; Shafer & Stocks, 2012). If all local hospitals and treatment centers decide to move from a normal standard of care to a crisis standard of care together, it then contributes to the perception and practice of fairness. As stated, circumstances change quickly and accurate information is often at a premium, so a degree of flexibility must be maintained. Changes made to decisions and protocols established earlier should be made only with careful deliberation.

Proportionality

Proportionality speaks to the development of policies, protocols, and decisions that are proportional to the size of the event and the surrounding circumstances (Abbasi et al., 2018; Academies, 2012b; Shafer & Stocks, 2012). Proportionality may involve the extent of damage to infrastructure, the number of expected victims and the severity of the injuries or illness, the availability of resources, or, in the case of a pandemic, the virulence and how easily the illness is spread. Decisions expected in a disaster may be extremely burdensome and should reflect the size of the event itself and be limited in scale and scope to what is necessary and no more (Abbasi et al., 2018; Academies, 2012b). Again, in the case of a pandemic, this may include policies concerning social distancing, school closures, the cancellation of large events, and possibly establishing quarantines. Decisions such as these must serve the public's interest and needs, for example, to limit the spread of disease.

This raises questions of its own. Who has the responsibility to make and enforce these decisions and what are the rules of engagement? How will they be enforced; what are the limits on law enforcement (LE) in enforcing the policies? Who will care for those quarantined? If a whole area is affected, who becomes responsible for utilities, food deliveries, medical care, and more? These become public health decisions that may go far beyond local public health facilities.

Accountability

Finally, those who make relevant decisions and establish policies are accountable for them. All of those involved in any aspect of planning must take responsibility for those decisions

(Abbasi et al., 2018; Academies, 2012b; Braunack-Mayer et al., 2010; Shafer & Stocks, 2012). Questions and concerns about the decisions should be raised prior to an event and not during an emergency. Adjustments can be made as the event progresses but should only be made with a large degree of situational awareness and based on new information as it becomes available.

Taking all of these principles into consideration while planning protocols for use in a disaster is challenging. Often, a planning committee may consider a principle that is in direct or indirect conflict with another group. Involving the community is perhaps the most challenging aspect of disaster planning. Finding agreement among diverse lay people and healthcare providers/disaster responders concerning the allocation of scarce resources is likely not possible. It has been found, however, that open dialogue between the groups can build trust (Daugherty Biddson et al., 2018).

Case Study

High numbers of injured have started to present to the ED and you begin to wonder how the hospital can possibly care for all of them. Most of the beds throughout the hospital are full.

The Organization and Phases of a Disaster

Disaster preparation and response can be divided into phases that make up the disaster cycle. The disaster cycle consists of (1) planning and mitigation, (2) response, and (3) recovery and returns to planning and mitigation. All aspects of each of these phases are dependent on available resources. In a perfect world, we have all of the necessary resources, including money, people, time, supplies, knowledge, information, and a safe place to prepare, respond, and recover from an event. We rarely have a perfect world.

Command and Control

Disasters are confusing and all responses to disasters involve a degree of disorganization. A clear command and control structure can minimize these concerns (Academies, 2012a; Acosta & Chandra, 2013; Admi et al., 2011; Al Thobaity et al., 2017; Glow et al., 2013). In a disaster, the hospital or clinic should establish one person with the authority, designated the incident commander (IC) to ultimately make decisions concerning the response. The IC works with the command staff within the incident command center (ICC). The command staff consists of a deputy commander, safety/resilience officer, and an information officer. See Table 18.2 for a summary of the parts of the incident command system.

A lead would be established in each of the departments within the hospital. Under these leads, departments would be further broken down into small manageable sections, each with their own leads and one given specific task. The chain of command is maintained by leads reporting to the leads above them, with department leads reporting to the IC. Major decisions regarding the response are discussed and cleared with the command staff while functional decisions of limited scope are made within the department by the lead (Academies, 2012a; Al Thobaity et al., 2017).

When this system breaks down, or is not established, confusion and poor decision-making may occur. An unfortunate example of this is the Memorial Baptist Hospital

TABLE 18.2 THE INCIDENT COMMAND SYSTEM

CATEGORY	POSITION	DESCRIPTION
Command Staff	Incident commander (IC)	The IC is the person with the authority and knowledge to make decisions concerning operations during a disaster. The IC is often the highest-ranking officer in the hospital but the position may be delegated to another.
	Deputy commander (DC)	The DC assists the IC throughout the event. They are in charge when the IC is not present. There may be multiple DCs designated during an event with specific areas of responsibility.
	Safety officer (SO)	The SO is the person focused on the well-being of the responders in areas such as environmental concerns, hydration, nourishment, and staff injuries. In the hospital setting, this person is often called the resilience officer.
	Information officer (IO)	The IO is the contact point between the response and the media. Their task is to assure that the necessary and correct information is provided to the media at the appropriate time.
Section Lead	Logistics	Logistics deals with supplies, resupply, transportation, and similar areas. It may be divided into smaller groups, each with its own task and lead.
	Planning	Planning deals with the specific plans to achieve the mission—in this case, caring for the victims. Planning would include the clinical care and disaster committees. Decisions concerning the transition from a normal standard of care to a crisis standard of care would be made at this level in conjunction with command staff.
	Operations	Operations may be the largest group in the response, particularly in the hospital setting. It consists of triage, treatment teams, ICU, step-down, other units, surgery, the emergency department, general nursing, medicine, aspects of pharmacy, housekeeping, security, social work, and more. Each group would be broken into smaller groups with their own leads and, if possible, one specific task. For instance, surgery may have an overall lead, while each operating room would have its own lead.
	Administration	The administration group is responsible for tracking what is used in a disaster response. This would include man-hours, staffing, supplies, and other expenses. They make sense of and keep order in the chaotic response.

The ICS is flexible. It can expand and contract as necessary. The leads from each group report to the section leads. The section leads report to the command staff, specifically the IC and DC. This system should be adapted to the needs and specific structure of the hospital.

incident in the immediate aftermath of Hurricane Karina. Although there was a designated IC and a preparedness plan in place, multiple decisions were made by other groups without regard to decisions made by the IC. This affected the communication and response both within the hospital and with the regional ICC, impacting evacuation efforts and patient care (Fink, 2013). Strong command and control structure are essential to effective disaster response (Academies, 2012a; Al Thobaity et al., 2017; Glow et al., 2013).

Case Study

You have moved to the command center to facilitate the hospital disaster plan. Your significant other is a lead member of the team caring for incoming admissions in the ED. You quickly review the disaster plan and protocols and establish the level of available supplies as well as the communication plan. A major concern is the loss of power. What capacity does your facility have? Will you need to consider moving patients within or out of the facility? Is it safe to do so at this time?

Planning and Mitigation

Planning and mitigation take place long before an event occurs. The basic rule is that you and your family should be prepared to survive an event for 72 hr to 5 days, on your own, without any outside help. This applies to individuals and institutions such as hospitals. While there is much that local, state, and federal agencies can to do help after a disaster, this usually takes time; the response at this level is often not quick.

There are significant factors to consider during planning, including supplies, communication, mutual aid agreements, committees to establish protocols for treatment and triage, emergency staffing, crisis standards and triggers for implementation, security, and communication. Detailed planning for institutions is beyond the scope of this chapter, but basic preparation for individuals is the first step.

It is difficult for healthcare providers to respond if they are not prepared (Evans & Baumberger-Henry, 2014; Lowe & Hummel, 2014; Whetzel et al., 2013), and it causes worry and concern about loved ones. Individuals or families should gather and store basic necessities for use during and in the immediate aftermath of a disaster. There are lists on several websites, including the Red Cross and CDC (Lowe & Hummel, 2014). Here is one list of basic necessities:

- Water: 1 gallon per day per person
- Food: nonperishable, easily prepared, nutritious food (and some comfort food as well), and necessary items to prepare the food
- Hygiene: towelettes and bucket for waste
- Shelter: tarps/tents, sleeping bags/blankets
- Clothing: appropriate spare clothing suitable for the weather, including rain gear, substantial footwear, hat, and warm jacket (appropriate for the weather)
- First aid supplies: including medications, both OTC and prescription
- Tools: various tools, flashlight, and knife

See Table 18.3 for additional recommendations for individuals and hospitals.

TABLE 18.3 PERSONAL AND HOSPITAL PREPAREDNESS

CATEGORY	PERSONAL PREPAREDNESS	HOSPITAL PREPAREDNESS
Food and water	Individuals and families should prepare and store at least 1 gallon of water per day per person. Nonperishable food should be stored in a cool dry safe location. Both should be enough to last for 3–5 days.	The hospital is responsible for providing food and water for all staff, patients, families, and, possibly, pets for 3–5 days in case the hospital is locked down and inaccessible by outside help.
Shelter	Individuals and families should consider the possibility that they cannot stay in their home during a disaster. Vehicles should be kept in good working order, and plans for staying with family, friends, or other considerations should be made.	Evacuation plans should be in place and practiced in the event that the structure of the hospital or the surrounding area is unsafe.
Communication	Getting information out and in is vital in a disaster. Redundant plans should be made to contact loved ones or contact emergency services as necessary as well as staying informed concerning the event.	Plans and redundant systems should be in place for both internal and external communication. The command structure, units, essential supply lines, and important committees should all be accessible to each other. Externally, the hospital will need to be able to contact the ICC for the area, EMS, fire, LE, and others.
Hygiene	If water and sewer utilities are not functioning, towelettes and buckets with plastic liners may suffice.	If water and sewer utilities are not functioning within the hospital, alternate facilities must be established. This may include chemical toilets or other plans.
Security	Individual and family safety is important. If evacuation orders are given, then plans should be in place to evacuate to a safe location. Consideration should also be made for safety when sheltering in place.	Hospital security should have plans for staff, family, and patient safety. Traffic and holding area control should also be considered.
Healthcare	Individuals and families should have first aid supplies, including both over-the-counter and prescription medications.	Hospitals need to have sufficient supplies and resources to care for patients and victims.

Personal Communication

Plans for communication should be established to gather information from external sources and get information out to loved ones and others. Cell phones and as laptop computers should be charged often as they can be an excellent resource for both gathering information and communicating. A battery-powered radio may become a valuable source of information if cell towers and the internet are not functioning. Simple two-wire phones (not requiring a power source other than the two-wire connection) connected to landlines are becoming rare, but as long as there are wires standing, they will connect.

Getting information out is important. Communication companies work hard to repair and replace cell towers in the immediate aftermath of a disaster. Nonetheless, service can be spotty and circuits overloaded. Establish a plan to call loved ones at regular intervals, such as the same time each hour. Conserve power by turning the phone off between times. Texting requires less power and may go through when voice calls do not.

Evacuation and Transportation

Plans for personal transportation are important in the case of a needed evacuation. If a vehicle is available, it should be kept in good working order with a half tank or more of fuel. A smaller version of the supplies listed for the home should be kept in or ready to be placed in the vehicle. A small cache of personal items (important items you cannot live without) should be readily available. Important papers such as driver's license, passport, marriage license, birth certificates, and an amount of emergency cash should be easily and quickly available. For those without a vehicle, an even smaller version that is easily carried should be created. Everyone should pay careful attention to evacuation plans established by the city or county, and if an evacuation order comes through, everyone should follow it.

Hospital Preparedness

On an institutional level, hospital preparedness is both more complex and on a larger scale. Institutions, such as hospitals, must be prepared to function without outside help for the same 72-hr to 5-day period as individuals. They must prepare for everyone in the hospital: staff, families and pets of staff, patients, and those who may present because of the disaster (see Table 18.3).

Supplies

Supplies are an obvious concern. Maintaining enough pharmaceuticals, linens, extra trauma supplies, food, water, and more to keep a hospital of any size functioning without outside help is a huge task. With enough notice (such as a hurricane), just in time shipments prearranged from suppliers could fill gaps, but sudden events without notice (such as earthquakes) can destroy infrastructure and stop emergency as well as regular shipments. Storage of supplies can also be a significant concern. Nonetheless, in a disaster, staff and patients may be "locked in" and the local hospital may be seen as a safe haven for family and pets of staff, patients, and victims displaced by the disaster. Waves of victims will also present with trauma or illness related to the event as well as the normal illnesses of the day. Preparations must be made well in advance of an event to care for this increased number of victims.

One aspect of planning, which may help with supplies and is essential for the consistency of care throughout an area, involves mutual aid agreements and agreements concerning the standard of care (Ablah et al., 2010). Mutual aid agreements are common among fire and EMS and provide coverage when one department is overwhelmed or needs additional help. Mutual aid agreements between local hospitals can help ensure supplies are shared and victims are treated consistently. Treatment teams from each local hospital should communicate regarding numbers of patients, open beds, services available, and, most importantly, triggers for the need to change from a normal standard of care to a crisis standard of care. While neighboring hospitals may be competitors on a normal day, during a disaster, victim care is most important (Academies, 2012a; Rambhia et al., 2012; Walsh et al., 2015).

Federal assistance in the form of the Strategic National Stockpile (SNS) is available for distribution in the event of a disaster. The SNS consists of airway supplies, ventilators, pharmaceuticals, and so forth. These are palleted and ready for transport by air to regional and military airports across the country. From there, they are distributed to areas of need. An assessment team accompanies the supplies to ascertain further specific needs (Esbitt, 2003).

Security and Communication

Security and communication are significant concerns for an institution during a disaster. Security plays a major role in keeping order during the chaos of disaster response. Planning for security should establish plans for traffic control and maintaining order for staff, patients, and their families. Families who present with victims or who may be trying to locate lost loved ones are under a significant amount of stress. Not everyone responds to a disaster in a calm and reasonable way. By teaming security and social workers together, this process may be easier and less disruptive. While it is often thought that everyone always works together in a disaster, there still may be people who take advantage of the situation. Security is responsible for keeping staff and victims safe.

Institutional Communication

In a disaster, communication is essential (Al Thobaity et al., 2017), even though the information is often incomplete and, at times, may be completely wrong. Communication can be divided into external communication and internal communication. External communication includes LE, fire, EMS, other hospitals, victim triage collection points, the ICC, and the press. Internal communication includes the hospital command structure, communication between units, hospital security, housekeeping, engineering, and more. Normal utilities may fail and emergency generators may also eventually fail, causing normal communication systems to fail as well. What communication does occur may be rushed, unclear, or misinterpreted. Without adequate communication, the response breaks down.

External Communication

Often, emergency rooms (ERs) have radio communication with EMS. Some are county-wide systems, which are able to contact all emergency services in the area, while others are limited to the ambulance services. In a disaster, communication must extend to all aspects of the response. The ICC should be in control of the response in the community. Ambulances should not simply pick up victims and take them to the nearest hospital. It is essential that the right injuries present to the right facilities. Burn victims are best treated at a burn center. Severe traumas should present to level 1 trauma centers. No one hospital should be overwhelmed when others are available. The ICC or the triage collection center (if it should exist) needs to be in contact with all of the hospitals in the area to confirm how many victims can be taken and what types of injuries are best treated at the facility. This central point of communication should also inform the hospital of the number of victims, their injuries and severity, and when they would be arriving.

Healthcare facilities need to be able to contact fire services and LE at all times, even more so in a disaster (Academies, 2012b; Al Thobaity et al., 2017). Disasters are often evolving incidents. Damage to the facility or continued deteriorating conditions, large crowds, unruly behavior, and other concerns may require the intervention of LE or fire services. Often these services are not on normal hospital/EMS radio systems and instead require using regular phone lines. Depending on the type and size of the disaster, these may not be functioning and other redundant measures should be planned.

Healthcare will often need to contact the press to get important information out to the public. This may include which hospitals and clinics are open and what kind of services are available. In the case of pandemics and epidemics, certain illnesses may be best treated at home. These patients may be asked not to come to the hospital. Lastly, hospitals and clinics should be able to talk to other hospitals and clinics. Information concerning hospital transfers, vital information concerning the disaster, supply shortages, and ways each may help the other will improve the response (Academies, 2012b).

Protocols and systems should be established with all parties for communication during a disaster and should include backup systems for when they fail (Al Thobaity et al., 2017). Standard landlines work well as long as the system is up. While this basic system functions with or without power, many landline phones require a power source. There are very few of the old two-wire phone systems left operational. Other options may include expanded radio systems, but they require extensive training and expense. Some systems are capable of multiple channels or groups within the system. This may avoid some of the confusion caused by several parties trying to communicate important information all at the same time.

Cell phone towers are often the first to come back online after a disaster and most people have a cell phone. A plan to distribute the cell phone numbers of key personnel involved with the ICC, field triage, other emergency services, and the hospital ICC may provide adequate communication or backup when other plans fail. Lastly, volunteers from local amateur radio groups may help. These groups are often functional even when all outside power is lost. Volunteers placed at key points can relay information as needed.

Internal Communication

Hospitals need internal communication to function (Al Thobaity et al., 2017). In a disaster, there should be a central ICC with one IC. Each department or section of the hospital would have a designated leader who falls under the command of the IC. Each department may designate smaller groups for specific tasks such as triage. Each of these smaller groups would have a designated leader as well. Communication between each section is essential and may include patient transfers or discharge to a holding area, resupply, space availability, changes in victim condition, numbers of patients, and more (Al Thobaity et al., 2017). While the standard phone system works well when power is available, outside utilities may be down and generators may fail eventually. Radio communication may work well depending on the size of the hospital. Cell phones also may work, although reception may be limited. Texting requires less power and signal strength and may help avoid the confusion of multiple calls. In all cases, wording must be concise and clear. It is important to say only exactly what is meant to be said. Repeating back the information may avoid confusion.

These redundant communication systems as well as elevators essential for patient movement, ventilators, intravenous pumps, computers, emergency lighting, and more need electricity to function. While some have backup batteries, these will only last a short period of time. Most, if not all, hospitals have emergency backup generators. These must be maintained in good working order, be tested often, and have an amount of fuel necessary to operate for the recommended 3–5 days before outside help can arrive.

Staffing

Staffing is another important consideration. Plans should be made for calling out additional hospital staff in the event of a disaster and its immediate aftermath. Staff family and pets need to be considered. Staff may be reluctant to report to the hospital if doing so leaves children, elderly parents, and even their pets alone and uncared for. Additional personnel, not credentialed by the hospital or possibly licensed by the state the hospital is located in, may wish to volunteer or may be needed as temporary hospital personnel. Plans for quickly validating licenses and credentialing should be made (Academies, 2012a).

It may not be possible to do this during the event due to a lack of an available internet connection. Potential volunteers can be listed prior to the event with license and temporary credentialing updated periodically. Local Medical Reserve Corps and federal response teams may also provide staff (McCormick et al., 2017). The National Disaster Medical System (NDMS) can provide healthcare personnel, temporary treatment facilities, and medical, veterinary, and mortuary services (Academies, 2012a). These must be requested on a state level and require time to respond. They are rarely first responders.

Hospital Evacuation

An essential aspect of hospital planning is the worst-case scenario, hospital evacuation. In the event that damage to the hospital is such that it can no longer function or if the area surrounding the hospital is no longer safe, plans must be made for evacuation of patients and staff. This is most complex. All local emergency services will likely be overwhelmed and other local hospitals will also be functioning at maximum capacity. While firm arrangements may not be possible prior to an event, this is something that should be discussed with other hospitals and emergency services.

Consideration also needs to be given to the evacuation procedures. Patients and victims will need to be moved from upper floors possibly without the help of elevators. Some of this patient movement will be complicated by the patient's health, medical equipment, and dark stairwells. Planning for moving these patients safely for the staff and the patient is essential.

Practicing evacuations is important and should include local EMS and fire and rescue teams (Admi et al., 2011; Austin et al., 2013; Baack & Alfred, 2013; Broach & Smith, 2017; Georgino et al., 2015; Jacobs-Wingo et al., 2019; Labrague et al., 2018; Livingston et al., 2016).

Standard of Care, Committees, and Protocols

Planning on the hospital level requires a significant amount of forethought. Even the smallest institution with limited personnel should have a disaster planning committee. This committee should include members from all hospital functions. Within this committee, subcommittees would deal with each area. All areas of the hospital are affected by disasters, so all the aspects should be involved with planning (Academies, 2012a; Al Thobaity et al., 2017). While all areas are important, those involving the treatment of victims take on an increased significance. These include the clinical care and triage committees. At some point in a disaster response, it should be assumed that the number and severity of injuries and illnesses would overwhelm the hospital's ability to respond with normal treatment protocols. It is up to these committees to establish treatment protocols based on a crisis standard of care and triggers for their implementation (Academies, 2012a, 2012b).

Nursing and medical staff are familiar with operating under a normal standard of care in which supplies are not rationed or reused and all patients, even the sickest or most injured, with little to no chance of long-term survival, are treated (under most circumstances). However, these same staff may not be familiar with or be comfortable making decisions in a crisis. A crisis standard of care differs from a normal standard of care in that certain supplies may need to be reused and it may be necessary to make difficult life-and-death decisions concerning treatment. These decisions may include the rationing of medications and ventilators and choosing palliative care for some victims in grave condition who may not benefit from the available resources (Academies, 2012a, 2012b; Hale, 2008).

Those involved with treatment should not make these decisions. They should only concern themselves with the treatment of the victim presented to them (Academies, 2012a, 2012b; Hale, 2008). The clinical care committee, in conjunction with the triage lead or committee and with input concerning available beds, space, supplies, and personnel from other members of the disaster committee, should decide when the hospital switches from a normal standard of care to a crisis standard. They should also be in contact with other hospitals in the area to ensure that victim care is consistent throughout the area (Academies, 2012a, 2012b).

The triggers and extent to which the standard of care changes should be decided long before the confusion of a disaster response. On a normal day, the availability of supplies and equipment fluctuates. During a disaster, the availability of supplies, equipment, and other resources may be overwhelmed. The clinical care committee should be aware of what is normally available and how quickly these resources are being used during the response. Trigger points, or points when resources are quickly becoming unavailable, should be decided upon prior to the event (Academies, 2012b). Members of the clinical care committee should monitor the response and institute the crisis standard of care and specific changes in treatment when these thresholds are reached. Triage should be notified of these changes in treatment and the classification of victims, including those now assigned to palliative care, and treatment teams should be notified of criteria for treatment decisions. This may include criteria for assigning ventilators to victims or determining how long a victim may stay on a ventilator based on the rate of improvement, the rationing of medications, alternative antibiotic use, and palliative care treatment for those who cannot be saved with the limited resources (Abbasi et al., 2018; Academies, 2012a, 2012b; Hale, 2008).

Key Points

The decision to change from a normal standard of care to a crisis standard is significant and difficult. Healthcare professionals live by the code of *do no harm* which often translates to *do everything that can be done to save the patient*. When moving to a crisis standard of care, every victim is treated, but the treatment may not be the ideal treatment and, for some who cannot be saved, the point of treatment is only to make the victim comfortable.

Establishing trigger points can also provide an important protection from legal actions taken after the event has resolved. Having specific protocols for treatment and triggers for the implementation of these protocols can show that a hospital and its personnel acted in a reasonable and responsible manner and avoid litigation or other legal actions (Abbasi et al., 2018; Academies, 2012a, 2012b).

All of the planning falls apart if those involved are not aware of the role that each person plays. The disaster plan should be disseminated throughout the hospital clearly indicating command and control and the roll of various personnel. Lastly, these procedures and protocols must be practiced. Annual drills with additional table-top exercises should be the norm. These drills and exercises should involve all aspects of the hospital and services provided by the community, such as EMS, LE, and fire (Academies, 2012b; Admi et al., 2011; Al Thobaity et al., 2017; Austin et al., 2013; Baack & Alfred, 2013; Broach & Smith, 2017; Georgino et al., 2015; Jacobs-Wingo et al., 2019; Labrague et al., 2018; Livingston et al., 2016; Morrison & Catanzaro, 2010; Pesiridis et al., 2015; Ruskie, 2016).

Case Study

You and your partner take a deep breath. You have planned for this. As a few cell towers come back online, you text the family member caring for your child—both are fine. Knowing your family is fine gives you the ability to focus more on the events occurring in the hospital. The disaster plan of the hospital goes into effect. Inpatients from the ICU and step-down units are being downgraded as appropriate. Patients are being seen in both the ER and the clinic. The clinical care committee, of which you are a member, has met and a crisis standard of care is being considered. The triage committee, of which your partner is a member, has been appraised of the clinical committee's concerns.

Response

Response begins immediately after the start of the incident. It is both simple—everyone does what they need to do as circumstances present—and complex. The first to respond in a disaster are the victims themselves. They perform self-rescue and begin to rescue those around them. Following this, local EMS, LE, and fire services respond. They perform more complex rescues and provide initial care for complex injuries. If the disaster is large enough, a victim collection point may be established. This is where large numbers of victims are gathered and prioritized for transport and treatment. The triage officer in charge of these collection points needs to be in contact with all local treatment facilities. This helps to ensure that the right patient is sent to the right facility. Severe traumas should go to trauma centers, burns to a burn center, and so on. This is true even if the appropriate facility is not the closest facility. The victim will receive the most appropriate care at the appropriate facility rather than being transferred after being taken to a closer facility. Of course, disasters are fluid and there are always exceptions to every rule.

While EMS will transport victims from the victim collection points and points of injury, others will also bring victims to hospitals and treatment centers. Victims will self-transport and good Samaritans will often provide transportation. This can be problematic for a few reasons. These victims may present to the closest facility, which may not be the best facility for the victim. Additionally, if there is contamination from the event, the victim, the good Samaritan, their vehicle, and possibly the emergency department at the hospital are now all contaminated. This is especially problematic if the contamination is highly toxic.

After local emergency services respond, emergency personnel from surrounding counties and the state respond. Many states now have compacts with surrounding states to provide additional aid in a disaster (Academies, 2012a). The state governor can also request a declaration for a state of emergency from the federal government. The president of the United States can also declare a national emergency event without a request from the governor. During a national emergency, all of the resources from the Federal Emergency Management Agency (FEMA), NDMS through the Department of Health and Human Services, and other agencies become available for the response (Hale, 2008).

On a personal level, it is important to remain calm, use the contents of the preparedness kit, and wait for the event to pass or for further instructions. Use communication plans to stay informed about the status of the disaster and available services. Call loved ones to let them know your condition or call for help as needed. Be situationally aware and stay safe.

On the hospital level, this again is more complex. Hospitals have an inherent duty to care for the community they are located in (Academies, 2012a; Kaji et al., 2010; Shirali et al., 2016).

Injured victims and those in need will begin to present to the ER. Injuries will include those physical and mental injuries related to the event as well as normal day-to-day concerns. The hospital should institute its disaster plan (Admi et al., 2011; Hale, 2008).

If the hospital is structurally unsafe as a result of the event, evacuation plans should be instituted. If the hospital is safe, plans for triaging and treating patients should begin. Initial response should involve a normal standard of care, although this may be stretched a bit. The clinical care committee should track supplies, personnel, and equipment carefully. Inpatients able to receive a lower level of care should be transferred to less acute beds in order to free up intensive care and step-down beds. All elective surgeries should be canceled. The surge capacity of the hospital should be established.

At this time, most patients presenting to the emergency department would be treated as they would on a normal day, although some consideration should be given to the survivability. Once trigger points are reached and other treatment facilities in the area are consulted, the crisis standard of care should be instituted (Academies, 2012a, 2012b; Admi et al., 2011).

Case Study

Patients began to overwhelm the ED. As the lead provider, you are responsible for triage. You quickly review your disaster triage protocol and direct your staff on disaster categories. You establish the triage areas within the facility based on these levels: ED resuscitation rooms are cleared for the critically ill, the waiting room is established as the triage area for those who need treatment but are relatively stable, and the ambulance bay is opened for the walking wounded. You work with the hospital operations team to open an unused floor for those who are dead on arrival or dying.

Triage

Key Points

Triage during a disaster, even within a normal standard of care, differs from normal day-to-day triage.

The AGACNP is also uniquely qualified for triaging victims or managing the triage team. On a normal day in the ER, it is nursing's task to triage patients. During a disaster, triage is complicated by an increase in the number of patients/victims and by a larger number of acute injuries (Firouzkouhi et al., 2017; Hale, 2008), Yet, triage remains the assessment of a victim's stability and extent of their injuries. The AGACNP brings the experience of the nursing triage and an understanding of medicine to this task (Al Thobaity et al., 2017; Wolf et al., 2017). They can establish the correct level of stability and add potential diagnosis (differential diagnosis). With this, the victim can be assigned the best place in the queue for treatment.

On a normal day, patients are triaged into 1 of 5 categories: 1 is for life-threatening injuries or imminent death, and 5 is for patients needing limited resources for their care.

During a disaster, EMS and treatment facilities begin using a triage tag system involving a color-coded tag with limited space to document victim information and treatment. These tags each have a unique number, which may be all that is available to identify the victim. Some tags come in pairs with the same unique number—one for the victim and one for the victim's belongings.

Each tag has a series of color tear off strips that are green, yellow, red, and black (there may be an additional blue strip before the black strip). Green is given to those victims with minor injuries who are often referred to as the walking wounded. Yellow is for those victims who require treatment, but are stable enough to delay care. Red is for those who are unstable and require treatment first, although circumstances may delay their treatment as well. Black is for those who are dead or dying and cannot be saved. On some tags, blue is the color assigned to those who are dying. While this color-coding system is used by both EMS and the hospital, hospital triage is often more complex and may consider more than the victim's level of stability.

Field Triage

Triage in the field often will utilize one of the several triage systems, such as START and JumpSTART (for children), SAVE, or SALT systems; of these, the START and JumpSTART systems are possibly the most common (Jenkins et al., 2008; Benson et al., 1996). Each system looks at simple parameters to judge the stability of the victim. They are based on a few simple vital signs and the patient's ability to follow commands. For the START system, all those who can walk are asked to walk to a specific point for further care. These patients are tagged green. Then, the person or persons triaging move to the closest victim. If the person is not breathing, the provider opens the airway. If the victim begins to breathe, they are tagged red; if not, they are tagged black and the provider moves on to the next victim. If the victim is already breathing at a rate greater than 30 respirations per minute, they are tagged red.

Next, the provider assesses the radial pulse and capillary refill. If no pulse is detected or if the capillary refill is greater than 2 s, the person is tagged red and quickly assessed for severe bleeding. The radial pulse is used since, in general, if a person has a radial pulse, their systolic blood pressure is at least 80. Next, the victim is asked to follow two commands. If they are able to do so, they are tagged yellow; if not, they are tagged red and the provider moves on to the next victim.

Aspects of this assessment can and should be done simultaneously, such as the assessment of breathing and pulse. No more than 60 s should be taken with each victim. Even with as little as 60 s with each victim, with 60 victims, it may take about an hour to get to the last victim. Minimal treatment should be done to the victim during the triage process. Only severe bleeding and other life-threatening conditions may require initial treatment. Additional treatment is done by those who follow (Jenkins et al., 2008; Benson et al., 1996).

The JumpSTART system for children is similar. Children who can walk are tagged green. For those who are not breathing, open the airway and give five rescue breaths. If the child starts to breathe, they are tagged red; if not, they are tagged black. Breathing and pulse are similarly assessed, using the normal respiratory rate for children. If a child is breathing at a rate <15 or >45 per minute, they are tagged red. Last, instead of following two commands, the child is assessed according to AVPU (appropriate/inappropriate, posturing, responding only to pain, or unresponsive). In both systems, those tagged as red are transported for treatment first, followed by yellow, and finally green (Jenkins et al., 2008; Benson et al., 1996).

Hospital Disaster Triage

Triage in the hospital setting is more complex. Triage in the field considers the stability of the victim only. In the hospital setting, the victim's injuries must also be considered (Hale, 2008). Victims with red tags, particularly those requiring further stabilization, or those with yellow tags who have deteriorated should be taken immediately to the ED. Those who are stable and require surgery should be placed in line for surgery and may be housed in the ED. Testing may be ordered, but only when such testing would dictate treatment. For example, a possible broken arm, with good distal neurovascular function, would likely be splinted without an x-ray, while a head, thoracic, or abdominal injury would require a CT scan to rule out bleeding and possible surgery. Victims with yellow and green tags should be sent to separate holding areas. These victims receive treatment after victims with red tags are treated and space is available.

The clinical care committee must work closely with triage. Treatment areas should only concern themselves with treatment. Only if treatment should fail, would the treatment team reclassify the victim as black. Classifying a victim who cannot be saved as black should be done in triage according to policies set forth by the clinical care committee. These victims should also be moved to a separate holding area and cared for with palliative care measures. All victims receive treatment (Admi et al., 2011; Hale, 2008).

While victims may deteriorate and move from green to yellow, yellow to red, or red to black/blue, they should never be retriaged to move from red to yellow or yellow to green. Moving in this reverse direction is dangerous and may cause providers to miss something important that the first triage provider noticed but is now hidden or unknown. If the victim is more stable than others in the same classification, then less stable victims should be treated first, but if classified as red or yellow, the victim should be treated as a red or yellow victim. Only when all victims with red or yellow tags are treated should those receiving palliative care be treated more aggressively and only after consideration of resources and the potential for more victims to arrive.

Overtriage and undertriage must also be considered. Overtriage can be defined as classifying a victim as less stable or more seriously injured than they are. Undertriage is the classification of a victim as more stable or less seriously injured than they are. Undertriage is far more serious than overtriage. Overtriage can be as high as 25%, while undertriage should be kept to less than 5%.

Retriage should be done often to note changes in victim's condition.

Holding areas for yellow, green, and blue/black should be staffed at a minimum with registered nurses (RNs) or, ideally, with advanced practice nurses (APNs) or physician assistants (PAs). If staffed only at the level of RNs, protocols and policies should be established to allow the RNs to start fluids, provide pain medications, order testing as appropriate, and otherwise care for the victims. The APNs or PAs may treat and discharge victims as appropriate.

Recovery and Mitigation

The recovery phase of the disaster cycle begins slowly after more acute needs have been met.

Key Points

Recovery is the slow return to normal or, more likely, a new normal.

In the recovery phase, an alternate infrastructure is established. The acute needs of victims are met. While some injuries resulting from clean up and rebuilding, such as chainsaw injuries and falls, will present, most victims presenting have more primary care needs. These may result from the disaster limiting access to PCPs, which in turn can cause a lack of regular medications and exacerbation of chronic illnesses. During the recovery phase, hospitals begin to move toward a more normal patient load and a normal standard of care.

After the disaster, there is a slow move toward planning and mitigation, thus bringing the disaster cycle to a close. Those who have led the response—the clinical care, triage, and disaster committees—begin to assess what worked well or what failed. EMS, LE, fire and rescue, and those in the ICC examine their response and ask the same questions. While people, the area, and hospitals are still recovering, the process begins again, and everyone involved determines what they can do better next time.

THE ROLE OF THE ADVANCE PRACTICE PROVIDER

Nurse APPs specifically AGACNPs have a unique perspective. They are trained both as a nurse and in the art and practice of medicine. They work collaboratively with physicians but have an independent license. They have their own prescriptive authority and, possibly, a DEA number and can diagnose, write orders, perform procedures, write histories and physicals (H&P), and admit and discharge patients. Training as a nurse allows the AGACNP to bring nursing as a compliment to medicine. This enables a more wholistic view of the victim during triage and treatment. They bring this unique perspective to planning as well. This dual perspective becomes very important when a crisis standard of care is implemented as it brings these perspectives into play for the difficult decisions a disaster may require. Because of this unique perspective, AGACNPs should be a part of all aspects of disaster planning and mitigation, response, and recovery, with the subsequent return to mitigation (Hanes, 2016).

They should sit on disaster planning committees for the hospital and the community as well as the clinical care and triage committees during planning and response, and they should be an active part of decision-making during recovery and subsequent planning and future mitigation (Admi et al., 2011; Al Thobaity et al., 2017; Hanes, 2016). Often, the decisions made by these committees and groups are difficult and rely on very hard and practical realities. Planning and mitigation are expensive. Stockpiling supplies and extra equipment must be balanced against the potential of a disaster. While disasters do happen, the question may be raised of when it might happen. Spending must be balanced against a disaster that may not come—at least, not for a while. Nurses and the AGACNPs are a trusted part of the community. Their perspective is one of caring for the whole patient, family, and community. They view the patient and family as one unit with needs that must be met. Nurses and AGACNPs advocate for their patients on a daily basis and bring this advocacy to disaster planning and response. They advocate for the potential needs of victims, families, and the community during a disaster (Mather, 2010; Wolf et al., 2017).

During the response, nursing and the AGACNP should again serve in all aspects of the response (Al Thobaity et al., 2017; Evans & Baumberger-Henry, 2014; Goodhue et al., 2012; Hanes, 2016; Wolf et al., 2017). Experienced clinical and administrative nurses are a vital aspect of the command and control system in the hospital. While advocating for the victims, they also speak to the needs of the providers and nursing staff.

The AGACNP should be a part of the clinical care and triage committees. Decisions made there are particularly difficult. The decisions concerning the rationing, reuse of supplies, and life-and-death triage decisions that come with a crisis standard of care need the unique combination of nursing and medicine of the AGACNP to help assure that the decision is not made too early or too late.

All providers, from nurses to physicians, may be required to work beyond the normal scope of their education and license. Nurses may be the only providers seeing and treating victims with green tags before discharge. Nursing staff may be required to manage holding areas of victims with yellow and green tags and, based on protocols, provide fluids and pain medication, order testing, and more. The AGACNP adds a deeper level of care to these areas. They bring the ability to fully manage victims in these areas and direct nursing if SOP is stretched. If the victim load is reasonable, the AGACNP should work within their education and license. However, in a disaster, the AGACNP may need to see victims outside their normal scope. If circumstances require the treatment of a child, consult with a physician and, if possible, have the chart signed off by a physician. When this is not possible, the crisis standard of care as defined by the institution should enable the AGACNP to work with full practice authority for all victims. The principle *do no harm* must guide care. Proper planning with triggers and protocols will offer some protection to the provider under these circumstances.

Case Study

Other departments of the hospital staff have stepped up. Pharmacy has set up a satellite center in both the clinic and ER. Housekeeping is ready to establish a decontamination area if needed. Holding areas are established for green and yellow victims and staffed. Protocols have been reviewed by the staff. Word is that the generator will be fixed within the hour. It will be a long night, but you, your partner, the hospital, and local response teams are prepared to work together and care for those in need. You are prepared and that has made the difference.

CLINICAL PEARLS

- Disasters are, well, a disaster. The mitigation phase is long and filled with committee meetings, compromise, decision-making, training, more compromise, and more training. Response is confusing, filled with hurried actions and waiting, followed by more hurried actions and more waiting. It is exhilarating and heartbreaking, sometimes at the same moment. It is exhausting and wonderful (if you are an adrenaline junkie). Recovery is slow and sometimes—quite often, really—painful, and that leads us back to preparation. As one who has been involved with all of this for quite some time, I can tell you it is rewarding and amazing. It changes you and, if you let it, the change is for the better.
- Without adequate preparation, response is haphazard, more disorganized than it needs to be, and inadequate. Preparation begins long before an event and involves all aspects of the institution and all personnel. It involves LE, emergency services, other local healthcare institutions, and other aspects of the community. Decisions and protocols must be based on fairness, a duty to care, and a duty to steward resources. They must be transparent and applied consistently and

proportionally to the incident. Those involved with planning and response are account-able for the good as well as the bad.

- Community engagement and discussion concerning preparations and protocols used in a disaster can be difficult and time-consuming, but are essential. Protocols used in a disaster response must be viewed by the community as fair. Engaging the community can establish trust that responders are doing everything that can be done even though not everyone can be saved.
- The AGACNP is qualified and has a unique and essential perspective concerning plan-ning and response. They should be members of key planning committees and, during a response, members of the clinical care and triage committees. They bring nursing's experience and understanding of triage (even if they have not worked triage as a nurse) and a deep understanding of medicine. These perspectives make them ideal candidates for heading up the triage team.
- Communication and information are essential. Know that the information you receive in a disaster may be incomplete or completely wrong. Responders must act on the infor-mation they receive but must remain flexible as new information becomes available. Communication systems fail. All systems must have redundant systems to back them up. Again, remain flexible for when the backup systems also fail.
- Be prepared! It starts with you and then expands to the community, the state, and finally the federal government. If you are not prepared, your ability to care for others around you will be compromised.
- Be strong and do not panic. Disasters happen, and chances are that you will be okay. In fact, chances are that most people will be okay. If you panic, your ability to make good decisions is diminished and, worse, your chances of morbidity and mortality increase. Stay calm and flexible. Make the best decisions you can under the circumstances.

REVIEW QUESTIONS

1. Community engagement will assure that there is agreement on protocols and priorities used in disaster response and the allocation of scarce resources.
   a. True
   b. False

2. Good Samaritan Laws and laws like them protect providers when they act outside their SOP in a disaster response.
   a. True
   b. False

3. The Command and Control structure of the Incident Command System has one Incident Commander, a deputy commander, other command staff, and leaders in Logistics, Operations, Planning, and Administration/Finance.
   a. True
   b. False

4. The disaster cycle consists of mitigation, response, and recovery only.
   a. True
   b. False

Answers: 1, b; 2, b; 3, a; 4, b

REFERENCES

Abbasi, M., Majdzadeh, R., Zali, A., Karimi, A., & Akrami, F. (2018). The evolution of public health ethics frameworks: Systematic review of moral values and norms in public health policy. *Medicine, Health Care, and Philosophy*, 21(3), 387–402. https://doi.org/10.1007/s11019-017-9813-y

Ablah, E., Konda, K. S., Konda, K., Melbourne, M., Ingoglia, J. N., & Gebbie, K. M. (2010). Emergency preparedness training and response among community health centers and local health departments: Results from a multi-state survey. *Journal of Community Health*, 35(3), 285–293. https://doi.org/10.1007/s10900-010-9236-7

Institute of Medicine. (2012a). *Crisis Standards of Care: A Systems Framework for Catastrophic Disaster Response.* The National Academies Press.

Institute of Medicine. (2012b). *Crisis Standards of Care: A Systems Framework for Catastrophic Disaster Response. Volume 1 Introduction and CSC Framework.* The National Academies Press.

Acosta, J., & Chandra, A. (2013). Harnessing a community for sustainable disaster response and recovery: An operational model for integrating nongovernmental organizations. *Disaster Medicine and Public Health Preparedness*, 7(4), 361–368. https://doi.org/10.1017/dmp.2012.1

Adini, B., Israeli, A., Bodas, M., & Peleg, K. (2019). Increasing perceived emergency preparedness by participatory policy-making (Think-Tanks). *Disaster Medicine and Public Health Preparedness*, 13(2), 152–157. https://doi.org/10.1017/dmp.2018.8

Admi, H., Eilon, Y., Hyams, G., & Utitz, L. (2011). Management of mass casualty events: The Israeli experience. *Journal of Nursing Scholarship*, 43(2), 211–219. https://doi.org/10.1111/j.1547-5069.2011.01390.x

Al Thobaity, A., Plummer, V., & Williams, B. (2017). What are the most common domains of the core competencies of disaster nursing? A scoping review. *International Emergency Nursing*, 31, 64–71. https://doi.org/10.1016/j.ienj.2016.10.003

Austin, E. N., Hannafin, N. M., & Nelson, H. W. (2013). Pediatric disaster simulation in graduate and undergraduate nursing education. *Journal of Pediatric Nursing*, 28(4), 393–399. https://doi.org/10.1016/j.pedn.2012.12.004

Baack, S., & Alfred, D. (2013). Nurses' preparedness and perceived competence in managing disasters. *Journal of Nursing Scholarship*, 45(3), 281–287. https://doi.org/10.1111/jnu.12029

Benson, M., Koenig, K. L., Schultz, C. H. (1996). Disaster triage: START, then SAVE - a new method of dynamic triage for victims of a catastrophic earthquake. *Prehospital and Disaster Medicine*, 11(2), 117–124.

Braunack-Mayer, A. J., Street, J. M., Rogers, W. A., Givney, R., Moss, J. R., & Hiller, J. E. (2010). Including the public in pandemic planning: A deliberative approach. *BMC Public Health*, 10, 501. https://doi.org/10.1186/1471-2458-10-501

Broach, J., & Smith, M. E. (2017). Emergency preparedness training preferences and perceived barriers to training among various healthcare providers and public health practitioners in Massachusetts. *American Journal of Disaster Medicine*, 12(2), 85–106. https://doi.org/10.5055/ajdm.2017.0264

Carrier, E., Yee, T., Cross, D., & Samuel, D. (2012). Emergency preparedness and community coalitions: Opportunities and challenges. *Research Brief*, (24), 1–9.

Daugherty Biddison, E. L., Gwon, H., Schoch-Spana, M., Cavalier, R., White, D. B., Dawson, T., Terry, P. B., London, A. J., Regenberg, A., Faden, R., & Toner, E. S. (2014). The community speaks: Understanding ethical values in allocation of scarce lifesaving resources during disasters. *Annals of the American Thoracic Society*, 11(5), 777–783. https://doi.org/10.1513/AnnalsATS.201310-379OC

Daugherty Biddson, E. L., Gwon, H. S., Schoch-Spana, M., Rengenberg, A. C., Juliano, C., Faden, R. R., & Toner, E. S. (2018). Scarce resource allocation during disasters; A mixed method community engagement Study. *Chest*, 153(1), 187–195. https://doi.org/10.1016/j.chest.2017.08.001

Esbitt, D. (2003). The strategic national stockpile: Roles and responsibilities of healthcare professionals for receiving the stockpile assets. *Disaster Management & Response*, 1(3), 68–70.

Evans, C. A., & Baumberger-Henry, M. (2014). Readiness: How prepared are you? *Journal of Emergency Nursing*, 40(5), 448–452. https://doi.org/10.1016/j.jen.2014.03.006

Fink, S. (2013). *Five days at memorial: Life and death in a storm rasvaged hospital.* Crown Publishing Group a Division of Random House Inc.

Firouzkouhi, M., Zargham-Boroujeni, A., Kako, M., & Abdollahimohammad, A. (2017). Experiences of civilian nurses in triage during the Iran-Iraq War: An oral history. *Chinese Journal of Traumatology*, 20(5), 288–292. https://doi.org/10.1016/j.cjtee.2017.07.002

Georgino, M. M., Kress, T., Alexander, S., & Beach, M. (2015). Emergency preparedness education for nurses: Core competency familiarity measured utilizing an adapted emergency preparedness information questionnaire. *Journal of Trauma Nursing*, 22(5), 240–248, quiz E1–E2. https://doi.org/10.1097/jtn.0000000000000148

Glow, S. D., Colucci, V. J., Allington, D. R., Noonan, C. W., & Hall, E. C. (2013). Managing multiple-casualty incidents: A rural medical preparedness training assessment. *Prehospital and Disaster Medicine*, 28(4), 334–341. https://doi.org/10.1017/S1049023X13000423

Goodhue, C. J., Burke, R. V., Ferrer, R. R., Chokshi, N. K., Dorey, F., & Upperman, J. S. (2012). Willingness to respond in a disaster: A pediatric nurse practitioner national survey. *Journal of Pediatric Health Care*, 26(4), e7–e20. https://doi.org/10.1016/j.pedhc.2010.11.003

Grimes, D. E., & Mendias, E. P. (2010). Nurses' intentions to respond to bioterrorism and other infectious disease emergencies. *Nursing Outlook*, 58(1), 10–16. https://doi.org/10.1016/j.outlook.2009.07.002

Grimm, D. (2014). Whole community planning: Building resiliency at the local level. *Journal of Business Continuity & Emergency Planning*, 7(3), 253–259.

Hale, J. F. (2008). Managing a disaster scene and multiple casualties before help arrives. *Critical Care Nursing Clinics of North America*, 20(1), 91–102, vii. https://doi.org/10.1016/j.ccell.2007.10.012

Hanes, P. F. (2016). Wildfire disasters and nursing. *Nursing Clinics of North America*, 51(4), 625–645. https://doi.org/10.1016/j.cnur.2016.07.006

Jacobs-Wingo, J. L., Schlegelmilch, J., Berliner, M., Airall-Simon, G., & Lang, W. (2019). Emergency preparedness training for hospital nursing staff, New York city, 2012-2016. *Journal of Nursing Scholarship*, 51(1), 81–87. https://doi.org/10.1111/jnu.12425

Jenkins, J. L., McCarthy, M. L., Sauer, L. M., Green, G. B., Stuart, S., Thomas, T. L., Hsu, E. B. (2008). Mass-casualty triage: Time for an evidence-based approach. *Prehospital Disaster Medicine*, 23(1), 3–8.

Kaji, A. H., Coates, W., & Fung, C. C. (2010). A disaster medicine curriculum for medical students. *Teaching and Learning in Medicine*, 22(2), 116–122. https://doi.org/10.1080/10401331003656561

Labrague, L. J., Hammad, K., Gloe, D. S., McEnroe-Petitte, D. M., Fronda, D. C., Obeidat, A. A., Leocadio, M. C., Cayaban, A. R., & Mirafuentes, E. C. (2018). Disaster preparedness among nurses: A systematic review of literature. *International Nursing Review*, 65(1), 41–53. https://doi.org/10.1111/inr.12369

Livingston, L. L., West, C. A., Livingston, J. L., Landry, K. A., Watzak, B. C., & Graham, L. L. (2016). Simulated disaster day: Benefit from lessons learned through years of transformation from silos to interprofessional education. *Journal of the Society for Simulation in Healthcare*, 11(4), 293–298. https://doi.org/10.1097/sih.0000000000000173

Lowe, L. D., & Hummel, F. I. (2014). Disaster readiness for nurses in the workplace: Preparing for the zombie apocalypse. *Workplace Health & Safety*, 62(5), 207–213, quiz 214. https://doi.org/10.3928/21650799-20140422-05

Mather, M. E. (2010). A personal reflection: Nursing in times of disaster. *Dimensions of Critical Care Nursing*, 29(6), 284–287. https://doi.org/10.1097/DCC.0b013e3181f0c16f

McCormick, L. C., Fifolt, M., Mercer, C., Pevear, J., III, & Wilson, J. (2017). Mississippi medical Reserve Corps: Moving Mississippi from emergency planning to response ready. *Journal of Public Health Management and Practice*, 23(1), 47–53. https://doi.org/10.1097/phh.0000000000000451

Morrison, A. M., & Catanzaro, A. M. (2010). High-fidelity simulation and emergency preparedness. *Public Health Nursing*, 27(2), 164–173. https://doi.org/10.1111/j.1525-1446.2010.00838.x

Pesiridis, T., Sourtzi, P., Galanis, P., & Kalokairinou, A. (2015). Development, implementation and evaluation of a disaster training programme for nurses: A switching replications randomized controlled trial. *Nurse Education in Practice*, 15(1), 63–67. https://doi.org/10.1016/j.nepr.2014.02.001

Rambhia, K. J., Waldhorn, R. E., Selck, F., Mehta, A. K., Franco, C., & Toner, E. S. (2012). A survey of hospitals to determine the prevalence and characteristics of healthcare coalitions for emergency preparedness and response. *Biosecurity and Bioterrorism*, 10(3), 304–313. https://doi.org/10.1089/bsp.2012.0022

Ruskie, S. E. (2016). All the resources was gone: The environmental context of disaster nursing. *Nursing Clinics of North America*, 51(4), 569–584. https://doi.org/10.1016/j.cnur.2016.07.011

Schoch-Spana, M., Sell, T. K., & Morhard, R. (2013). Local health department capacity for community engagement and its implications for disaster resilience. *Biosecurity and Bioterrorism*, 11(2), 118–129. https://doi.org/10.1089/bsp.2013.0027

Shafer, M. R., & Stocks, L. (2012). Conducting ethically sound disaster nursing research. *Annual Review of Nursing Research*, 30(1), 47–66. https://doi.org/10.1891/0739-6686.30.47

Shirali, G. A., Azadian, S., & Saki, A. (2016). A new framework for assessing hospital crisis management based on resilience engineering approach. *Work*, 54(2), 435–444. https://doi.org/10.3233/wor-162329

Smith, E., Burkle, F. M., Gebbie, K., Ford, D., & Bensimon, C. (2018). Acceptable limitations on paramedic duty to treat during disaster: A qualitative exploration. *Prehospital and Disaster Medicine*, 33(5), 466–470. https://doi.org/10.1017/s1049023x18000857

Walsh, L., Craddock, H., Gulley, K., Strauss-Riggs, K., & Schor, K. W. (2015). Building health care system capacity to respond to disasters: Successes and challenges of disaster preparedness health care coalitions. *Prehospital and Disaster Medicine*, 30(2), 112–122. https://doi.org/10.1017/s1049023x14001459

Wells, K. B., Springgate, B. F., Lizaola, E., Jones, F., & Plough, A. (2013a). Community engagement in disaster preparedness and recovery: A tale of two cities--Los Angeles and New Orleans. *Psychiatric Clinics of North America*, 36(3), 451–466. https://doi.org/10.1016/j.psc.2013.05.002

Wells, K. B., Tang, J., Lizaola, E., Jones, F., Brown, A., Stayton, A., Williams, M., Chandra, A., Eisenman, D., Fogleman, S., & Plough, A. (2013b). Applying community engagement to disaster planning: Developing the vision and design for the Los Angeles county community disaster resilience initiative. *American Journal of Public Health*, 103(7), 1172–1180. https://doi.org/10.2105/ajph.2013.301407

Whetzel, E., Walker-Cillo, G., Chan, G. K., & Trivett, J. (2013). Emergency nurse perceptions of individual and facility emergency preparedness. *Journal of Emergency Nursing*, 39(1), 46–52. https://doi.org/10.1016/j. jen.2011.08.005

Wolf, L. A., Delao, A. M., Perhats, C., Moon, M. D., & Carman, M. J. (2017). The experience of advanced practice nurses in US emergency care settings. *Journal of Emergency Nursing*, 43(5), 426–434.E16. https://doi. org/10.1016/j.jen.2017.04.007

19 Pain Management and Palliative Care

Sarah E. Loschiavo

Case Study

You are the APRN on the hospitalist service. Mrs. M is a 40-year-old female with a history of metastatic breast cancer who presented to the emergency room this morning with a 1-week history of back and abdominal pain, fatigue, nausea and vomiting, yellowing of her skin, and poor appetite.

Her past medical history includes migraines diagnosed at age 16 and right-sided breast cancer diagnosed at age 37 s/p multiple failed lines of treatment including chemotherapy. She had two cesarean sections at ages 32 and 34 and bilateral mastectomy at age 37 with reconstruction followed by external beam radiation therapy.

She is widowed; her husband died in an motor vehicle accident 2 years ago. She has two children (ages 6 and 8) and is a stay-at-home mom. She denies alcohol, tobacco, or illicit drug use.

Her current medications include Escitalopram 10 mg daily, Zofran 8 mg every 8 hr as needed, multivitamin daily, morphine 15 mg PO every 4–6 hr PRN, Xeloda 1,500 mg PO every 12 hr 1 week on/1 week off. She has no known drug allergies.

In her review of systems you find that she is negative for fever, chills, and night sweats and positive for progressive fatigue, and has poor appetite, a 15-lb weight loss over 2 weeks, nausea and vomiting, dark urine, yellowing of skin, headache, and pain in the mid back and right abdomen intermittently radiating to her shoulder.

Her physical examination reveals the following: temperature, 98.6 °F; pulse, 104 bpm; respiratory rate, 16 breaths/min; blood pressure, 96/60 mm Hg. She is restless, diaphoretic, and moderately distressed due to complaints of pain, stating, "I need to get back home to get my children off of the bus." Scleral icterus is present. Pulmonary examination reveals diminished right lower base with dullness to percussion to the RLL field. Cardiovascular examination reveals tachycardia without murmur, rub, or gallop. Her abdomen is slightly distended, with tenderness on palpation of the right abdominal quadrant and hepatomegaly. Her skin is jaundiced. The remainder of her physical examination is normal.

Laboratory testing included a normal CBC with differential; her complete metabolic panel was normal except for the following: total bilirubin, 9.2 mg/dl; ALP, 754 U/L; ALT, 480 U/L; AST, 346 U/L.

You request several radiology scans. The MRI of her cervical, thoracic, and lumbar spine shows widespread osseous metastases throughout the cervical, thoracic, and lumbar spine. An MRI of her brain shows numerous enhancing masses with a 3.5-cm mass in the right frontal lobe most compatible with metastatic disease. A CT of her abdomen and pelvis shows innumerable foci within the liver suspicious for metastatic disease. Multiple upper abdominal and mesenteric lymph nodes are suspicious for involvement of the tumor.

You need to evaluate Mrs. M for admission, which includes performing a comprehensive pain assessment and developing an appropriate plan of care. What does this include?

INTRODUCTION

The Center to Advance Palliative Care defines palliative care as specialized health care for people living with serious illness. Palliative care emerged with the hospice movement of the 1970s, but it was not until 2006 that hospice and palliative medicine became a defined medical specialty. This type of care is focused on providing relief from the symptoms and stress of a potentially serious or life-threatening acute or chronic illness. Palliative care can be provided at any stage of an illness and alongside curative treatments. The National Consensus Project for Quality Palliative Care defines palliative care as both a philosophy of care and an organized, highly structured system for delivering care. Palliative care not only manages pain and other symptoms but also includes psychosocial and spiritual care for the patient and the family (Dahlin, 2013). Primary palliative care is an essential part of nursing care focusing on the "whole person." The American Nurses Association Code of Ethics for Nurses states that nursing care focuses on alleviating suffering and seeks to provide interventions to relieve pain and other symptoms. Palliative nursing approaches care from both a scientific perspective and a humanistic perspective, and the process is facilitated through a combination of science, presence, openness, compassion, mindful attention to detail, and teamwork (Ferrell & Coyle, 2010). APRNs care for patients across a variety of healthcare settings and are ideally suited to provide primary palliative care to patients throughout their disease.

Key Points

Palliative care can be initiated at any stage of life-threatening disease and encompasses symptom management and addresses individual and family needs across physical, psychological, social, and spiritual domains.

Medical advances in diagnosis and treatment of serious and life-threatening illness have resulted in patients living longer with physical symptoms such as pain (Dahlin, 2013). Pain is one of the most common and distressing symptoms described by palliative patients. Even though pain can be controlled in 85%–95% of patients through pharmacological or nonpharmacological methods, poor pain relief continues to be reality for many patients (Mehta & Chan, 2008; Scarborough & Smith, 2018). Patients with advanced cardiovascular disease, COPD, end-stage renal disease, and other end-stage diseases suffer similar levels of pain to those found in patients with malignant disease (Dahlin, 2013). The International Association for the Study of Pain defines pain as an unpleasant sensory and emotional experience associated with actual or potential tissue damage (Mehta & Chan, 2008), but it is subjective. The quality and location of the pain are determined entirely by the patient (Moses, 2014).

Key Points

It is important to remember that specific populations of people including the disabled, the elderly, children, minorities, the underinsured, women, and those with a history of drug abuse are at risk for undertreatment of pain.

COMPONENTS OF PAIN

Dr. Cicley Saunders founded the first modern hospice and pioneered the field of palliative care. She developed the concept of "total pain" or "whole person pain" to characterize the multidimensional nature of the patient's pain experience. Dr. Saunders believed that pain has physical, psychological, social, emotional, and spiritual components, each contributing to a patient's perception and tolerance of pain. Healthcare practitioners have a tendency to focus on the physical component of pain excluding other aspects that can negatively impact adequate pain management. The mnemonic PAIN (Table 19.1) is helpful to remember each component.

Physical pain is a major component of "total pain." It can be caused by physical injury; a tumor pressing on organs, nerves, or bones; anticancer treatments, such as surgery, chemotherapy, or radiation therapy; general debility; and benign causes or comorbidities (Holmes et al., 2008).

Spiritual pain is often overlooked in clinical assessments. Patients living with a serious illness often search for meaning and purpose in their lives. They can experience anger at their illness or their fate. Specific religious certainties are often questioned, and patients may have thoughts such as "What did I do to deserve this diagnosis? Why me? What did I do to upset my god?" Spiritual assessments are underutilized and can be challenging for providers for a variety of personal and professional reasons. APRNs are ideally trained to provide compassionate care and kindness to patients who are experiencing spiritual distress

TABLE 19.1 TOTAL PAIN COMPONENTS

P	Physical pain: may be related to disease process and/or treatments and can influence other symptoms
A	Anxiety (emotional component) and depression
I	Interpersonal (sociocultural component): may experience guilt, loss of trust, self-worth/identity, or stressors including family, friends, employment, finances
N	Not accepting (spiritual component), existential distress, uncertainty, hopelessness

Data from Moses B. D. (2014). *Tarascon palliative medicine pocketbook.* Jones & Bartlett Learning Company.

or uncertainties. There are several spiritual screening assessment tools available. Simple questions such as "Is religion or spirituality important to you as you cope with illness?" or "Are you at peace?" can open the dialogue for further assessment.

Social pain is an unpleasant experience that is associated with actual or potential damage to one's sense of social connection or social value. This pain can result from a loss of close relationships or rejection (Holmes et al., 2008; Total Pain Concept, 2009). For example, breast cancer patients can become sensitive to body alteration from surgery which causes them to withdraw from social interactions, intimacy, and relationships. Serious illness can also significantly impact a person's financial security due to loss of employment, high co-pays and deductibles, and cost of medications.

Finally, psychological pain causes and is affected by fear, anxiety, and depression. Serious illnesses can lead to anxiety about the future, prompting patients to ask questions such as "Am I going to die?" or "Is this curable?" When a serious illness impacts a patient's sense of self, some patients feel a painful sense of isolation, brokenness, and loss of identity.

Figure 19.1 summarizes the interaction of these four types of pain.

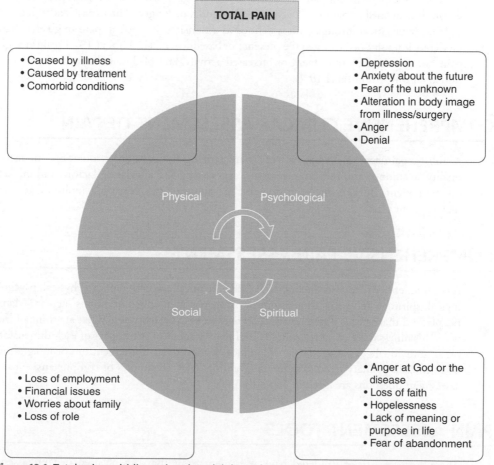

Figure 19.1 Total pain multidimensional model. (Data from Mehta A., Chan L. S. (2008). Understanding of the concept of "total pain." *Journal of Hospice and Palliative Nursing, 10*(1), 26–32 and The Total Pain Concept. (2009). https://www.oncoprof.net/Generale2000/g15_Palliatifs/gb15_sp42.html.)

PATHOPHYSIOLOGY OF PAIN

The APRN must understand and identify the pathophysiology of pain, which will assist in developing a targeted plan of care. Nociceptive pain is the most common type of pain. It is caused by potentially harmful stimuli being detected by nociceptors around the body. It is subdivided into somatic pain and visceral pain. Neuropathic pain is caused by damage or disease affecting the peripheral and/or CNS. Psychologic pain is an unpleasant feeling or suffering from a nonphysical origin.

> ## Key Points
>
> Suspect psychologic pain in patients complaining of "whole body pain."

Assessing the patient's pattern of pain is also essential. Acute pain is often severe, comes on quickly, and lasts a fairly short time. It usually has a precipitating cause (Dahlin, 2013). Chronic pain or persistent pain can come on quickly or slowly and can range from mild to severe. It is defined as pain that persists for 3 months or longer (American Cancer Society, 2019). Finally, breakthrough pain is defined as a transient increase in pain to greater than moderate intensity, occurring in the presence of baseline pain (Dahlin, 2013). Breakthrough pain can be caused by movement or increased activity, end-of-dose failure, or poorly controlled chronic pain (Table 19.2).

COMPREHENSIVE CLINICAL ASSESSMENT OF PAIN

A holistic pain assessment begins with characterizing the pain onset, duration, intensity, quality, location(s) and radiating elements, aggravating and alleviating factors, and impact on the patient. By assessing each domain, the clinician can develop a multimodal pain management plan.

COMPREHENSIVE PAIN ASSESSMENT

A comprehensive pain assessment by the APRN requires evaluation of the physical, psychological, spiritual, and social dimensions of pain. Ask open-ended questions such as "Many people find that serious illness affects their lives in unexpected ways. What are some of the ways this illness is affecting your life?" Careful assessment of the impact of each dimension on an individual's pain experience will guide selection of pain interventions or integration of an interdisciplinary team as required (Dahlin, 2013). Examples of comprehensive pain assessment questions are listed in Table 19.3.

PAIN ASSESSMENT TOOLS

There are a variety of validated pain assessment tools that can be used in your assessment. The Memorial Pain Assessment Card, the Wisconsin Brief Pain Inventory, and the McGill Pain Questionnaire are all tools that assess the patient's pain intensity, pain relief,

TABLE 19.2 PATHOPHYSIOLOGY OF PAIN

TYPE OF PAIN	CHARACTERISTICS	DESCRIPTION	DIFFERENTIAL DIAGNOSES	INTERVENTIONS
Nociceptive (somatic)	Well localized: deep musculoskeletal and cutaneous tissues	Dull, achy, throbbing, soreness	• Bone metastases • Surgical origin • Myofascial or musculoskeletal infiltration or spasm	1. Opioids 2. NSAIDs
Nociceptive (visceral)	Poorly localized: stretching, infiltration, compression, distension of thoracic or abdominal viscera	Deep, squeezing pressure or cramping Can be associated with nausea, vomiting, and diaphoresis	• Cirrhosis • Pancreatic cancer	1. Opioids 2. NSAIDs
Neuropathic	Injury to peripheral nerve or central nervous system	Burning, radiating, numbness, tingling, sharp, constant dull ache, electric shock, pins and needles, pricking, radiating	• Postherpetic neuralgia • Chemotherapy-induced peripheral neuropathy • Nerve involvement from tumor • Radiation-induced	1. Anticonvulsants 2. Antidepressants 3. Steroids 4. Nerve blocks 5. Benzodiazepines 6. Opioids 7. Local anesthetics
Psychologic	Mental, emotional pain from a nonphysical origin	"Whole body pain," "pain everywhere"	• Psychologic disorders	1. Mental health interventions and treatments 2. Support and counseling 3. Nonpharmacologic approaches

psychological distress, and functional impairment (Dahlin, 2013). Scales commonly used to measure only pain intensity include the Numerical Rating Scale, Visual Analog Scale, and Likert Verbal Rating Scale. In patients who are unable to provide a pain intensity score, it is important to assess the nonverbal signs of pain including facial grimacing, restlessness, diaphoresis, moaning, or tachycardia. It is also important to assess for signs of uncontrolled pain, which can affect every system of the body. Table 19.4 includes common systemic effects of uncontrolled pain. Patients with chronic pain may not manifest autonomic features of uncontrolled pain such as elevated heart rate, high blood pressure, or rapid, shallow breathing because their body has acclimated to the presence of pain. However, chronic pain is often associated with anxiety, depression, and sleep disturbances.

RISK ASSESSMENT FOR ABERRANT BEHAVIOR

Risk assessment for aberrant behaviors is an essential part of the comprehensive pain assessment. Because of the opioid epidemic and its impact on patient care, the APRN must include risk stratification for aberrant drug-taking behaviors as routine practice when

TABLE 19.3 COMPREHENSIVE PAIN ASSESSMENT QUESTIONS

ASSESSMENT CATEGORY	SAMPLE QUESTIONS
Quality	Can you describe your pain? What does it feel like?
Intensity	On a scale of 0–10, with 0 being no pain, 5 being moderate pain, and 10 being severe pain, what pain score describes your level of pain right now? What number describes your worst pain? What number describes your best pain? What number pain do you live at on a daily basis?
Region and radiation	Where is your pain? Where does the pain originate? Does the pain move or radiate to another site?
Aggravating/ alleviating factors	Does anything make the pain worse? Does anything make it better? What pharmacological and nonpharmacological interventions have you tried?
Temporal characteristics	When did the pain start? Does your pain come and go or is it constant? How long does the pain last?
Functional impact	How has the pain affected your life? How has it affected your mood, energy level, appetite, and sleep? How does pain affect your work or relationships?

Data from Center to Advance Palliative Care. (n.d.). *About palliative care.* https://www.capc.org/about/palliative-care/ and McPherson M. L. (2010). *Demystifying opioid conversion calculations: A guide for effective dosing.* American Society of Health-System Pharmacists.

prescribing opioid therapy. In addition to opioid overdose, opioid misuse, opioid abuse, and opioid use disorder must be addressed. APRNs are encouraged to use validated screening tools such as the Opioid Risk Tool to assess risk and address harms of opioid use before initiating opioid therapy and intermittently during continuation of therapy (Webster & Webster, 2005). In response to the need for opioid prescribing guidelines, the CDC released guidelines that provide clear and concise recommendations to providers to improve patient access and avoid diversion and abuse (Manchikanti et al, 2012). These include conducting thorough assessments, considering all possible pharmacological and nonpharmacological treatments, closely monitoring risks, and safely discontinuing opioids when

TABLE 19.4 EFFECTS OF UNCONTROLLED PAIN ON THE BODY

BODY SYSTEM	EFFECTS
Brain	Anxiety, depression, poor concentration
Cardiovascular	Increased heart rate, increased blood pressure, increased oxygen needs
Endocrine	Increased blood glucose, increased cortisol production
Gastrointestinal	Reduced gastric emptying and motility, nausea and vomiting, constipation
Immune	Increased susceptibility to infection
Musculoskeletal	Increased muscle tension, shaking, facial grimacing, furrowed brow
Nervous	Changes in pain processing
Respiratory	Increased respiratory rate, shallow breathing
Urinary	Increased urge to urinate

appropriate. Some providers obtain a urine drug screen and/or blood toxicology test before starting opioid therapy and at intervals during treatment. Finally, many states have adopted prescription drug monitoring programs (PDMP) to enhance safe opioid prescribing for the prescriber and patient.

> **Key Points**
>
> Practice laws for checking the PDMP are state-specific; therefore, the APRN must understand individual state statutes concerning SOP.

MANAGEMENT OF PAIN

Effective pain management plans incorporate pharmacological and nonpharmacological modalities to manage the patient's multidimensional pain. APRNs play a crucial role in pain assessment and management throughout the course of a disease process from diagnosis to death.

PHARMACOLOGICAL

The WHO developed a "three-step ladder" (Figure 19.2) for cancer pain relief in adults that is applicable to all disease states. It provides the framework for pharmacological management of pain based on the patient's level of pain. It is important to remember that this is a guide based on the pain severity; therefore, a patient does not need to start at step 1 (Dahlin, 2013).

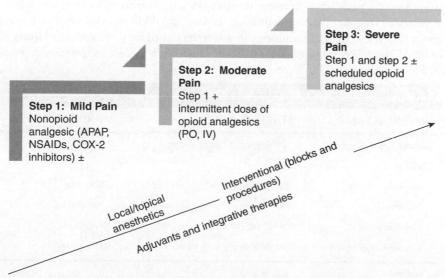

Figure 19.2 Analgesic pain management ladder. (Data from Scarborough B. M., & Smith C. B. (2018). Optimal pain management for patients with cancer in the modern era. *CA: A Cancer Journal for Clinicians, 68,* 182–196 and World Health Organization. (n.d.). *WHO's cancer pain ladder for adults.* https://www.who.int/cancer/palliative/painladder/en/.)

NONOPIOID MEDICATIONS

NSAIDs, acetaminophen, and aspirin are the most commonly used medications for mild to moderate nociceptive pain (Table 19.5). They exert their analgesic effects mainly at the peripheral nervous system (Dahlin, 2013). NSAIDs have antiinflammatory, analgesic, and antipyretic properties. Exercise caution with NSAID use in patients with renal impairment, heart failure, liver toxicity, atherosclerotic disease, and history of gastrointestinal bleeding, and in oncology patients due to interference with platelet aggregation (Dahlin, 2013; Moses, 2014). Acetaminophen can be used as a first-line treatment in patients with mild pain; however, it should be avoided in patients with liver disease. Chronic daily dosing of greater than 2–3 g/day (less in elderly, frail, or patients with liver disease) is not recommended due to risk of hepatotoxicity.

OPIOID MEDICATIONS

Morphine, oxycodone, hydromorphone, and methadone are the most commonly used medications for moderate to severe pain. They exhibit their analgesic effect by binding to opioid receptors inside and outside the CNS (Dahlin, 2013). Monitoring for opioid-induced side effects including constipation, nausea/vomiting, urinary retention, drowsiness, itching, hyperalgesia, delirium, and respiratory depression is essential.

> **Key Points**
>
> Opiate-induced constipation is the most common side effect, so opioids should be prescribed in conjunction with a daily bowel regimen (stool softener and stimulant).

Opioids can cause drowsiness and nausea upon initiation of treatment that typically subside over 1 week when tolerance develops. Finally, patients naïve to opiate therapy are at increased risk of respiratory depression. Patients should be assessed for obstructive sleep apnea (OSA) and vigilant monitoring should be instituted for those with any history or risk of OSA. The APRN must assess for sedation which often precedes respiratory depression.

TABLE 19.5 NONOPIOID PAIN MEDICATIONS

GENERIC (BRAND)	STARTING DOSE	MAXIMUM DOSE
Acetaminophen (Tylenol)	325–650 mg PO every 4–6 hr	4 g/day
NSAIDs[a]:		
Ibuprofen (Advil)	100–200 mg PO daily to every 12 hr	400 mg/day
Naproxen	250–500 mg PO every 8–12 hr	1,500 mg/day
Meloxicam	7.5–15 mg PO daily	15 mg/day
Celecoxib (Celebrex)	100–200 mg PO daily to every 12 hr	400 mg/day

PO, by mouth.

Data from Dahlin C. M. (2013). *Core curriculum for the advanced practice hospice and palliative registered nurse*. Hospice and Palliative Nurses Association; Moses B. D. (2014). *Tarascon palliative medicine pocketbook*. Jones & Bartlett Learning Company; and University of Florida Health. (2019). *Pain management and dosing guide*. http://pami.emergency.med.jax.ufl.edu/resources/dosing-guide/.

[a]Exercise caution in the elderly and avoid in renal dysfunction, peptic ulcer disease, and congestive heart failure.

ADJUVANT MEDICATIONS

Antidepressants, anticonvulsants, topical anesthetics, and corticosteroids are commonly used for the treatment of neuropathic pain. Table 19.6 lists several adjuvant medications commonly used for the treatment of neuropathic pain, including anticonvulsants, serotonin-norepinephrine reuptake inhibitors, and anesthetics. These adjuvants can be used safely in combination with opioids. Cannabinoids including medical marijuana are growing in popularity to treat symptoms of illnesses or other conditions. The most common use for medical marijuana in the United States is pain control. As of 2018, 33 states and the District of Columbia have approved the medical use of cannabis. Despite this fact, at the federal level, marijuana remains a Schedule 1 drug under the Controlled Substances Act, defined as a drug with no currently accepted medical use and a high potential for abuse (Malcom, 2019).

NONPHARMACOLOGICAL INTERVENTIONS

Nonpharmacological interventions play an important role in effective pain management. Integrative therapies that have the strongest evidence to support their role in pain management include acupuncture, therapeutic massage, counseling, meditation, guided imagery, music therapy, positioning, and spirituality (Dahlin, 2013). Procedures such as trigger point injections, nerve blocks, or epidural infusion should also be considered. Using nonpharmacological interventions as part of the comprehensive pain treatment plan requires careful assessment and a multidisciplinary team-based approach.

OPIOID CONVERSION

Opioids are indicated for the management of moderate to severe pain. Morphine has been used to treat pain dating back to the Civil War. It was originally advertised as "a wonder drug" because of its success in pain relief. APRNs who work with seriously ill patients are generally comfortable prescribing morphine due to its long history of

TABLE 19.6 NEUROPATHIC PAIN MEDICATIONS

CATEGORY	GENERIC (BRAND)	STARTING DOSE	MAXIMUM DOSE
Anticonvulsants	Gabapentin (Neurontin)	300 mg PO QHS then TID	3,600 mg/day
	Pregabalin (Lyrica)	50 mg PO TID	300 mg/day
SNRIs	Duloxetine (Cymbalta)	30 mg PO daily	60 mg/day
	Venlafaxine ER (Effexor ER)	37.5 mg PO daily	225 mg/day
Anesthetics[a]	Lidocaine (Lidoderm)	5% transdermal patch 12–24 hr/day	3 patches

PO, by mouth; QHS, every night at bedtime; SNRIs, serotonin-norepinephrine reuptake inhibitors; TID, three times a day.
Data from Dahlin C. M. (2013). *Core curriculum for the advanced practice hospice and palliative registered nurse*. Hospice and Palliative Nurses Association; Moses B. D. (2014). *Tarascon palliative medicine pocketbook*. Jones & Bartlett Learning Company; and University of Florida Health. (2019). *Pain management and dosing guide*. http://pami.emergency.med.jax.ufl.edu/resources/dosing-guide/.
[a]Avoid in liver failure.

existence, availability of multiple dosage formulations, low cost, and proven effectiveness (McPherson, 2010). However, morphine is not always the best opioid medication for every patient. There are several reasons providers chose to rotate opioids, including lack of therapeutic response, adverse side effects, change in health status, availability of a particular opioid, concern about abuse/diversion, cost and insurance coverage, or stigma associated with opioids (McPherson, 2010). APRNs must understand how to rotate patients to another opioid medication and/or formulation safely and effectively. Table 19.7 compares different opioids and routes of administration that produce the same analgesic effect. This table can be used to review equivalent doses between opioids and routes

TABLE 19.7 OPIOID PRESCRIBING AND EQUIANALGESIC DOSING TABLE

DRUG (EQUIANALGESIC TO 10 mg MORPHINE IV)	INJECTION (IV)	ORAL	ONSET	DURATION (hr)	NOTES
Morphine	10 mg	30 mg	IV: 5–10 min PO (IR): 30–60 min PO (SR): 30–90 min	PO (IR): 3–4 PO (SR): 8–12	Avoid in renal insufficiency, elderly due to active metabolite buildup
Oxycodone	N/A	20-30 mg	IR: 10–15 min ER: 10–20 min	IR: 3–4 ER: 8–12	Caution in renal insufficiency and total acetaminophen dose in combination products
Hydromorphone	1.5 mg	7.5 mg	IV: 5 min PO: 15–30 min	IV: 3–4 PO: 3–4	Caution in renal or hepatic dysfunction (dose reduce)
Fentanyl (Duragesic)	100 µg (0.1 mg)	N/A	12–24 hr	72 hr/patch	Opioid-tolerant patients ONLY Preferred in renal or hepatic failure
Hydrocodone	N/A	30 mg	PO: 10–20 min	PO: 3–4	Caution in hepatic dysfunction and total acetaminophen dose in combination products
Tramadol	N/A	300 mg	PO: 1 hr	PO: 4–6 (IR)	Weak opioid, active metabolite, avoid using with MAOIs

ER, extended release; IR, immediate release; MAOIs, monoamine oxidase inhibitors; PO, by mouth; SR, sustained release.
Data from Dahlin C. M. (2013). *Core Curriculum for the Advanced Practice Hospice and Palliative Registered Nurse*. Hospice and Palliative Nurses Association; Moses B. D. (2014). *Tarascon Palliative Medicine Pocketbook*. Jones & Bartlett Learning Company; UConn Health Department of Pharmacy. (2016). *Pocket Reference for Opioid Management of Pain[Brochure]*; and University of Florida Health. (2019). *Pain Management and Dosing Guide*. http://pami.emergency.med.jax.ufl.edu/resources/dosing-guide/.

HOW TO CALCULATE A NEW OPIOID DOSE

Formula:

Actual drug dose		**Equianalgesic data (see Table 19.7)**

$$\frac{\text{X mg TDD new opioid}}{\text{TDD mg current opioid}} = \frac{\text{Equianalgesic dose of new opioid}}{\text{Equianalgesic dose of current opioid}}$$

Example: Mrs. M is taking morphine sulfate immediate release 15 mg PO every 6 hr. TDD morphine = 60 mg. She has good pain control but experiences side effects. You plan to rotate her to hydromorphone.

Step 1: Set up equations with parallel ratios
Step 2: Calculate new dose by cross-multiplying

$$\frac{\text{X TDD oral hydromorphone}}{\text{60 mg TDD oral morphine}} = \frac{\text{7.5 mg oral hydromorphone}}{\text{30 mg oral morphine}}$$

Step 3: Divide to get X TDD

$$\frac{450}{30} = \frac{30X}{30}$$

Answer: 15mg = X TDD hydromorphone

Step 4: Reduce dose for cross tolerance by 25–50% (controlled pain); we will use 25%.
          Answer: 11 mg TDD hydromorphone

Step 5: Determine dosing interval based on individual needs.
          Answer: 11 mg TDD hydromorphone divided by 6 (every 4 hr dosing) = 1.8 mg or ~2 mg
          RX: Hydromorphone 2 mg tablet by mouth every 4 hours as needed for pain

Step 6: Monitor closely for therapeutic response, side effects, and safety

Figure 19.3 How to calculate a new opioid dose.

of administration (McPherson, 2010). There are several steps needed when converting opioids. First, complete your comprehensive pain assessment, including review of current medications. Remember that patients may not be taking the opiate medication as prescribed or even at all. Next, decide which opiate medication to switch to. This decision is influenced by kidney/liver function, previous side effects to certain opiates, allergies, route of administration, and safety concerns, including children in the home or diversion. Finally, calculate the new opioid using the formula in Figure 19.3. The literature recommends to reduce the newly calculated dose by 25%–50% unless the patient has uncontrolled pain. "The patient will have greater sensitivity to the new opioid which is a welcomed effect" (McPherson, 2010). Finally, monitor the patient closely for side effects, uncontrolled pain, and therapeutic effectiveness.

Case Study

Mrs. M reports mid back pain that is "aching, constant, and radiating." Her current pain score is 7/10, her worst is 10/10, and her best is 5/10. The pain is affecting her sleep. There are no associated symptoms. Her right upper abdominal quadrant pain is described as "deep, dull, and intermittently radiating to the right shoulder." You review the results of her imaging and she starts crying and says "God, what did I do to deserve this? I can't die. My children need me because they already lost their father."

You correlate your comprehensive pain assessment and defend or remove each from your differential diagnosis.

- Physical pain: Mrs. M was found to have widely metastatic disease throughout her cervical, thoracic, and lumbar spine on MRI imaging. Using Table 19.3, her back pain description is consistent with somatic and neuropathic pain. Her CT abdomen and pelvis and her abdominal pain description are consistent with visceral and neuropathic pain. Her physical examination reveals restlessness, tachycardia, and diaphoresis.
- Spiritual pain: Mrs. M is exhibiting spiritual pain evidenced by questioning her faith.
- Social pain: Mrs. M is worried about her children and her role with their family, and she is expressing fear about dying.
- Psychological pain: Mrs. M appears anxious and verbalizes fear and anxiety about the future along with worries about who will care for her children.

Your comprehensive pain assessment reveals that Mrs. M's pain is multidimensional. Using this information, you formulate a comprehensive plan of care to address her pain.

1. Physical pain: Scheduled opioids are recommended in this case due to the severity and etiology of her pain. Morphine is chosen for pain control because she is tolerating the morphine sulfate immediate release without side effects, verbalizes a decrease in her numeric pain rating 30 min after taking medication, and has normal kidney function. Mrs. M has been taking the morphine sulfate immediate release 15 mg every 4 hr around the clock and reports that her pain returns right before she is due for her next dose. You order MS Contin 30 mg PO every 12 hr and morphine sulfate immediate release 15 mg PO every 4 hr as needed for breakthrough pain. Adjuvants including anticonvulsants, antidepressants, steroids, or topical analgesics should be incorporated to address the neuropathic component. You order duloxetine 30 mg PO every night at bedtime for neuropathic pain. You also recommend that she optimize nonpharmacological interventions such as heat, repositioning, or meditation.
2. Spiritual pain: You ask simple questions to assess if her spirituality is a source of comfort or distress. Mrs. M identifies as religious and accepts a referral to the hospital chaplain.

3. Social pain/psychological pain: The APRN plays an integral role in exploring this dimension of pain and integrating the interdisciplinary team. You refer her to a social worker to explore social barriers, provide patient and family support, provide counseling, and assist with financial concerns and advance care planning. Psychiatry can assist in addressing situational anxiety and depression along with counseling and interventions such as CBT.

During her week-long admission, Mrs. M declined despite aggressive supportive care. She was evaluated by the interdisciplinary palliative and supportive care team. After many discussions surrounding her goals of care, she decided to transition to comfort-focused care and was discharged home from the hospital with hospice services. One week later, the hospice nurse calls you (the prescriber) stating "Mrs. M reports she is in pain and I have some concerns about her medications after completing a pill count." Review Table 19.8 and formulate the differential diagnoses.

According to the pill count, Mrs. M has used twice as many of the long-acting pain medication (MS Contin) as prescribed, yet the short-acting medication for breakthrough pain has been used as directed. In attempting to understand this situation, you will want to start by asking about the patient's pain, how she has been taking the medication, and how it has been securely stored. Further investigation by the APRN is warranted in this clinical situation. Your differential diagnoses must include total pain presentation, opioids poorly responsive to pain, opioid misuse/abuse/diversion, opioid-induced hyperalgesia, tolerance, or disease progression. Mrs. M has been keeping a journal of her pain severity and interference over the past week and documented that her pain severity had significantly increased in the morning when she awoke and in the evening, so she started taking two of the MS Contin twice daily. The fact that she has been the only person handling her medication, she has kept them secure, and she admits to taking more than prescribed based on the rationale of her increased pain level guides you to discuss the side effects and potential for overdose with high-dose opioids, as well as the importance of communicating with the healthcare team. Although it is not unusual for patients to form dependence on opioid medications to obtain the same analgesic effect over time, it would be unlikely to occur this quickly and you are concerned about disease progression in the face of her rapid decline. You also ask about how she has been handling her anxiety about her children, and she tells you that the social worker has been helping to communicate with her extended family to provide arrangements. Her sister is also living with her now as her caregiver. She is feeling more calm and secure about her children and would just like to spend as much time with them as possible during her remaining time. With her own concerns about the increased dosage of morphine

TABLE 19.8 CASE STUDY: MRS. M'S PILL COUNT

MORPHINE PRODUCT	NO. OF DOSES DISPENSED	NO. OF DOSES REMAINING	NO. OF DOSES ON HAND (VERIFIED BY RN)
MS Contin 15 mg	60	46	23
MSIR 15 mg	180	138	138

that is now at 150 mg/day, she agrees to switch to a fentanyl (Duragesic) patch, which will provide a more constant analgesic level. A fentanyl patch will take approximately 24 hr to reach its full therapeutic effect, so she and her caregiver will require specific instructions on when to stop taking the MS Contin and use of the morphine sulfate immediate release over the transition period. Providing verbal and written instructions as well as instructions on when she or her caregiver should communicate with the healthcare team will help to prevent adverse effects. The patient, caregiver, and hospice nurse each understand and agree with the pain management plan and have an honest discussion with Mrs. M about her fear of dying. With her children and family beside her, Mrs. M is comforted by knowing that her healthcare team will continue to oversee her pain management at the end of her life and will be there to console her loved ones with her final passing.

CONCLUSION

Primary palliative care is an essential skill that APRNs should acquire, cultivate, and incorporate into their daily practice. Understanding the complexities of "total pain," including the relationship between the physical, spiritual, social, and psychological dimensions, is critical for APRNs to understand when caring for patients with serious illnesses. A comprehensive pain assessment is a continuous process that includes a complex network of different factors. As seen in Figure 19.4, the comprehensive pain assessment and determination of differential diagnoses of pain help to inform realistic pain goals and the pain treatment plan. It is important that this process is patient-centered, involving the individual and family in options, preferences, and needs at each stage, and reassess pain and other symptoms frequently while monitoring the effectiveness of the treatment plan holistically. Mrs. M's case demonstrates the importance of a total pain assessment and highlights the importance of interdisciplinary care to address multidimensional pain and improve quality of life. It is essential for the APRN to identify components of pain that are not amenable to opioids such as fear of the unknown, loneliness, financial distress, or body image disturbances, all of which require alternative management strategies such as stress reduction, counseling, and support services for handling social and economic issues. Careful listening is an important

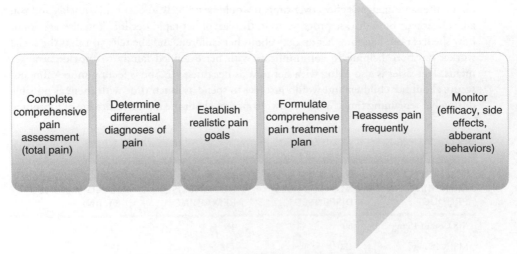

Figure 19.4 Alternative pain management strategies.

skill in determining the best way to reduce patient discomfort and address total pain. The United States is experiencing the effects of the opioid epidemic with an alarming increase in the number of deaths from overdoses over the last several years. Therefore, it is crucial that APRNs balance treating patients with pain while minimizing risks, including overdose, misuse, abuse, and diversion.

CLINICAL PEARLS

- Palliative care is focused on providing relief from the symptoms and stress of a potentially serious or life-threatening acute or chronic illness.
- Palliative care can be provided at any stage of an illness and alongside curative treatments.
- Pain has physical, psychological, social, emotional, and spiritual components, each contributing to a patient's perception and tolerance of pain.
- A comprehensive pain assessment by the APRN requires evaluation of the physical, psychological, spiritual, and social dimensions of pain.
- Using open-ended questions will help you accomplish a comprehensive assessment.
- Use a validated pain assessment tools in your assessment.
- Risk assessment for aberrant behaviors is an essential part of the comprehensive pain assessment.
- Effective pain management plans incorporate pharmacological and nonpharmacological modalities.
- Antidepressants, anticonvulsants, topical anesthetics, and corticosteroids are commonly used for the treatment of neuropathic pain and can be used safely in combination with opioids.
- Using nonpharmacological interventions as part of a comprehensive pain treatment plan.

REVIEW QUESTIONS

1. Which statement about palliative care is FALSE?
   a. Palliative care offers compassionate care to patients with serious illness at any point in their disease process.
   b. Palliative care can be provided along with curative treatments.
   c. Patients receiving palliative care elect to forgo life-prolonging treatments.
   d. Palliative care focuses on the "whole person."

2. APRNs caring for patients experiencing pain need to recognize and avoid common misconceptions about pain. Which of the following is correct?
   a. The patient is the expert in their pain experience.
   b. Opioid use always leads to drug addiction.
   c. The patient's perception of pain is always accurately related to the extent of tissue damage.
   d. Chronic pain is always psychological in nature.

3. Which physical symptom could the APRN expect in a patient who is complaining pain?
   a. Bradycardia
   b. Decreased respiratory rate
   c. Decreased muscle tension
   d. Diaphoresis

4. Which of the following statements about pain is true?
   a. Multidimensional pain should never be considered in a patient experiencing opiate refractory pain.
   b. Total pain refers to the physical, psychological, spiritual, and social pain experienced by patients.
   c. The distress associated with spiritual pain rarely exacerbates physical symptoms.
   d. Well-controlled physical symptoms interfere with a patient's ability to interact with loved ones.

Answers: 1, c; 2, a; 3, d; 4, b

REFERENCES

American Cancer Society. (2019). *Acute, chronic and breakthrough pain.* https://www.cancer.org/treatment/treatments-and-side-effects/physical-side-effects/pain/other-types.html

Center to Advance Palliative Care. (n.d.). *About palliative care.* https://www.capc.org/about/palliative-care/

Dahlin, C. M. (2013). *Core curriculum for the advanced practice hospice and palliative registered nurse.* Hospice and Palliative Nurses Association.

Ferrell, B. R., & Coyle, N. (2010). *Oxford textbook of palliative nursing* (3rd ed.). Oxford University Press, Inc.

Holmes, H. M., Stein, R., & Knight, C. (2008). *Alleviating psychological and spiritual pain in patients with life-limiting illness.* In *Hospice and palliative care training for physicians- a self-study program* (3rd ed., pp. 1–85). American Academy of Hospice and Palliative Medicine.

Malcom, K. (2019). *What drives patients to use medical marijuana: Mostly chronic pain.* University of Michigan. https://labblog.uofmhealth.org/lab-report/what-drives-patients-to-use-medical-marijuana-mostly-chronic-pain

Manchikanti, L., Abdi, S., Atluri, S., Balog, C. C., Benyamin, R. M., Boswell, M. V., Brown, K. R., Bruel, B. M., Bryce, D. A., Burks, P. A., Burton, A. W., Calodney, A. K., Caraway, D. L., Cash, K. A., Christo, P. J., Damron, K. S., Datta, S., Deer, T. R., Diwan, S., …Wargo, B. W., & American Society of Interventional Pain Physicians. (2012). American Society of Interventional Pain Physicians guidelines for responsible opioid prescribing in chronic non-cancer pain: Part 2-guidance. *Pain Physician*, 15, S67–S116.

McPherson, M. L. (2010). *Demystifying opioid conversion calculations: A guide for effective dosing.* American Society of Health-System Pharmacists.

Mehta, A., & Chan, L. S. (2008). Understanding of the concept of "total pain". *Journal of Hospice and Palliative Nursing*, 10(1), 26–32.

Moses, B. D. (2014). *Tarascon palliative medicine pocketbook.* Jones & Bartlett Learning Company.

Scarborough, B. M., & Smith, C. B. (2018). Optimal pain management for patients with cancer in the modern era. *CA: A Cancer Journal for Clinicians*, 68, 182–196.

UConn Health Department of Pharmacy. (2016). *Pocket reference for opioid management of pain* [Brochure].

University of Florida Health. (2019). *Pain management and dosing guide.* http://pami.emergency.med.jax.ufl.edu/resources/dosing-guide/

Webster, L. R., & Webster, R. M. (2005). Predicting aberrant behaviors in opioid-treated patients: Preliminary validation of the opioid risk too. *Pain Medicine*, 6(6), 432–442.

World Health Organization. (n.d.). *WHO's cancer pain ladder for adults.* https://www.who.int/cancer/palliative/painladder/en/

INDEX

Note: Page numbers followed by "f" indicate figures, "t" indicate tables and "b" indicate boxes.